Your Good Health

Your Good Health

How To Stay Well, and What To Do When You're Not

Edited by

William I. Bennett, M.D.

Stephen E. Goldfinger, M.D.

G. Timothy Johnson, M.D.

Harvard University Press
Cambridge, Massachusetts
London, England

Quotation on page 437 from THE FAMILY REUNION by T. S. Eliot
copyright 1939 by T. S. Eliot; renewed 1967 by Esme Valerie Eliot.
Reprinted by permission of Faber and Faber, Ltd., and
Harcourt Brace Jovanovich, Inc.

Library of Congress Cataloging in Publication Data

Your good health.

Includes index.
1. Health.   2. Environmental health.   3. Health
behavior.   I. Bennett, William, 1941–   .
II. Goldfinger, Stephen E., 1935–   .   III. Johnson,
G. Timothy, 1936–   . [DNLM: 1. Medicine—popular
works.   2. Self Care—popular works.   WB 120 Y81]
RA776.Y64   1987   613   87-19671
ISBN 0-674-96631-7 (alk. paper) (cloth)
ISBN 0-674-96632-5 (paper)

Contents

Introduction

A few years ago, we asked our colleagues at Harvard Medical School 25 questions about how they take care of their own health. Do they take vitamins? Do they go out and exercise? Do they avoid red meat? Do they smoke? How much alcohol do they drink? Do they eat eggs, drink coffee, floss their teeth?

Doctors are always giving advice; that's their business. We wanted to know what advice these reasonably well-informed physicians were following themselves. The answers were interesting. (You can find them, along with the questions we asked, and some interpretation, at the end of this book.) There was a lot of agreement on the main points. For example, the doctors tended to avoid taking medications unless the need was very clear. The answers to some other questions (mostly about dietary fat and fiber consumption) revealed something less than unanimity.

There's no shortage of advice in this world—especially when it comes to health. Some of this advice is good. Some of it is, at best, uncertain and can be expected to change in a year or a decade. A lot of it is pointless. And, once in a while, a recommendation is downright harmful. The problem, for all of us, is deciding which category a particular bit of advice belongs to.

We wrote this book in the same spirit that led us to develop the questionnaire. Doctors and patients aren't two different species. Because of their training, physicians may find it easier to evaluate ideas about health. But they have to make the same personal decisions that anyone else does: Will I really feel better and live longer if I make myself go jogging (even though it's drizzling and I'd rather turn on the stereo and read the newspaper)? Is it worth the effort to cut down on dietary fat, or alcohol, or overwork?

And when a pain, or an injury, or a fever strikes, we all, in a very real sense, serve as our own first doctors. This is not always an easy task, even for a physician. It's a medical axiom that decisions about

1

triage (who needs to be treated right away and whose treatment can be delayed) should be made by the most experienced physician present. Ironically, in daily life everyone, experienced or not, serves as his or her own triage officer, deciding whether or not to pursue a symptom or a problem.

In this book we have tried to serve as "double agents" for the reader. On the one hand, we draw on the knowledge and experience we and our colleagues have acquired as physicians. On the other, we have looked at this material from the point of view of nonphysicians. We've attempted to pass along what we see as worthwhile information and workable recommendations to people who don't plan on getting a medical education but who do want to make informed choices about their own health.

In doing so, we've made some assumptions about you:

- You value your independence. You don't want just to be told, "Do this, do that." You want to know the evidence and the reasoning, then make your own choices.
- You want solid information, but don't want to get bogged down in a lot of detail. Even though you care about health, you don't have time to turn yourself into a full-fledged authority.
- You would like to live a long life, but you'd also like to enjoy it along the way. Of course, you want to take the best possible care of yourself, but not at the price of putting everything that's fun, or tasty, on a "forbidden" list.
- When you are ill, or in need of medical care, you want to be able to ask the right questions and evaluate the answers for yourself. When a medical decision needs to be made, you want to be a partner in making it.
- Your interest in personal health extends to the larger picture—the environment and the social and political factors that affect your well-being and that of your family, friends, or neighbors.
- You want your information served straight, without superfluous anecdotes and ornamentation.

This book is not an encyclopedia of medical diseases. It is a companion to healthy living. The main focus is on what you can do for yourself: habits you can develop or modify, choices you can make in day-to-day life. Encouraging evidence from the past 10 or 15 years suggests that good choices *do* make a difference. The life expectancy of American adults has increased during this period.

There does not appear to be any one reason, and it is quite clear that medical care alone is not the only reason people are living longer.

Consider the example of heart disease. American hearts are healthier now than they were even 20 or 30 years ago. The reasons are not exactly known, but several trends have been important. The intake of animal fat is lower now than in the past, and the cumulative effect of even small decreases appears to be very large. The number of cigarette smokers in the population has declined—and the risk of heart attack declines almost the day someone quits smoking. Finally, an important role has been played by one medical intervention: treatment of high blood pressure. Hypertension is a major cause of heart disease, and even modest gains in controlling blood pressure are reflected in improved survival rates. Perhaps more important, longer lives are also healthier lives. The person who doesn't smoke, for example, will live, on average, 7 or 8 years longer than the smoker, and in the process will have fewer symptoms, fewer days lost to illness—*and,* the dermatologists tell us, younger-looking skin.

What's in this book

We begin with a look at some of the basics of fitness and nutrition. In the first chapter we talk about practical ways to keep the heart and blood vessels working well, and we summarize recent theories about nutritional influences on health—from fiber, fish oil, and fat to sugar and supplements. We take a long look at weight control—an area where misinformation and exploitation are vastly more abundant than reliable data.

Then we discuss some of the most commonly used recreational drugs, ranging from coffee to cocaine. Tobacco and alcohol have a profound effect on health and life expectancy in our society. Together, they probably cause as much illness and early death as all other environmental factors taken together. Any pleasure they give must be balanced against this enormous toll.

In the third chapter we go on to look at some of the other environmental factors influencing well-being—hazards of the home, the workplace, and the world around us. We look at some fairly simple methods for controlling or responding to asbestos, radon, noise, shift work, and radiation exposures, to name a few. And we discuss a couple of things that are not worth worrying about.

Chapter 4 provides a close look at the part of us most exposed to the environment: skin and other components of the body's surface—hair, nails, teeth, and eyes. Appearance and health go together in the enjoyment of life, and we pay attention to both in this chapter.

Chapter 5 is about sex and its complications. To a surprisingly large extent, many adults' health worries center on sexual function or reproduction. Perhaps that's not so astonishing. How we feel about ourselves, and how good we feel, is often associated with our intimate relationships, our feeling of sexual fulfillment in an emotionally satisfying context.

Of course, feeling good depends on a variety of other elements of daily experience—ranging from getting a good night's sleep to handling emotional upsets, to coping with the headaches, back pains, and other irritations of daily life. In Chapter 6 we look at some of these factors—chiefly from a medical and biological point of view. We emphasize the physical aspect because it's what we know most about, and because that is the focus of this book, not because we think psychological or spiritual factors are unimportant.

Sooner or later, most people have to cope with a major illness. In Chapter 7 we consider the "big three"—heart disease, stroke, and cancer. We provide an overview of how these conditions develop in the body, how they can be detected early in the course of the disease, and how new treatments—such as balloon surgery for coronary artery disease and lumpectomy for breast cancer—are changing the way physicians combat these life-threatening illnesses.

At various stages of life, everyone comes to deal with doctors. We all must be patients from time to time. Chapter 8 offers suggestions to people who are on the receiving end of medical care: how to ask questions, how to think about cost and quality of care, how to use the preventive services that medicine has to offer—flu shots, mammograms, tonometry for glaucoma detection, blood cholesterol measurements, Pap smears, glucose tolerance tests, electrocardiograms, and many more. Here especially, we take on our role as double agents—offering "insider information" on ways to get the most health care for your dollar.

As editors of the *Harvard Medical School Health Letter*, we are strongly committed to finding the best possible evidence on which to base our interpretations and recommendations. But this goal has to be tempered with the recognition that there are many zones of uncertainty in every realm of science or medicine. One of the pleasures of putting out a monthly publication is the opportunity to report on new developments, the opportunity to change our minds from time to time as better evidence appears. For this book, however, we have selected material that seems most likely to withstand the test of time and be of practical value in people's daily lives.

1 | Basic Maintenance: Fitness, Weight Control, and Nutrition

No one should ever underestimate the amount of abuse the human body can tolerate—and even thrive on. The body is not a bank account, a passive balance between what comes in and what goes out. It actively regulates itself; it is wonderfully resistant to many forms of deprivation, and equally resistant to many of our efforts to "improve" it. A little more or a little less of this or that vitamin or mineral usually doesn't make much of an impression on the tough, intricate, autonomous, living system in which we make our home for the better part of a century.

The object of a basic maintenance program for this miraculous machine is not to adjust and regulate every part, but to give it enough of the raw materials on one hand, and enough stimulation on the other, to keep it running itself. We urge you—as we discuss exercise, weight control, and nutrition—to feel a little relief in the recognition that you don't have to manage every detail of your own metabolism. (If you did, you would never be able to think about anything else.) Your best bet, and basic obligation to your body, is to provide it with enough latitude for its natural self-caring and self-protective mechanisms to do their job. At the extremes of indolence versus athletic intensity, starvation versus dietary opulence, this can't happen. But in between is a wide range in which you can live your life that is both healthy and enjoyable.

In this book we give first place not to what you take in but what you put out, in the form of physical activity. It is becoming more and more clear that exercise—which doesn't have to be fanatical, unpleasant, or obsessive—tones up not only the muscles but many basic biochemical processes. In a very real sense, the more active you can be, the less concerned you need to be with what you eat. Indeed, body fat, which has long been regarded as a problem to be solved by eating less, is more effectively controlled through regular, mild exercise than through dieting. But in a society blessed with an abundance of food, it is possible to suffer from both nutritional deficiencies and excesses. This chapter closes with some discussion of the major themes in contemporary nutrition.

Fitness

Gasoline may well be one of the most hazardous substances in our environment. Not because it's poisonous, flammable, and explosive—though all those things are true—but because we use it. And therefore we don't use our bodies.

Throughout the twentieth century, levels of physical activity have been declining—so much so that most people living in modernized, urban areas are surely as inactive as anyone has ever been in history. The result is emerging as something we might call the "disuse syndrome": an increasing susceptibility to certain diseases, such as atherosclerosis, high blood pressure, and diabetes; a tendency to gain weight with age; and vulnerability to injuries and back problems.

These drawbacks of sedentary life should neither be ignored nor overstated. Although the prevalence of so-called "degenerative" conditions is very high, the fact is that American adults are living longer than ever before. But "living longer" and "feeling better" are not necessarily synonymous. Without a certain amount of attention and use, bodies may endure to old age, but not very gracefully. On the whole, bodies that are exercised wear better—though it has yet to be definitively proved that they last longer.

The central benefit of exercise is to the heart and blood vessels. Nobody can seriously question this effect. Whether it's bus drivers in London, longshoremen in San Francisco, farmers in Iowa, or office workers in New York, the evidence is highly consistent: the more active people are, the less likely they are to develop heart disease or die of a heart attack.

How does exercise protect the heart?

Less demand

Muscles that are exercised change. With repeated use, they develop the ability to extract more oxygen from the blood that flows through them. This means that they can get by with slower blood flow. So they don't signal the heart to pump as hard for any given level of activity. To appreciate what this means, think about someone who is late for a plane. With a camera over his shoulder and a carry-on bag in his hand, he half runs, half walks what seems like a mile to get to the gate. If his leg muscles have not been getting regular use, say from habitual fast walking, they are perfectly capable of doing what they're asked to do, but only by demanding rapid, hard pumping from the heart. With more practice they would take the situation in stride (so to speak), and the heart would only have to increase its output by a modest amount.

Because the leg muscles are the largest and hardest-working of the body, the heart gets most protection if these muscles have been trained. But one muscle does not benefit from the training of another. If our traveler has exercised only his leg muscles with a regular evening walk or morning jog, the muscles of his arms and upper chest will still cry out for help as they lug the added weight of carry-on baggage.

There is a definite additional benefit to working the arms, even though arm muscles are relatively small. Part of the reason is that the arms are attached to the chest and waist. Muscles of the upper torso must work to stabilize the body when you are carrying a grocery bag or a cello. These muscles make demands on the heart, just like all the others. In cardiac folklore, shoveling snow is often used as the example of an activity that can precipitate a heart attack. If there is substance to this belief, it is probably because muscles of the upper body tend to be even more out of shape—and thus put even more demand on the heart—than leg muscles, which get at least a little use in almost everyone.

Less pumping

A second way that exercise protects the heart is by allowing it to pump less rapidly even at rest. This results mainly from training the *sympathetic nervous system,* which is responsible for managing many of the body's most basic (and automatic) functions. Among other things, the sympathetic nerves influence the rate and intensity of the heart beat. For a reason that is not clearly understood (but intuitively makes sense), regular exercise trains the sympathetics to take it easy during rest. A measurable consequence of this effect is that the resting heart rate tends to slow down as a result of physical activity. People who have been exercising may have a resting pulse that is 10–20 beats slower than it would be if they were sedentary. The lowered resting pulse may or may not be important in itself. But during moments of anger or other emotional turmoil, lowered "sympathetic tone" probably limits stress on the heart.

Cleaning up the coronary environment

A third, and very important, protective effect of exercise is on the chemistry of the blood—particularly the way cholesterol is handled. Cholesterol is an essential raw material used in several ways by the body. It is incorporated into cell membranes, where it contributes stability, and it is used as the basic substance from which half a dozen crucial hormones are elaborated. But when too much of this waxy substance is present in the blood stream, it has a fatal tendency to invade the walls of arteries and damage their structure. In time, the arteries become narrowed and eventually even blocked by build-up of cholesterol.

This process occurs most frequently in arteries that must carry a rapid flow of blood. Presumably minor damage to the inner surface of the vessel occurs more frequently in high-flow areas. Such damage leads platelets to accumulate. These cell fragments are normally responsible for repairing breaks in the circulatory system; they initiate the complex process of clotting. But when platelets overreact to minor disruptions of the vessel lining, they are no help at all; they make matters worse. Among other things, they stimulate the process by which cholesterol invades the artery wall and initiates the sequence of events known as atherosclerosis (*see Chapter 7*).

Where does exercise come in? It has at least two effects. First, it makes platelets less "sticky" than usual, and thus less likely to start the atherosclerotic process. And exercise also stimulates the body to put blood-borne cholesterol into a form known as *HDL-cholesterol*, which does not get deposited in artery walls. Indeed, HDL (a protein carrier for cholesterol, technically termed *high density lipoprotein*) actually tends to pull cholesterol away from tissues where it doesn't belong and carries it to the liver, where it can be "disposed of properly." Exercise appears to be the most effective way of activating the system for disposing of excess cholesterol. The combination of these two effects—reducing platelet stickiness and converting cholesterol from the invasive to the noninvasive type—is extremely powerful in protecting people from heart disease.

Blood cholesterol is not the only risk factor for heart disease that is modified by regular exercise. Both high blood pressure and the most common form of diabetes can be at least partially prevented or treated with exercise. Regular physical activity does not lower normal blood pressure, but most studies of people with mild to moderate high blood pressure have observed this effect—especially a lowered peak, or *systolic* value (*see Chapter 7*). It really isn't clear why exercise helps to reduce high blood pressure. But because the sympathetic nervous system plays a major role in regulating blood pressure, an obvious guess is that this is where the action is.

Exercise also helps suppress the type of diabetes that appears in adult life and that does not require insulin injections to achieve control. This form of the disease, known as type-2 or non-insulin-dependent diabetes, is basically a genetic disorder. Long before diabetes becomes apparent, people with the genes for type-2 diabetes have subtle but detectable abnormalities in the way their bodies handle both carbohydrates and fats. An important feature of this condition is that some tissues, such as muscles, become insensitive to the effects of insulin. To compensate, more insulin is produced— in an apparent effort to maintain normal levels of blood sugar (specifically *glucose*). During the early phases of the disease, this leads to accumulation of body fat, which just makes matters worse, because fat increases the body's resistance to insulin. A vicious cycle is set in motion. In time, blood glucose levels begin to rise as well, and then the diabetes becomes severe enough to cause symptoms.

One theory holds that a variety of tissues, including the blood vessels, are damaged by high blood glucose, mainly because glucose in high levels becomes chemically bonded to all sorts of proteins, which function abnormally as a result. Perhaps most sensitive, and certainly most crucial, are certain proteins in the walls of small arteries. As glucose becomes attached to these proteins, the blood vessels become distorted and fragile. Another theory is that the excess of glucose forces unusual chemical reactions to take place inside cells.

Physical activity combats diabetes in two important ways. Exercise automatically increases the muscles' sensitivity to insulin. Thus, normal blood sugar can be maintained with less secretion of insulin—and this may in itself protect the insulin-producing cells from what amounts to "overwork" and eventual failure. Exercise also keeps body fat from accumulating. Less body fat means greater sensitivity to insulin, less total demand for production of the hormone, and more normal levels of blood sugar.

Even from this very rapid review, it should be evident that exercise might protect arteries from two kinds of invasion:

- The shift of cholesterol into the protective HDL form keeps cholesterol out of the walls of larger arteries with rapid blood flow.
- The lowering of blood sugar—a result of increased sensitivity to insulin—may protect proteins in smaller arteries from becoming chemically denatured by glucose.

It should also be apparent that exercise is more valuable before, rather than after, these abnormalities appear. Once arteries have been damaged, a return to normal is much more difficult—though not absolutely out of the question.

Extra credit

The way exercise enhances the work of the heart and circulatory system is the clearest health reason for including some kind of regular exercise program in one's life. Other less easily defined and studied benefits of physical activity are probably equally important ways of making life more enjoyable (or less painful). A good deal of evidence suggests that exercise reduces mood swings—acting to limit both depression and anxiety (see Chapter 6). Physical activity very clearly reduces body fat, as we'll discuss in a later section. Many people feel that appearance is improved in a body that gets some work, but this is obviously a much harder aspect to quantify, and one that depends as much on personal values as anything else. Certainly, being in good physical condition opens more opportunities to people at all ages to participate in activities ranging from athletics to walking tours of interesting cities.

Exercise and chronic illness

People with a variety of diseases may fear that exercise will make them worse—or they may wish to exercise but not know what kinds of activity are open to them. In reality, there are few chronic diseases that rule out all forms of physical activity. Many of the more common ones may actually improve with the right kind of exercise.

Arthritis, for example, often benefits from an activity that moves the affected joints without putting too much strain on them. Swimming or underwater exercises in warm water can be both soothing and helpful. Asthma is sometimes made worse by outdoor exercise, but swimming, at least partly because one is automatically breathing humidified air, can produce a noticeable improvement. For some strange reason, symptoms of hay fever are often somewhat relieved by exercise. In some conditions, such as multiple sclerosis, it is essential not to become fatigued, but mild exercise, within the person's capacity, appears to be beneficial.

The rules of the game

In using the word "exercise," we have had something fairly specific in mind. All forms of exercise are not created equal. The type that most helps the heart is called *aerobic exercise*. This shouldn't be confused with the more-or-less commercial term "aerobics," which has come to be associated with people wearing shiny tights and jumping around to loud music—for a fee.

The word "aerobic" comes from the word "air" and for all practical purposes, when applied to exercise, means something like "heavy breathing"—the sort of breathing that goes with steady activity, such as fast walking, that is kept up for more than a few minutes.

To be specific, exercise is aerobic when it involves some regular, repeated activity that is intense enough to make the heart beat faster than usual and breathing get deeper. An activity is not aerobic if it is so intense that it can only be kept up for seconds to minutes before a rest is needed. Lifting a really heavy weight, for example, is too intense to be called aerobic. In fact, it is so intense that muscles can't use oxygen to supply the needed power; the chemical processes for doing this are simply too slow. Instead, the muscles use up temporary stores of energy within their cells and must then wait until the exertion is completed to replenish them via the slower oxygen-based system.

Aerobic exercise basically relies on the oxygen system to supply energy—but pushes it. So if you set out for a fast walk, and keep it up for half an hour, your heart rate and breathing speed up to supply the necessary fuel and oxygen. But the supply lines are never really taxed to the point that they give out.

If an aerobic activity is repeated frequently—at least every other day—the muscles involved seem to "remember" that they are having to meet an increased demand for work. They proceed to improve their ability to meet it. Mainly, they increase their ability to extract oxygen from the blood, and they also equip themselves with a richer supply of small blood vessels to improve the delivery system. The heart also responds by increasing its capacity to deliver large volumes of blood with less effort (mainly by enlarging the amount it pumps with each stroke and thus reducing the rate at which it has to beat).

These changes in the muscles of the heart and limbs begin very rapidly and continue for quite a long while as the body becomes "trained." Within a week, marked differences may be noticed as a sedentary person begins a simple program of walking or walk-jogging. Within a few months, more indirect metabolic changes can be measured: the shift of cholesterol to the beneficial HDL form, loss of body fat, perhaps lowering of blood pressure, improved handling of blood sugar, and so on.

What does it take to get these effects? There are some stock recommendations, which give a rough idea. But they should not be taken too literally, because an exercise program that doesn't take account of individual capacities, needs, and interests is likely to fail.

How often and how hard?

Very little effect comes from aerobic exercise that is done less than 3 times a week; 5 is preferable.

Each person should set his or her own rules for intensity of exercise; the beauty is that the benefits of exercise are geared to how hard it *feels* for the person doing it. There are some practical ways, though, to set goals. The most common is to use heart rate. How fast *your* heart beats in response to a challenge is a measure of your condition, a nice sort of sliding scale.

For healthy people in youth to middle age, the rule of thumb is that maximum heart rate is 220 beats a minute *minus* your age. So a person of 40 would think of 180 as the highest possible heart rate that could be achieved during exercise. About 60% of that heart rate, say 110 beats a minute, is regarded as the minimum level to get benefit from aerobic exercise; 70% (126 beats) is a moderate level, perfectly adequate to see real improvement. Some people might wish to push harder—and may be able to go as high as 85%—but there is no overwhelming reason for most of us to do so. People who have been pretty sedentary should stay at the lower end of this range; they'll get plenty of benefit from a heart rate around 60% of their maximum, and there's no real need to push to higher levels, unless the spirit is willing and the flesh isn't too weak.

As fitness improves, so does the amount of work needed to raise the heart rate. So this formula—fixed as it looks—is automatically adjusted upward as time goes by.

Taking your pulse is relatively easy. It requires a finger and a watch with a hand or counter for seconds. Lightly touch the finger to your wrist, just back from the base of the thumb, or else rest it against your neck, a little to one side of the windpipe and right under your chin, while turning your head to the opposite side. Don't press—especially not at the neck—but move your finger around until you can feel a beat underneath it. Your heart rate will slow quite rapidly after you finish an activity, such as jogging. So you want to take your pulse immediately after stopping and then only for a few seconds, so as to estimate what it was immediately before you stopped. The easiest system is to count for 6 seconds and then multiply by 10 to get the count for a full minute, which is how heart rates are usually expressed.

It isn't absolutely necessary to wear a watch and go through the business of trying to take your pulse while in the midst of exercise to get an idea of how hard you're working. It turns out that people who pay attention to the way they're feeling can judge pretty accurately how hard they're exercising. A standard 15-point scale, known as the *perceived exertion scale* (or Borg scale, after its developer; *see p. 16*), has been devised to help people think about their level of exertion. Using this device requires that you keep the whole

• Perceived exertion scale •	
6	
7	Very, very light
8	
9	Very light
10	
11	Fairly light
12	
13	Somewhat hard
14	
15	Hard
16	
17	Very hard
18	
19	Very, very hard
20	

scale in mind and then place yourself on it according to the way you *feel*. The ratings apply to the "total, inner feeling of exertion," not to any one factor, such as pain in the legs or shortness of breath. To use the scale effectively, you need to be honest with yourself, not overestimating or underestimating how hard the exercise feels.

Most people get solid aerobic benefit from exertions they place around 11–13 on the scale (and, as it happens, their heart rates are likely to be around 110–130, or roughly 10 times the point value they assign to the feeling of exertion). Perception of intensity tends to be closest to measured intensity in the range from about 8 to about 15; it's not so accurate at the extremes. About 10% of people, because they consistently overrate or underrate their sense of exertion, can't really use this scale. Most others get pretty close. Those who have a specific health problem that makes exercise difficult may have to distinguish between the discomfort caused by the problem and the actual sense of exertion they are experiencing.

People who have health problems should not undertake exercise programs without medical supervision. Often, in a cardiac rehabilitation program, the intensity of exercise will begin at very mild levels—bringing heart rate only 10 or 20 points above the resting level. As time goes on, the levels reached by people with coronary artery disease may increase well above these heart rates—but that is a goal to be aimed at, not a place to start.

How long?

Many people mutter a soft "Oh Lord" to themselves after this question. In reality, each session of aerobic exercise doesn't have to last for a terribly long time to get some appreciable benefit. At a minimum, 15 minutes of continuous activity is sufficient to provide noticeable benefit; one hour, for most people, is probably the upper limit that offers any benefit to health. Over that, the training is more for athletic or competitive reasons.

But bear in mind that more than 15 minutes are needed for the full session. Exercise should always be preceded by a warm-up period before full intensity begins. Cold muscles are inefficient and very likely to be injured. Warm-up doesn't need to consist of vigorous stretching. Indeed, cold muscles don't stretch very well. But light stretching, which involves rotating the trunk, swinging the arms up and over the head, bending forward at the waist, kneeling and bending way forward (to stretch the lower back), pulling up on the ankle with the hand (to stretch the front of the leg), and similar activities work well.

At least as important is a cool-down period after the exercise. This can consist simply of walking at a comfortable rate for 5 minutes or so after fast walking or jogging. This activity prevents post-exercise fainting (which may result if blood pools in the legs, as it is inclined to do when activity is abruptly stopped). Stretching may actually be easier at this point, because the muscles have been warmed up.

So the "how long" question is really answered: a *minimum* of 15 minutes of the brisk activity, preceded by 10 of warming up and followed by at least 5 more for cooling off.

What works?

The general rule is: any activity consisting of regular, repeated, rhythmic movement of the whole body (or a large part of it), for more than 15 minutes.

On the whole, putting in about 2,000 calories' worth of activity a week—the equivalent of walking or jogging 3 miles a day—seems to confer about the maximum amount of cardiac benefit. More exercise than this clearly produces greater "fitness" but doesn't further reduce the risk of heart disease (which is already pretty minimal in most people putting in 20 miles a week of walking or jogging).

Starting slow: the fundamental program

Ironically, the athletic mentality may be the greatest enemy of lifelong fitness. The belief that exercise must be organized, intense, and competitive gets people off on the wrong foot to begin with. In most schools, physical education programs still, after years of criticism, focus on activities that cannot be continued into adult life. Whatever *other* benefits may be attributed to football, field hockey, lacrosse, or wrestling, lifetime fitness isn't one of them. Even swimming tends not to be a lifetime activity, if only because most people live too far away from a pool of any reasonable size to keep at what is otherwise a superb exercise.

And to the extent that adults remain involved in organized sports as their main activity, they are likely to lose out on fitness (while preserving companionship and entertainment, to be sure). There's nothing like an occasional weekend game of anything to make many people feel sore and unmotivated for the rest of the week. With the best of intentions, adults commonly begin to avoid physical activity or confine it to occasional weekends by the time they are in their mid to late twenties. And if your model of physical fitness is a hard-fought football or hockey game, it's far more likely that you'll wind up watching it on television than attempting to do it yourself.

The main thing to recognize about physical fitness in contemporary America is that it has become more difficult to achieve because most of us are much less active than we think. In the decades since World War II, social changes in the United States have contributed to a marked decline in the amount of physical exertion that life *requires*. Typical amounts of voluntary, recreational activity may not fully compensate for the fact that daily life requires so much less exertion.

The suburbanization of America, with progressively longer commuting times and more commitment to the automobile, not only cuts into recreational time but reduces the amount of walking that would be involved in getting to and from work on public transportation. The shift of occupations from industry to service has reduced the level of physical activity for huge numbers of people. The mechanization of labor has not been confined to construction sites; even office work, which has always been pretty sedentary, probably requires even less motion than before as a result of computerization. Escalators were a novelty thirty years ago; now they are commonplace. Television has been all too effective as entertainment for children—at the price of confining them to a 5-yard radius of the screen. The net result is that energy output in daily life is phenomenally low in this country.

But what about the fitness craze of the past decade or so? It probably has made a difference—though mostly among people of relatively young age and high social class. And even in this group, except for real fanatics, the value of the activity is often smaller than you'd expect. A tennis game two or three times a week may do fairly little to offset the fact that the person playing the game drives to and from work as well as to and from the tennis court.

One of the biggest benefits of exercise, as we have mentioned, is the way it shifts blood cholesterol from the harmful, or invasive, form to the beneficial HDL variety. A 1983 survey of some 66 published studies on the relationship between exercise and cholesterol found that the *amount of time* spent exercising has much more influence on this process than the intensity. Whether a given amount of time was spent in high-intensity or moderate exertion did not seem to make much difference. In other words: slow and steady—and *often*—are the watchwords. A brisk walk or slow jog for half an hour or so every day is more valuable than a heavy workout over the weekend.

The moral is that almost everyone should start a fitness program by not thinking about a programmed, recreational activity. Instead, attention should be directed to finding small, routine ways to increase output during the day.

Simply walking more can make a significant difference to fitness. Dr. Ralph Paffenbarger of Stanford University has shown that the equivalent of walking an hour a day can markedly lower the risk of a heart attack. In England, Geoffrey Rose showed that walking 20 minutes or more to work was associated with a 30% reduction in certain important abnormalities of the electrocardiogram. In many studies, it appears that the biggest difference in cardiac risk is between the people who move very little and those who simply walk a few more blocks or climb a few more stairs every day. Adding more vigorous activity on top of this does lead to even greater improvement, but the difference is not quite as marked.

For someone who lives in a high-rise apartment building and drives to an office that is in a skyscraper, even this amount of activity cannot be regarded as "routine"—some amount of programming becomes necessary. Purposely parking the car a few blocks away from one's destination, choosing stairs instead of elevators, planning a lunch-time stroll—these are some of the obvious options. The basic point is that at least *some* exercise in every

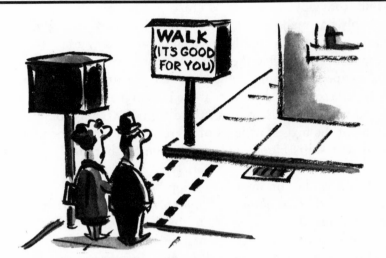

If you buy the hard-sell diet programs, books, or pills on the market, you'll lose more dollars than pounds in the long run. Long-term weight control appears to require regular, frequent physical activity. A pair of good walking shoes will take off more pounds than any other purchase you make.

day should be of the sort that doesn't require any change of clothing or basic routine to perform.

Walking, for most people, is the ideal choice. The skill required is minimal, the potential for injury is negligible, and the benefits are considerable. Even someone who routinely does more intense exercise benefits from walking, because this mild but steady and sustained exercise helps to keep muscles warmed up and increases their tone—thus, in all likelihood, helping to protect them from injury when they shift into high gear.

Some people, because of a physical disability, cannot comfortably walk for long distances. They may not be able to treat walking as the routine exercise that serves as background for others. Consultation with a physical therapist or exercise specialist may be helpful in finding ways to exercise without walking (such as underwater routines, or arm exercises carried out with small hand weights or other equipment developed to provide the upper body with aerobic activity).

Moving on

So why do anything more than walk for a while each day? Because low-intensity exercise has a limited ability to prepare the body for moments of high demand: the snowy morning when the car just has to be dug out, the sprint to a departing train, or the afternoon spent hauling stuff down from the attic (at last). Also, maintaining the capacity for relatively intense exertion makes it possible to enjoy lighter activities with less effort.

Does that mean jogging? Let's face it: Not everyone wants to jog, not everyone can jog, and furthermore not everyone *should* jog. (More on this in a moment.) Jogging works, to be sure, but so do many other forms of aerobic exercise. Even walking can become a high intensity activity when done rapidly (as in race walking) or while carrying small hand weights (a strategy formalized as "Heavyhands" by Dr. Leonard Schwartz). Hiking, especially on hilly terrain, adds intensity to walking, and for the really committed there are sports such as orienteering (a kind of cross-country search for clues, carried out with a map and a compass).

Swimming is a fine activity, if you're the sort of person who has a year-round pool, or is organized enough to get to a pool several times a week.

Skipping rope is excellent exercise—but is often too intense for many beginners to keep it up. (You have to swing the rope fast enough to keep it in the air; this puts a lower limit on the rate of skipping.) But if this is what you really *want* to do, you can get some flexibility by using rope of different weights. Jumping on a mini-trampoline has the opposite limitation. It's fine for exertion at mild to moderate levels. But the physics of the trampoline put an upper limit on how fast and high you can jump. Again, if this is something you just love to do, as you get into better condition you can make it harder by holding small hand weights or doing various kinds of more elaborate jumping.

Most forms of dancing work well—especially vigorous folk, modern, or ballet—but an evening of rock 'n roll or ballroom dancing is also remarkably aerobic. "Aerobics" or "aerobic dancing" of the sort that has come to be identified with Jane Fonda is appealing to a lot of people and can be made very vigorous.

Bicycling is a bit of a problem. Outdoor bicycling can be a very low-level exercise, simply because it's often possible, or necessary, to coast. In many areas, you just can't bicycle at high speed without running the risk of an accident. If you're not riding a heavy bike uphill and into the wind, outdoor bicycling may be mild exercise indeed. Stationary indoor exercise bicycles, on the other hand, can be adjusted to provide a good workout—though they have the drawback of boredom. On the other hand, using a bicycle for routine transportation can make a significant contribution to fitness. In many areas, commuting on a bicycle hardly takes longer than going by public transportation or car. Even at a slow and comfortable speed, the time spent bicycling makes a useful contribution to total exercise time.

Making a choice

There's no way around one basic fact. For exercise to be good for you, it has to feel like exercise—at least a little more than "fairly light," in the terms of the Borg scale, up to "somewhat hard." For a lot of people that's a problem. They don't like punishment, and if exercise feels like punishment—or if it simply requires a lot of folderol and equipment just to begin—they won't do it. Perhaps the most important aspect of choosing an exercise, more than its theoretical value, is (1) whether the activity is psychologically appealing, that is, whether it is both pleasant and somehow meaningful to the person doing it, and (2) whether it is reasonably easy to get started.

An interesting study describes the experience of sedentary police officers who were started on a 20-week exercise program. Half of them were asked to go to a central facility 3 times a week; the others received instruction but then continued on their own. Members of the unsupervised group were less likely to quit the program, and a major reason seemed to be that they did not have to spend time traveling to and from the place where they exercised. In sum: the higher proportion of time that can actually be spent exercising, the more likely people are to continue exercising.

Yet another instructive piece of research was conducted with obese children. These kids were brought into a weight-control program that (correctly) stressed physical activity as the main method to be used. Half of the children were encouraged to pick exercises or sports from a list, to learn them, and to continue their involvement after the formal program was over. The other half were asked what they liked to do (as long as it was some kind of exercise) and then simply told to do more of it. A year later, it was the children in this second group who were more likely to have continued their activity, and to be lower in weight.

The rating game

In choosing between various activities, of course, it's worth having some idea of how intense they are likely to be. The easiest way to compare activities is to use a unit of measure nicknamed the "MET" (from "metabolic rate"). When you are sitting stock still, your level of activity can be defined as 1 MET (the basic minimum of exertion required by breathing, and so on, to keep you alive). Other kinds of activity can be rated by the amount they increase this expenditure of energy. At 5 METs (a value typical for social dancing) you are putting out 5 times the energy you would if you were sitting on the sidelines.

The table on page 24 lists some common (and not so common) activities, rated in METs. Bear in mind that the rating only applies while you're actually engaged in the activity (but for a sport like golf, this includes the time going from hole to hole, so the ratings are different depending on whether one rides a golf cart or walks with the clubs).

One thing you'll notice about walking is that it starts out in the lower range, but by the time you're pushing a 10-minute mile (which is very brisk walking) the amount of effort increases considerably. The reason for this is that the main resistance to walking comes from the tissues of the body itself. At slow rates, there's almost no tissue resistance, but somewhere around 4–5 miles an hour, that changes. As speeds get even higher, the effort starts to increase very sharply. That's one reason why it's natural to break into a jog somewhere around a 12-minute mile. At that speed, the effort of running (which is really a series of small jumps) is less because the stride lengthens, giving legs more time to swing back and forth.

Tread with caution

Whether you should see a doctor before you start to exercise is one of those questions only you can really answer. In principle, it seems like a good idea. In practice, many people would *never* get started exercising if they had to get a doctor's approval first. The best rule

• Energy demands of exercise •

Activity	METS
Sitting quietly	1
Walking, 30-minute mile	2
Shuffleboard	2–3
Golf (power cart)	2–3
Horseshoe pitching	2–3
Bowling	2–4
Fishing (bank, boat, ice)	2–4
Sailing	2–5
Stationary bicycle (adults can adjust in this range)	3–18
Walking, 20-minute mile	3
Table tennis	3–5
Softball	3–6
Volleyball	3–6
Social and square dancing	3–7
Hiking (mostly level ground)	3–7
Bicycling (recreation, transportation)	3–8
Canoeing, rowing, kayaking	3–8
Calisthenics	3–8
Horseback riding	3–8
Shooting baskets	3–9
Walking, 16-minute mile	4
Golf (without power cart)	4–7
Climbing stairs	4–8
Swimming	4–8
Badminton	4–9
Tennis	4–9
Walking, 15-minute mile	4.6
Water skiing	5–7
Downhill skiing	5–8
Mountain climbing	5–10
Backpacking	5–11
Dancing (aerobic, folk, jazz)	6–9
Touch football	6–10
Cross-country skiing	6–12
Walking, 12-minute mile	7
Snowshoeing	7–14
Rope skipping	8–12
Paddle/racket ball, squash	8–12
Handball	8–12
Running, 10-minute mile	10
Running, 8.5-minute mile	11.5
Running, 7-minute mile	13

of thumb is that if you think you should see a doctor, you probably should. If you're not certain, here are some thoughts.

Somebody with no symptoms and no known risk factors can start a program of increasing fitness without seeing a doctor. But the choice of activity should begin at the lower end of the range of energy demand. Above the age of 40–45, men would be wise to consult with a physician and consider further evaluation before embarking on a new exercise regimen. For women the age is around 50–55. If someone under 50 has a family history of sudden death, or a personal history of fainting spells, chest pain, unusual shortness of breath, or cardiac problems, a careful history and physical examination are warranted.

In some cases, a "graded exercise test" or "exercise tolerance test" may be recommended. These tests usually take the form of walking on a treadmill or pumping a stationary bicycle. This sort of testing is also being offered by a lot of health clubs and other private fitness enterprises.

The logic of an exercise tolerance test is fairly straightforward. If the coronary arteries are diseased, they may fail to respond to the stress of vigorous exercise with a sufficient supply of blood. Result: heart attack. A milder, controlled stress can be used, however, to test for this possibility. The technique is reasonably simple. The subject is attached to an electrocardiograph (ECG), an electronic device that often detects malfunction of the heart. As a rule, blood pressure is also monitored, and the subject is asked to report any chest pain.

Then a period of gradually increasing exercise begins. Usually, it takes the form of walking on a treadmill at progressively faster rates (or increasing grades) until the subject feels unable to continue. If the heart's rhythm or the pattern of the ECG tracing changes, the coronary arteries *may* be diseased. And the occurrence of chest pain along with these other abnormalities is strong evidence that there is a problem with circulation to the heart.

Although the exercise tolerance test is relatively simple and safe to administer, it is not infallible. Interpretation is subject to two kinds of error. A person with coronary artery disease may be missed (a "false negative"), or apparent abnormalities in the results may lead to the assumption that a healthy heart is diseased (a "false positive").

In the latter case, an extensive series of tests may be undertaken in an attempt to establish the innocence or guilt of the arteries under suspicion. But even additional tests may not be able to write a clean bill of health with any certainty. The ultimate result may be that a perfectly well person of 30 or 40 winds up with a curtailed life-style—and finds it difficult or impossible to purchase life insurance—all because of a false-positive test. There is also a risk that treatment may be recommended—even in the absence of symptoms clearly warranting it.

The point is that these tests, even when they are safe to administer, carry real risks. Sometimes there is clearly a reason to perform an exercise tolerance test—a need to check out suspicious symptoms, to establish the level of exercise tolerance in someone who is known to have coronary artery disease, or to evaluate the progress of therapy. But unless there is such a definite purpose, the exercise tolerance test may create as many problems as it solves.

The value of an exercise tolerance test in people who are under 50, have no family history of premature heart disease, and are in good health is open to debate—*wide* open. Whether to go through with such a test should be discussed with one's personal physician. Medical tests are not automatically a good thing, and misinformation is never a bargain.

Beefing it up

Aerobic exercise is more popular than body building, but Nautilus and Universal machines, not to mention free weights, have picked up their share of devotees. There are some good reasons for indulging in a certain amount of strength conditioning. Done with moderation, strengthening exercises protect bones, muscles, and joints from injury. Indeed, strength training in moderation is now recognized as an important component of exercise programs not only for adolescent athletes (whose growing tissues can suffer from overuse injuries inflicted by rigorous training programs in swimming, track, and so on) but for older people as well. The older adult who has been sedentary and returns to active life can benefit from the toning and increased muscle bulk that comes from periodic strengthening exercises.

There are currently 4 basic varieties of body building:

ISOMETRIC EXERCISE This involves contracting the muscles without moving the body part that is stressed. Standing still and pushing against a wall is an example. Tensing the muscles of an arm or leg without moving it is another.

ISOTONIC EXERCISE   This is exemplified by weight lifting. The body part moves against resistance while maintaining a constant tension in the muscle involved. Usually, though, it's not possible to lift the same amount of weight through the whole range of motion. In flexing your arms, for example, you can move the greatest weight when your elbows are partially bent, not when they are most bent or nearly straight. People using free weights tend to jerk or "cheat" in order to overcome this problem when lifting weights that are appropriate for the middle of their range.

VARIABLE-RESISTANCE EXERCISE   These exercises attempt to overcome the problem of uneven strength through the range of motion. The popular Nautilus machines, for example, have been designed to smoothly change the resistance you feel as you take a weight through your range of motion. As you pull on the lever of one of these machines, the weight usually starts out somewhat reduced and then increases to a maximum at the middle of the motion, only to reduce again near the end. Theoretically, this pattern of movement gives the maximum workout while minimizing the risk of injury. In practice, of course, it's possible to get injured by overdoing a Nautilus workout, just as it's possible to get injured by other forms of exercise.

ISOKINETIC EXERCISE   This type of strength training is relatively new in concept, and has required the development of new machines to deliver it. Like the Nautilus equipment, these machines try to deal with the problem of the muscles' varying strength through a range of motion, but they differ in that both position and tension vary while the speed of motion is held constant. The advantage of this form of training, in theory, is that the well-motivated person could put his or her absolute maximum effort into the whole range of motion. Isokinetic training is also used in some rehabilitation programs for people recovering from injuries.

There are also some exotic variants of strengthening exercises, such as "eccentric" training, in which a very heavy weight is taken from the flexed to the extended position, and "plyometric" training, in which a heavy weight is pulled back from a fall. All of these forms of strength training have their advocates—and a rich supply of folklore—to back them up. On the whole, isotonic (and probably variable-resistance) methods seem to produce the largest increases in strength. Isometrics are somewhat less effective, and there isn't really enough comparative data on isokinetic methods to establish whether they have an advantage (except as a rehabilitation technique with a low potential for injury).

With the most common forms of strength training, isometric and variable-resistance, the basic routine is to put maximal effort into a motion (say lifting a barbell) at a level of resistance (or weight) that permits rapid repetition for 7 to a dozen times. After a brief rest, this routine may be repeated for a total of 3 sets. As the muscles become stronger, more repetitions of the motion become possible. At somewhere between 12 and 15 repetitions, the weight is increased by a few pounds, so that only 6 or 7 repetitions are now possible, and the exercise is repeated over a course of days or weeks until, again, this number has been approximately doubled. Then more weight is added until you start looking like Arnold Schwarzenegger—or a reasonable facsimile.

Isometric exercises, which were more popular 15–20 years ago, are most effective if a given contraction is maintained at maximal intensity for 6–10 seconds (so that virtually every fiber in a muscle is participating). The exercise should be repeated several times a day.

Trainers and athletes make endless fine distinctions between versions of these routines. For most people, the point is that lifting a modest and tolerable amount of weight—or performing the equivalent activity on a machine—at least half a dozen times leads to increasing strength. Doing 3 sets of the exercise is even better, and when the number or repetitions reaches 12–15, some weight may be added.

A noticeable feature of this kind of exercise is that one works very intensely for a few seconds, then stands around huffing and puffing for a while until ready to do the next exercise. On the whole, this form of activity makes very little contribution to the heart and circulation, and it does have the drawback of raising blood pressure.

A form of weight training that attempts to provide the advantage of *both* strength and endurance, or aerobic, exercise is called *circuit training*. In circuit training, which has its adherents in the fitness community, a series of "stations" is set up. At each one, you perform some kind of weight or resistance activity as often as possible for 30 seconds, then you move swiftly on to the next station and again do whatever is required for 30 seconds. Usually there are 6–8 stations, so after 5–6 minutes you start over and do another set, which may be repeated again so as to put in a minimum of 15 or 20 minutes exercising. This type of training can do a great deal for strength, endurance, and flexibility; it is also extremely effective in weight control.

Overdoing it

Exercise can, without a doubt, impair health. The greatest fear some people express is that the strain of jogging, or a similar activity, will cause a heart attack. It is perfectly true that this can happen. Someone who jogs regularly is slightly more likely to have a heart attack while jogging than at other times of the day. But this statistic is highly deceptive, because, on the whole, joggers (or people engaged in other fitness activities) have a much lower risk of heart attacks. Jogging is clearly beneficial to the heart—but if a person's heart is going to go ahead and get sick, he or she is most likely to discover that fact while jogging.

Stress fractures, sprains, and strains

A much more likely discovery while jogging is pain: usually in a knee, ankle, or foot. Running does have its down side. A survey of runners in the 10-kilometer (6.2-mile) Peachtree Road Race in Atlanta revealed that more than a third of the participants in that race developed some kind of problem with their bones or muscles within a year. As you might expect, increased mileage meant an increased rate of injury. Of those who ran less than 9 miles a week, about 20% reported some kind of injury; at 30 miles a week, about 50% were affected. Most common were knee and foot problems.

Pain in a committed runner is likely to elicit almost philosophical debates about whether to "run through" it or give it a rest. Both running philosophers and physicians agree that if the pain is caused by a *stress fracture,* rest is the order of the day, or, more accurately, several weeks.

Stress fractures are caused by repeated force acting on bone structure. These forces can be due to a blow or to the pull of muscles on the bone. In runners, stress fractures are most often found in one or the other of the two leg bones (the tibia and fibula). They are most likely to occur shortly after a new exercise program is begun, or after the runner makes significant changes—wearing new shoes, increasing distance, or using a different route or surface. Unfortunately, routine x-rays may not reveal a stress fracture right away. The crack is hard to see; it's only when new, and slightly thicker, bone grows in to repair the damage that a line can be seen. If a diehard runner won't cease and desist without proof, a bone scan can be done. In this procedure the patient is given a minuscule amount of radioactive material; abnormal uptake in the region of injury demonstrates the fracture. A relatively short period of rest in this case can quite literally save a lot of time and pain.

Sprained ankles are among the leading injuries responsible for days lost from work. What happens in a sprain is that an abnormal motion, most commonly bending or twisting, stretches or tears the fibrous tissue (ligaments) that hold the ankle bones together and give it stability. The severity of damage caused by sprains varies greatly. It is never correct to assume that an injury is "just" a sprained ankle. If the rupture of ligaments is extensive, there may be prolonged disability or a permanently unstable ("weak") ankle.

A *strain* is stretching or tearing of a tendon—the fibrous cord that attaches a muscle to bone. Like a sprain, a strain can result in severe pain or disability if it is not treated appropriately at the time of injury.

Immediate therapy for a sprain or strain is to get weight off the injured part (if it is a knee or ankle), elevate it (preferably above the level of the heart), and put ice on it. Keeping the ankle elevated and iced for 24 hours or so can make a big difference in the rate of healing. Injured wrists and elbows should receive essentially the same treatment—rest, elevation, and ice. These steps minimize the chance of further damage and reduce swelling to a minimum. An elastic bandage may make the injured joint more comfortable and may also help to reduce swelling, but it will not provide enough stability to avoid risk of further damage if the joint is stressed too soon.

These "soft-tissue" injuries can be remarkably slow to heal and can make trouble for long periods of time. Whether to see a doctor about an apparently minor injury is always a judgment call. Basically, if there is any doubt, it's worth a call and the inconvenience of a trip to the office while trying to keep weight off a painful limb.

Running and blood loss

At least 4 different studies have revealed that runners who regularly log great distances, such as those preparing for marathons, develop slow intestinal bleeding. The blood loss is subtle, but may be reflected in a mild anemia, known as *runner's anemia*. It appears that regular runners do have slightly lower levels of red blood (hemoglobin) and lower stores of iron, which is used as part of hemoglobin, the protein that makes red cells red. It's unclear whether runners would benefit from supplements of iron to favor replacement of their lost blood.

Another way that athletes may lose blood is in the urine. This condition was first recognized in 1881 by a German physician, who observed that infantrymen often had blood in their urine after a long march. The condition came to be known as *march hemoglobinuria*. The reason for the condition is quite interesting. It happens because red cells carried through the small blood vessels in the soles of the feet are damaged by repeated impact. As a consequence, they release their hemoglobin, and if enough of the protein gets out of the cells, it will pass into the urine as the kidney filters the blood. Today, the condition is most often seen in runners or walkers, if they go hard and long enough. Better padding in shoes, a softer stride, and resilient running surfaces can go a long way toward preventing marathon hemoglobinuria—as it should probably be called in the 1980s.

Amenorrhea and bone density

Enthusiasts often push themselves to ever higher levels of exercise in the belief they are strengthening their bodies. There are, in fact, some important exceptions to this rule—and women are particularly vulnerable. As women reach intense levels of training, they quite commonly lose their periods. The reasons are not completely clear, but at least part of the cause is loss of body fat. Below a certain level of stored energy, the female body apparently turns off reproductive cycles rather than risk a pregnancy with insufficient reserves for completion. Production of estrogen is reduced, and the result is known as *athletic amenorrhea.*

Athletic amenorrhea is reversible and not in itself any particular problem, unless a woman wants to get pregnant. But this form of amenorrhea appears to mimic menopause in one important respect: It favors thinning of bone, and for the same reason as menopause.

Low estrogen permits calcium to dissolve out of bones. Athletes with amenorrhea lose calcium especially from their lower (or lumbar) spines.

Bones usually respond directly to the stress of exercise by acquiring *more* calcium and growing stronger, but intense conditioning in women apparently has an indirect effect, through lowered estrogen, that works in the opposite direction. More studies are needed to establish whether female athletes with amenorrhea run the risk of symptomatic osteoporosis later in life.

On the other hand, postmenopausal women who are currently exercising to protect against osteoporosis should continue to do so. Exercise does strengthen bone, even when it reduces estrogen. This was demonstrated by a group of oarswomen with athletic amenorrhea. They had stronger vertebrae than equally trained runners—presumably because pulling on oars stimulates back bones to grow stronger, whereas running does not.

Weight Control

Few people find it surprising to be told that Americans, on average, have gained weight throughout the twentieth century. They are more likely to be surprised when they learn that Americans are also eating less, on average, than in the past. This nutritional paradox comes largely from the fact that most people are exercising less than ever before. Even those who perceive themselves as active, because they play racketball once or twice a week or participate in other recreational athletics, may be so sedentary the rest of the time that their total output of calories in physical activity is negligible. As a result, Americans, like other urbanized, industrial populations, have reduced their intake of calories.

The paradox is even more serious. While "eating too much," some people are also "eating too little." The average diet, even at the currently low levels of intake, is obviously sufficient to let people become fat, but it may not provide all the nutrients that people require. As the number of calories in a diet goes down, so do the quantities of vitamins and minerals. It can be extremely difficult on a diet of less than 2,000 calories a day to consume enough iron (supplied chiefly by meat and fortified breads or cereals) or calcium (from dairy products, dark green vegetables, some fish) to meet the body's requirements. These deficiencies are likely to be most significant in women, who need iron to replace menstrual losses and calcium for pregnancy, lactation, and their own bones in later life. And, currently, it is women who are most likely to be dieters.

In this section we will discuss weight control—a problem that has not been solved, despite the enormous number of claims that are made in popular magazines and books. In the next section we will go on to look at other aspects of nutrition as they affect well-being and aging.

The problem of overweight

In 1952 an influential article appeared in *Today's Health,* at the time a widely read magazine. The title of the article was "Overweight—America's Number 1 Health Problem." The author meant "health hazard," but in retrospect his choice of words seems justified. The connection between weight and health is an unsolved problem over 30 years later, and it is currently one of the more controversial subjects in medicine.

In 1985 a major conference on the subject was sponsored by the National Institutes of Health. A panel was charged with listening to experts present and discuss the published evidence. The members of this jury were then asked to come up with their assessment of the facts. They concluded, "The evidence is now overwhelming that obesity, defined as excessive storage of energy in the form of fat, has adverse effects on health and longevity." The statement is true—but it obscures some important uncertainties: "How much fat is harmful?" and "What exactly are the risks?"

The panel went on to recommend, in essence, that 34 million Americans—around one-sixth of the population—seek weight-reduction treatment to improve their health. This advice, if taken, could add 2–5 billion dollars to the annual health-care budget, assuming that professional visits and participation in some kind of active program were involved. Would such an effort and expense be effective? There are few firm answers in this area, much less is there a clear solution.

Setting the table

"Obesity" and "overweight" are arbitrary terms. There is no good definition of these words, and there never will be. Body fat is what is

▪ Height and weight tables ▪

Height	Metropolitan Life Ages 25–29		Gerontology Research Center Men and women by age (years)				
ft-in	Men	Women	25	35	45	55	65
4-10	—	100–131	84–111	92–119	99–127	107–135	115–142
4-11	—	101–134	87–115	95–123	103–131	111–139	119–147
5-0	—	103–137	90–119	98–127	106–135	114–143	123–152
5-1	123–145	105–140	93–123	101–131	110–140	118–148	127–157
5-2	125–148	108–144	96–127	105–136	113–144	122–153	131–163
5-3	127–151	111–148	99–131	108–140	117–149	126–158	135–168
5-4	129–155	114–152	102–135	112–145	121–154	130–163	140–173
5-5	131–159	117–156	106–140	115–149	125–159	134–168	144–179
5-6	133–163	120–160	109–144	119–154	129–164	138–174	148–184
5-7	135–167	123–164	112–148	122–159	133–169	143–179	153–190
5-8	137–171	126–167	116–153	126–163	137–175	147–184	158–196
5-9	139–175	129–170	119–157	130–168	141–179	151–190	162–201
5-10	141–179	132–173	122–162	134–173	145–184	156–195	167–207
5-11	144–183	135–176	126–167	137–178	149–190	160–201	172–213
6-0	147–187	—	129–171	141–183	153–195	165–207	177–219
6-1	150–192	—	133–176	145–188	157–200	169–213	182–225
6-2	153–197	—	137–181	149–194	162–206	174–219	187–232
6-3	157–202	—	141–186	153–199	166–212	179–225	192–238
6-4	—	—	144–191	157–205	171–218	184–231	197–244

Heights and weights are given in pounds for people without shoes or clothing.

Sources: Metropolitan "Height and Weight Tables," 1983, *Statistical Bulletin* January–June 1983; Gerontology Research Center tables from Andres, Bierman, and Hazzard, *Principles of Geriatric Medicine* (New York: McGraw-Hill, 1985), pp. 311–318.

known as a continuous variable—it's something you have more or less of, not something that you either have or don't have. There's no absolute way to show that gaining another pound will put a person over the limit of normal, but many authorities feel that an arbitrary standard is better than none at all.

If we knew more, we might be able to take another approach. We could tell one person, "The amount of fat on your body is taking 6 weeks off your life expectancy," and tell another, "Sorry, it's 6 years." Available information doesn't make these predictions possible. The common solution is to pick a point that seems practical and divide people accordingly as sheep or goats. With body fat, the main tool for making this decision has long been a set of tables prepared from data collected by the insurance industry.

By combining information about the weight and survival of their policy holders, the companies have developed a set of tables to predict mortality rates. These tables are used for setting insurance premiums. In their raw form, the tables fill many pages and are all but unreadable. As a service to the public, the Metropolitan Life Insurance Company has converted the raw material into convenient, and by now very familiar, tables defining the weight ranges that are supposedly compatible with longest life. In the 1942 edition, these weights were called "ideal"; in the 1959 edition they were downgraded to "desirable"; but by 1983 they no longer had an adjective. Now the tables are simply labeled "Height and Weight Tables." The implication, however, remains that people over the weight range listed in the table have a shortened life expectancy.

There are several reasons for questioning this implication. Applicants for individual insurance policies may not be typical of the American population as a whole. But even if they were, the process used to generate the Met Life tables involves some assumptions that may not be accurate. One feature of the tables is a pure fiction: the division into "frame sizes." Frame size has never been measured by the insurance companies. The notion that a big body frame entitles someone to 20 extra pounds, or that a small one lowers the limit, is based purely on theory. Thus, in reprinting the tables (see p. 34), we have omitted frame sizes.

Who, when, where?

Perhaps the main problem with the Metropolitan Life tables, as with a great many other approaches to the problem of body fat, is the assumption that overweight or obesity is a single condition, one that means the same thing to everybody. Accumulating evidence indicates that this just isn't so.

Who has the fat helps determine its effect on health. Genetic background is an important influence, for example. Certain groups of Native Americans develop more complications associated with obesity than do others with a different heredity.

When the fat is acquired also seems to make a difference. Weight gained in early adulthood may be associated with more ill health than weight gained later in life. The Metropolitan Life tables have always presented a single weight as best for all ages. But the same raw data on which these tables are based have been reanalyzed by scientists at the Gerontology Research Center in Baltimore, who find that age does make a difference.

Their results indicate that people with the lowest mortality rate tend to gain about a pound a year—give or take—from the age of 25 to the age of 65 (*see p. 34*). These results, it goes without saying, have inspired controversy. In general, the Gerontology Research Center's table suggests that young adults should be lighter than the Metropolitan Life table indicates, but as age increases, the newer table becomes more liberal. This table also gives the same values for both men and women. Because women have lighter bones and muscles, this implies that women can be relatively fatter than men for the same life expectancy. A notable feature of both tables, when frame size is not considered, is how wide the ranges are—often 20 to 40 pounds.

Where fat is deposited may be critical. Fat around the middle— the "spare tire" or "middle-age" spread—seems to be especially associated with health problems. For example, it has been shown that women whose fat is distributed more on the lower part of their bodies (hips and thighs) appear to run a lower risk of diabetes than women whose fat is located at their waistlines. And, according to at least one study, the man who has fat accumulated at his waistline is at higher risk of heart disease than a heavier man whose fat is more evenly distributed.

Weighing the hazard

Severe obesity is clearly associated with serious health risks. But is there a measurable risk to being only somewhat fatter than average? How you answer that question depends on how you weigh the evidence, so to speak. Statistically, high blood pressure and type-2

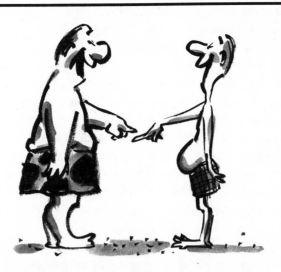

Recent research suggests that a pot belly, even in someone who is otherwise relatively thin, is more of a threat to health than fat distributed more evenly on the body or concentrated in the lower half. Pot bellies also appear easier to lose: try cutting down alcohol intake and increasing regular physical activity.

diabetes (adult-onset or non-insulin-dependent diabetes) are most strongly associated with being overweight. These are both serious—potentially lethal—illnesses. Both take their toll mainly through damage to the blood vessels, and ultimately by increasing the rate of heart attacks. A plausible inference is that any added amount of body fat, in and of itself, would raise the risk of dying from a heart attack, and this claim has often been made.

But research results published in the past decade or so give evidence on both sides of the question. The well-publicized Framingham Study, which has followed over 2,000 people since 1948, has been most frequently cited as showing a strong correlation between added pounds and early death—mainly from heart disease. However, different groups analyzing the Framingham data have disagreed on the interpretation of the findings. Meanwhile, other epidemiologic studies have indicated that moderate degrees of overweight are not associated with high mortality. The discrepancies between studies may ultimately be explained by the "who, when, where" factors discussed above: different kinds of people, with fat located in different places on their bodies and acquired at different times of life, may produce divergent statistics.

Given the strong association of overweight with at least two serious health problems, how can the statistics be so equivocal? There is little doubt that type-2 diabetes accounts for a large share of the mortality that overweight people suffer. The case with high blood pressure is beginning to look a little more uncertain. Some recent data suggest that high blood pressure found in association with obesity is not as likely to produce complications as high blood pressure in people of normal weight. Until more complete evidence is available, however, virtually everyone would agree that treating high blood pressure is the prudent approach.

If added body fat drives up total mortality less rapidly than cardiovascular mortality rate—and this appears to be the case—one reason could be that fatter people have a lower death rate from cancer. Some studies have found this to be the case. But there are also conflicting results in this area, and some types of cancer—especially those of the breast and reproductive organs—are thought to be more common in overweight people.

A variety of other conditions are said to result from overweight and to contribute to ill health and early mortality. A commonly cited example is gallstones. And in the case of gallstones, as well as other conditions requiring surgical correction, it is often said that the risk of surgery on overweight people is increased. This is true, but, again, the risks are relatively small and only encountered when the overweight is fairly extreme.

It is worth bearing in mind that the American people have been getting somewhat fatter, on the whole, during the past few decades, yet their life expectancy has continued to increase. This fact alone would argue that overweight is not a grave threat to public health, at least as crudely measured by these mortality rates.

Attitudes

A potential health hazard for many overweight people, but one that isn't well studied, results from the discrimination, prejudice, and exploitation that they often experience. For example, doctors may be inclined to disparage their overweight patients, seeing the failure to lose weight as a sign of unwillingness to cooperate with recommendations intended for their own good. To the extent that overweight people are stigmatized as "bad" or "uncooperative" patients, unsympathetic treatment could result in poor health care.

Overweight people encounter prejudice in employment and school admissions. One study has indicated that an overweight person is seen as a less desirable employee, even if he or she is acknowledged to have the same ability as a normal-weight person. Women appear to be more vulnerable to this kind of discrimination than men. Negative attitudes toward overweight people are very commonly expressed and are easy to elicit with almost any kind of questionnaire or other test. Overweight people are likely to respond to such tests with equally negative attitudes—presumably an indication of lowered self-esteem.

Yet, remarkably enough, considering all this, on measures of mental health the overweight come out essentially normal. No single type of personality has been discovered among overweight people, although most such people share a tendency to disparage their own bodies, to be depressed over their appearance and failure to lose weight, and to be apprehensive about their ability to succeed in work or in sexual relationships. All of these factors make overweight people easy prey to the enormous industry marketing weight-loss methods.

Some of the damage that is done by ill-advised weight-loss efforts is physical—the result of inadequate nutrition provided by popular reducing methods. It is at least possible that long-term dieting has contributed to the epidemic of osteoporosis now being observed. Women, particularly in adolescence and early adulthood, have proved vulnerable to disorders of eating behavior, and these are widely believed to be the result of attempts to pursue popular diets. (The 12-pound-in-2-week variety is probably the most damaging in this regard.) The current epidemic of eating disorders—anorexia and bulimia—must be regarded as an important adverse effect of misdirected efforts to control weight.

Leaving the table

It is more difficult to say now than it was 35 years ago that every added pound of body fat is a threat to health. Some evidence points to a "safe zone" of 10–20 pounds on either side of approximately average weight. Much below or above this level, early mortality is observed. However, some authorities remain committed to the view that *any* amount of excess body fat is a health liability. The controversy isn't going to be resolved easily, because important information is just too hard to obtain. There is no definitive experiment that can be performed. Instead, we can expect, in the next years or decades, to see an accumulation of studies that point one way or the other.

A very important gap in existing data has to do with the health of people who successfully reduce and keep the weight off. There is essentially no trustworthy evidence on this score, although it is very clear that, in the short run, weight loss improves both blood pressure and type-2 diabetes. In any case, tables of "desirable" weight should be used very cautiously. In making judgments about the significance of any particular body weight, the whole person should be considered. Family background, other medical conditions that may be present, and psychological factors should be weighed, along with the patient, before a final recommendation is made.

The options

Ask almost anyone how to lose weight, and the automatic answer is likely to be "go on a diet." And lots of people go on diets. By at least one estimate, roughly 10% of the population is on a "serious" diet at any one time. Indeed, the reducing diet is about as American a ritual as eating Thanksgiving dinner. An industry worth many billions of dollars is based on the marketing of diets—through books, programs, low-calorie lines of frozen food, magazine articles, pyramid schemes, and any other gimmick that a smooth-talking entrepreneur can think up. Yet, for a "therapy" that is taken so much for granted, dieting is supported by remarkably little evidence. What there is suggests that diets are far from an ideal strategy for managing long-term weight problems—and they may have some important drawbacks even as a short-term approach.

Calorie counting: does it work?

Contrary to what is often claimed, reducing diets cannot be used to "retrain" eating habits for successful long-term weight control. The reason is quite simple. The fraction of one's daily food intake that is converted to fat is usually very small. Let's say, for example, that you have gained 2 pounds a year for the last 5 years and that you normally eat around 2,500 calories a day (a little low for most men, a little high for most women, but a reasonable compromise). To gain these 10 pounds you would have eaten only 19 calories a day in excess of what your body used—less than the amount in a single lime or 5 unsweetened strawberries.

Since there's no way a normal person can accurately cut 20 calories out of his or her daily intake—even 300 is less than most people can accurately guess—the typical dieter cuts out a large number of calories. It's usually more than 500 and often as much as 1,000. Reducing intake by this much produces noticeable weight loss in fairly short order.

The loss is actually much more rapid than could result from loss of fat. Early in a diet, the largest amount of weight is lost in the form of body water—which simply goes out in the urine. For a couple of reasons, lowering food intake causes the body to release some fluid that is normally retained. This can amount to a few pints—and therefore a few pounds on the scale—as well as, maybe, half an inch at the waist band (since water, like fat, does have bulk). But the loss of water is not permanent, and in any case it doesn't mean anything.

Another, more important substance is also lost in the first weeks of a reducing diet: protein, which is taken out of muscles. The protein is converted to glucose, a sugar that is demanded by the brain. The human body lacks the biochemical machinery that would be capable of converting body fat into glucose (though it can convert glucose to fat). So, during starvation or a diet, the body turns to muscle protein as its source of glucose to feed the brain and to serve a few other needs that cannot be met in other ways.

Finally, like starvation from any cause, reducing diets lead the body to lower its resting metabolic rate. *Resting metabolic rate* simply means the bare minimum of energy the body requires to keep going. It is determined by having people sit still for a while and do nothing while their energy consumption is measured. For virtually everyone, resting metabolism accounts for the largest fraction of energy expended every day—usually more than half. It turns out that bodies appear to have some discretion in the amount of energy they burn in resting metabolism. You can think of it this way: The temperature of a room can be held at a given level if all the windows are tightly sealed and the heater is turned low, or the same result can be achieved by opening the windows a crack and burning a little more oil. The body on a diet is like the first room. Less fuel is burned in response to the perceived shortage of fuel (food). Obviously, this adaptation would be protective in time of scarcity. In a time of dieting, it simply means that after a few days the person who is determined to lose weight must reduce intake even more than at the beginning of the diet to continue losing at the same rate.

Diets: the record

In addition to these theoretical difficulties with dieting, there is the problem of evidence. Since 1931 many scientific studies of weight loss have been published. Of these, about 100 give enough information on the effects of lowering food intake to be interpretable. Many different techniques have been used. They have ranged from rigid, very-low-calorie diet plans, to programs combining education and encouragement, to behavior modification based in psychological theory. These various methods have been applied to many different kinds of people—from those who are only mildly overweight to those with severe degrees of obesity.

Most people who have been studied in such programs were 30–100% overweight, and they have typically lost less than 10% while enrolled in the program. In general, people have regained what they lost in a matter of 2–4 years, often much sooner. Thus, although there are clear exceptions—people who do manage to lose weight through dieting and then keep it off for long periods—this does not seem to be the general experience.

It is important to recognize that the published evidence on dieting for weight control does not include any information on people who "treat themselves," for example by purchasing a diet book. Some might do better than the research subjects, but there are reasons for doubting that they do. Also, there are no scientific data whatsoever on the results obtained by commercial enterprises offering weight-loss or weight-control programs. Most of them are careful not to make specific claims—but the implications that their methods or products work is not supported by published evidence.

Behavior modification, a new wrinkle

About 15 years ago, with wide agreement that standard reducing diets worked poorly for most people as a long-term method of weight control, behavior modification became a more popular approach. Generally speaking, behavior modification is a set of techniques for altering habits that people find hard to give up but consciously don't want to continue. In one form or another, behavior therapy may be used to alter drug use, a phobic response (say to snakes or spiders), procrastination, sexual dysfunction, and so on. As applied to weight problems, behavior modification almost always focuses on eating as the behavior to modify—though in the past few years exercise has come to play a more prominent role in these programs.

The underlying idea of most behavioral treatment of weight problems is that the person comes to eat too much as a result of responding to the wrong cues. Instead of just feeling hungry, the overweight person may use food in a variety of thoughtless ways. Perhaps the person eats on the run, fails to notice when hunger is satisfied, and keeps eating more than is needed. Perhaps the person uses food when the real craving is for company, or entertainment.

The usual program of behavior modification includes the following methods:

- Self-monitoring to identify the false cues stimulating the person to eat. Keeping a diary of food consumption is a basic tool.
- Limiting or controlling the cues that lead to eating. This means, for example, keeping high-calorie foods out of the house, eating only at specified times and in permitted locations, or devising other ways to limit "opportunities" to eat.
- Controlling the act of eating, mostly training people to eat more slowly and deliberately, and not to combine eating with other activities. Counting chews or putting down the knife and fork between each bite are some common devices to slow eating. Never eating in front of a television is often suggested as a way to make sure that eating does not become confused with other activities.
- Rewarding success. Two kinds of success are encouraged by behavior modification. One of them, of course, is weight loss. The other is achieving a prescribed change in eating or other habits targeted by the program. Sometimes these "rewards" are as minimal as giving oneself "points" for doing the right thing. Sometimes they may take the form of money paid back from a kitty established at the beginning of treatment. Sometimes they involve having a spouse or friend offer to do something nice after a certain

number of points have been accumulated or a certain number of pounds lost. In general, such rewards should be administered frequently—with every pound or two, not after 30 or 50 pounds are lost.

- Changing the foods that are chosen. Most behavior modification programs do not involve calorie counting. But they encourage systematic selection of foods that are not high in fat or calories. The emphasis is usually on complex carbohydrates.
- Altering attitudes. Behavior modification programs often try to help people modify patterns of thinking that are self-defeating. Instead of thinking, "I'm taking too long to lose weight," the client is encouraged to think, "I'm losing, and it's more important just to keep losing than worry about how much." Sometimes thought exercises may be given so that people can learn to block the self-defeating idea as soon as it appears.

Although programs of behavior modification originally focused almost exclusively on diet, there is an emerging consensus that exercise is at least as important as eating behavior. So behavior-modification techniques are now used, in some programs, to help clients begin and maintain a program of physical activity. This development is too new for its effectiveness to be assessed. On the other hand, there is now enough accumulated experience with behavior modification to permit some conclusions.

Behavior modification must be seen as a package. Nobody knows which item in this list is most effective, because the techniques have never really been evaluated one-by-one. Some psychologists have expressed doubts as to whether any of them is really working the way it is meant to. For example, by focusing attention on food, behavior modification might, in theory, increase rather than diminish a person's desire to eat.

Behavior modification does, in practice, "work," though in a rather limited way. On the whole, it produces slower weight loss than regular reducing diets. But weight loss is likely to continue for a year or so after treatment is begun. A typical amount is on the order of 12–20 pounds (in someone whose goal is to lose about 50). Indications are, however, that 4–5 years later, the weight will be regained.

Behavior modification is still recommended as the best single approach for people who have only mild weight problems. It seems unlikely, however, that behavior modification focused exclusively on eating behavior will make a significant long-term difference.

The argument for exercise

Even though exercise has not been as thoroughly tested for as long as one would like, there are reasons for being hopeful. Over and over again, research has shown that exercise leads to a reduction in body fat along with a shift to more muscle. This effect is observed even when people don't change their eating habits, and it is as true of people who are very obese as of the more mildly overweight. Indeed, results may be more striking in people who have a lot of weight to lose than in those who are closer to average weight.

Exercise produces weight loss in at least three ways.

First is the obvious fact that calories are expended during exercise. This is probably the least important effect. Food is a remarkably compact form of fuel, and most of us are perfectly capable of compensating for calories expended in exercise by eating an additional doughnut or ice-cream cone in the course of a day.

Second, exercise raises rather than lowers the resting metabolic rate for about 24 hours after the workout. In people who are *both* dieting and exercising, the two effects approximately cancel, so that metabolic demands continue at their same old level. Quantitatively, this may be a more important contribution to the calorie drain than the cost of exercise itself. However, even here, compensatory eating would be possible.

So the third effect is probably most important. Exercise seems to have a direct effect on the amount of fat a body "wants" to maintain. In effect, getting into condition sends signals to the brain that instruct it to lower the body's level of adipose tissue. (You can think of this effect as being somewhat analogous to the way *resting* heart rate is lowered as a result of regular exercising.) The effect is gradual, but very consistent. To achieve this effect, the person exercising must observe certain rules: (1) The exercise has to be aerobic, as discussed earlier in this chapter. (2) The exercise must be done frequently. Three days a week really isn't enough; 5–7 is closer to optimal. Obviously, if exercise is to be this frequent, it can't feel like torture; brisk walking may be the best choice. (3) Each period of exercise should continue for at least half an hour at a time.

A common misconception is that exercising leads to reduced

food intake. It doesn't necessarily, but that doesn't seem to matter. People may actually increase their intake while exercising—even as they begin to lose body fat.

On the other hand, people beginning an exercise program may, at least temporarily, *gain* weight. The reason is that, at first, muscle is sometimes built up more rapidly than fat is broken down. There may be an effect on body fluid as well, but this is less clear. Thus, even though the waist starts to shrink, the scale may show little change for several weeks or even months. People who worry about what the scale says may be inappropriately discouraged from continuing their exercise program and opt for a crash diet instead.

Many people ask how much weight they will lose on an exercise regimen. There's no way to predict, and it's clear that exercise will not remove all excess fat from all people. The fat deposits that exercise diminishes most effectively are those located around the waist. Because fat in this area seems most harmful to health, this is a highly desirable result.

Although exercise can't be used as a magic wand to remove all visible traces of fat, it has important invisible benefits. Even when a fair amount of fat is retained on the body, control of blood sugar, blood pressure, and blood cholesterol can be dramatically improved by regular exercise. From the standpoint of health, the person who exercises regularly is probably much better off than a thinner person who does not.

Changing what you eat

An idea that was fairly popular until about 30 years ago was that the real basis for weight gain was not eating "too much" but eating "the wrong things." Some foods have been identified as more "fattening" than others, and countless diets have been based on the notion that people would automatically lose weight by avoiding them.

For nearly a century, from the mid-1850s to the mid-1950s, the usual culprit in this scenario was carbohydrate: starch in the form of potatoes, bread, rice, pasta, and sweets. The most popular diets of this century, including *Dr. Atkins' Diet Revolution, Calories Don't Count*, and *The Scarsdale Diet*, have been based on this idea. Some, such as *Calories Don't Count*, only required the customer to switch to a diet that was mostly fat and protein; others, such as *The Scarsdale Diet*, also restricted intake of calories.

The success of these diets probably resulted mainly from the fact that they produce even more rapid loss of body water than typical reducing diets—and therefore seemed to have excellent results in the first few weeks. However, it is now clear that they have no other advantage, and there is good reason to think that using these diets often, or for a prolonged period, would be harmful because of their relatively high fat content.

Indeed, restricting carbohydrates is now thought to be exactly the wrong idea. If anything, a good reducing regimen should allow lots of starches, particularly in the form known as "complex carbohydrates"—meaning whole grain breads, rice, pasta, and so forth. Sweets, so long as they are low in fat content, probably do no particular harm—although some debate about the role of sugar in the diet remains (*see below*).

Currently, expert opinion is that fat in the diet is much more likely than carbohydrate to be responsible for weight gain. The reasons for this effect are not altogether clear. Pure fat is very high in calories—more than twice as high as carbohydrate or protein. But that almost certainly is not the whole reason that eating fat favors weight gain.

In any case, the trick is in learning to recognize important sources of fat in the diet. We'll discuss this more in the next section. Suffice it to say at this point that many foods are deceptive either in reputation or in name. For example, things we call "sweets"—such as pies or ice cream—often have more of their calories as fat than sugar. On the other hand, substances that are rather obviously full of fat—such as mayonnaise—may not be particularly important sources of fat in the diet, because such small quantities are eaten. Indeed, red meats, dairy products, and baked goods may be the most significant sources of fat, simply because we eat relatively large quantities of them.

In general, very little is known about other components of the diet as they affect fat storage. A fairly obvious one to consider is alcohol. Alcohol has calories, but it may also act, somewhat like dietary fat, to promote storage of body fat. One weight-loss strategy for the moderate drinker is to go on the wagon. It can't hurt, and it often seems to produce striking weight reduction without other dietary measures.

A promising, but not fully proven, theory is that some people experience a particular craving for carbohydrates. This craving may occur only at some times of day or at certain seasons, according to the theory. When it does occur, people are likely to overeat because their bodies are calling for carbohydrate but aren't "smart" or specific enough to go just for crackers or bread. So unneeded calories are ingested in the struggle to satisfy a particular craving.

Promoters of "health foods" and various dietary supplements have trotted out an endless stream of products supposedly favoring weight loss or weight control. Among the more recent are substances derived from grapefruit and a microbe known as *spirulina*. None of these has any support from scientific studies at the present time. There is no known material that can be added to a regular diet to produce weight loss.

Drugs

For about 20 years, amphetamines (dexedrine and others) were commonly prescribed as "appetite suppressing" drugs and were frequently dispensed to overweight patients as an aid to beginning a weight reduction effort. This use of amphetamines is no longer accepted for two reasons. First, these drugs have horrendous side effects, which can include addiction and a variety of psychiatric symptoms. Second, amphetamines and similar drugs have been shown to make weight control harder, not easier, after they are stopped. People who take amphetamines while participating in a weight-loss program regain their weight even faster than those who do not.

The reason is that amphetamines do not act to lower appetite. Instead, they influence the body's tendency to store a certain amount of fat. As long as the drug is used, fat stores are kept at a lower level. When it is taken away (as it must be to prevent addiction), the mechanisms of fat storage return to normal, and weight is rapidly regained.

The drug contained in various over-the-counter preparations for weight-control is PPA (phenylpropanolamine), which is chemically similar to amphetamine. It lacks the severe side effects, but it produces less weight loss. Presumably, rebound is as much a problem with PPA as it is with amphetamines.

Although amphetamines are out of favor, some other drugs are currently in research phases and are likely to appear on the market before long. They may have fewer or less severe side effects than amphetamines. But the new drugs are unlikely to be any more effective unless taken for indefinite periods of time. They would obviously have to be very safe, and produce an absolute minimum of unpleasant side effects, to be worth taking.

The basic point to understand about weight-control drugs is that they probably will have to be taken for a lifetime if they are to be taken at all. No currently available drug is clearly safe enough to be used this way. When used as short-term aids to weight loss, amphetamines, and probably other drugs in this class, are counterproductive.

Drastic measures

People who are severely obese clearly face much greater risks than those who are only moderately obese. How these terms are defined, of course, is a matter of debate. As a general rule, being "severely" obese is taken to mean weighing about twice the average. In view of the risks—and the unhappiness—that often go along with such an extreme degree of obesity, relatively high-risk treatments are sometimes recommended. We'll briefly discuss some of these—but any decision must be individualized, and candidates for any of these treatments would do well to seek an independent second opinion before beginning.

MODIFIED FASTING Just as regular reducing diets take off pounds, extremely restricted diets take off pounds even faster. But severe caloric restriction (to less than 500 calories a day) has been associated with distinct hazards, including sudden death. No such program should be entered without close medical supervision.

Very-low-calorie diets may cause loss of body protein. This protein is taken from various sources, including skeletal and heart muscle. However, if the patient eats a little bit of very high-quality protein each day, some of this protein loss can be prevented. This is the basic rationale of the so-called *protein-sparing modified fast* (PSMF). Some investigators maintain that the diet works best (and produces least hunger) if essentially no carbohydrate is given. Others argue that the amount of carbohydrate is not important, or even that it may help with the diet, and that adding carbohydrate prevents some unpleasant side effects, such as dizziness.

Very-low-calorie diets can produce rapid weight loss, but it has not been proved that most people treated this way will maintain their loss. Indeed, some concern has been expressed that such diets

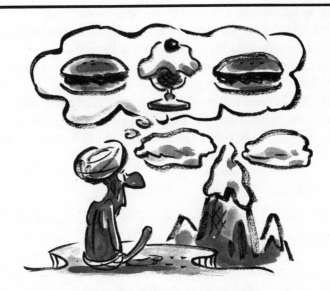

Fasting doesn't "purify" the body. Instead, fasting breaks down body tissue, including muscle, and thus contributes its own waste that has to be removed. The body needs regular supplies of food to stay in good working order.

lead to easier regain of weight—and a more difficult time with the next diet.

When people are on a very-low-calorie diet, their other nutritional needs (for vitamins and minerals) must be very carefully met. And even then the diet is not risk-free. Some sudden deaths have occurred in well-monitored patients. The most likely explanation appears to be that heart muscle was lost as a result of the diet, and this led to heart rhythm disturbances causing the death. Such deaths seem to occur when people adhere very rigorously to the diet for relatively long periods of time—months rather than weeks. Liquid-formula diets containing an inadequate supply of protein and other nutrients have led to a higher rate of casualties.

Very-low-calorie dieting is still in an experimental stage. Patients are probably safer undertaking such a program in a research setting rather than in a commercial weight-loss establishment.

SURGERY   In the last 20 years or so, a variety of surgical operations have been designed in an attempt to limit the ability of extremely obese people to consume food or absorb it once they have eaten it. It is really not at all clear why these procedures work, or how they work—when they do, indeed, work.

The first of these was known as *intestinal bypass surgery,* a very descriptive name. In this procedure, most of the intestine, though left in the abdomen, was bypassed. A direct connection was made between the upper part of the small intestine (the jejunum) and the end of it (the ileum), so that the length of digestive tract available for food absorption was made very short. If patients overate, it was assumed, they wouldn't be able to absorb the excess and would have diarrhea as a result. It turned out that many people had diarrhea anyway, though some eventually adapted and found that they were quite comfortable with the new arrangement. Unfortunately, the rate of metabolic complications, often involving severe liver damage, proved to be excessively high, and this form of surgery is not now recommended.

Technically more difficult than intestinal bypass surgery are the various procedures that limit the size of the stomach, so that it rapidly fills up when food is eaten. These *gastric limitation procedures* are currently the most popular form of surgery for obesity. There is not enough data on the rates of "cure" or of complications to be certain whether the operation produces more benefits than hazards. A certain amount of skepticism seems warranted.

THE BUBBLE   A fairly naive idea about hunger is that people stop eating because their stomachs are "full." It has been known for a long time that this isn't the whole story. But in the last couple of years many people have had an inflatable bubble installed in their stomachs. Placement is done through the mouth, as an endoscopic procedure; surgery is not required. The hope was that this simpler procedure would have much the same effect as gastric-limitation surgery. When the FDA originally approved use of the bubble, it was with the restriction that it could be left in place only 4 months, after which it would have to be removed.

However, the bubble has proved to have some significant complications. Sometimes it collapses, creating a risk that it will pass into the intestine and cause an obstruction. By the end of 1986, nearly 40 major abdominal operations had been required to retrieve bubbles that had passed into the intestine. Somewhat more often the bubble chafes the surface of the stomach and creates a kind of ulcer. Thus, the company producing the bubble, as of this writing, has recommended that it be left in place for no more than 3 months.

The bubble was approved by the FDA with minimal research back-up. Recent evidence suggests that success attributed to the bubble actually resulted from the diet and exercise program required of the recipients.

JAW WIRING   More used in England than the United States, jaw wiring is just what it sounds like. Braces are put on the teeth and wired together so that the person with this muzzle in place cannot open wide enough to eat normal food. He or she must subsist on a diet of liquids or very soft foods. Like the bubble, the wires are not left in place permanently, but are used to produce relatively rapid temporary loss. Dental complications are fairly frequent. There is also some worry that if the patient vomits, inability to clear the material might lead him or her to aspirate it into the lungs—with potentially fatal consequences.

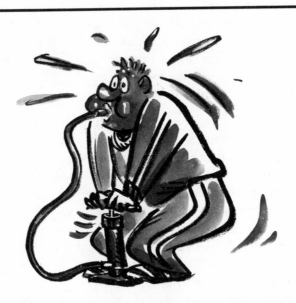

How "full" you feel is not just a matter of how much bulk there is in your stomach. Within limits, your body can figure out approximately how many calories you've eaten. The sensation of feeling full comes not only from the quantity of food you eat, but also the type.

Why weight control is so difficult

For a long time there has been a heated debate among researchers as to whether obesity is or is not under genetic control; 1987 may be recorded as the year in which genes began to emerge as the winner. At first glance, it may seem perfectly reasonable to think that genes are the reason why people get fat or thin. Family members often resemble each other at the waistline, as well as in other ways. Some authorities think that even if the *amount* of fat people acquire is not under genetic control, where it is located on the body probably is. A tendency to put fat on the hips rather than the waist, or vice versa, seems to be inherited—and could hardly be explained except as genetic.

Statistical studies have indeed confirmed that fatness runs in families. Where the controversy arises is in the interpretation. It's possible to inherit a Rembrandt from your parents—but nobody thinks owning a Rembrandt is genetic. One argument used to support the position that genes play little or no role in obesity is the observation that husbands and wives tend to be similarly lean or fat (unlike the nursery-rhyme Sprats). Since husbands and wives are almost always, for legal and social reasons, unrelated, this family resemblance would seem to have a nongenetic basis: the inclination of married people to acquire the same habits of living, to eat the same foods, and so forth.

There is, however, a major flaw in this interpretation: Husbands and wives resemble each other about as much at the *beginning* of their marriage as at the end. Such a resemblance probably results from the fact that like chooses like—and not because couples grow to be more alike the longer they live together (though that may also be true). There's quite a bit of evidence that people tend to select as partners others who resemble them in a variety of ways. So, married couples could have similar genes because that's how they chose each other.

The nature/nurture question, again

Two studies published in 1986, both by Albert Stunkard, a psychiatrist and professor at the University of Pennsylvania, and his colleagues, strongly support the genetic interpretation. These investigations, which received considerable publicity, exploited the two major methods for distinguishing genetic inheritance from environmental influence in human beings: comparison of adopted children with their two sets of parents, and comparisons of identical with fraternal twins. Although neither adoption nor twin studies give perfect data, there are few alternative ways to study the genetics of human beings, who can't be subjected to breeding experiments.

In the first report, Stunkard and his colleagues gave data on adopted children who had been compared with both sets of their parents, biological and adoptive. The excellent adoption records maintained in Denmark, where the study was done, made highly accurate research possible. In brief, the adopted children resembled their genetic parents much more closely than their adopted parents, who had provided their environment and, presumably, training in habits.

Stunkard's second study was conducted on pairs of identical and fraternal twins located from lists of American veterans of World War II and the Korean conflict. Their current weight and height were compared, as were these same measurements from enlistment records. Using a standard statistical method, the Stunkard group first computed the similarity between the identical pairs and that between fraternal pairs. They then matched the two sets of scores. It was very clear that identical twins resemble each other more strongly, and that the similarity increases with age. From these studies, Stunkard and his colleagues could estimate that when one person is fatter than another, about 80% of the difference is the result of their genes.

But we all know people whose weight changes over time, and most people gain weight with age. If this is so, how is it that fat stores are under genetic control?

"If . . . then . . ." genes

The reason may be that the genes controlling energy storage are different from the ones we're used to thinking about—the textbook genes that determine the coloring of skin or eyes, the shape of a head. In those cases, the genes write a very simple rule: "Junior will have brown eyes," and that ends the discussion. And there may indeed be some genes that dictate, quite simply, "John will be thin." At least, many experts think there are such genes. This is consistent with the observation that some people, no matter what they do, seem incapable of gaining weight at all.

But for most of us, the genes governing body fat probably write a more complex script. Instead of giving absolute instructions, they phrase their orders in an "if . . . then . . . " form: "If Fred doesn't walk at least a mile every day, he will get fat." These genes can be thought of as writing a set of rules for how Fred will react to his environment—and the rules might be very different for Hugo.

This theory at least would make a lot of sense of the scientific data that have accumulated over the years. To summarize: (1) It is clear on one hand that people do change their body fat stores, both as individuals and from generation to generation, (2) but it is also evident that body weight is exceedingly resistant to change when people actively attempt to alter it. Success is temporary, and often not all that significant. The reason may simply be that environmental influences outside our control are the main force, other than genes, acting on our body weight.

A historical example may help to make the point. Within the relatively recent past—a hundred years or so—the Pima, Native Americans who once lived a hard-scrabble farming existence along the banks of Arizona's Gila River, were quite normal in weight. They lived a harsh life, but one that was adequate to keep them going from generation to generation. In the past few decades, the Pima have shifted to a more contemporary lifestyle. They drive cars and trucks, they eat a typical southwestern diet of corn and beans that is also relatively high in fat—and the Pima have become a fat people, with a high rate of the illnesses sometimes associated with over-weight, notably diabetes and gallstones.

Two things are clear from this history. On one hand, the Pima are genetically different from other people who live in the same region and share much the same diet and living conditions but do not have nearly the same rate of obesity. On the other hand, the Pima are now in a radically different environment from that of their own recent ancestors. Whether you say the Pima are obese as the result of genetics or environment depends entirely on the perspective you choose. By comparison with their neighbors, they are genetically obese; by comparison with their great-grandparents, they are environmentally obese.

For most people living in Denmark and the United States, differences in habits and the environment may be too small to offset the powerful influence of genes. Overall, it is very unlikely that circumstances prevailing in a modern, industrialized, urban society will force people toward the thinner end of their genetic potential.

Nutrition

It is often said, "We are what we eat." It would be more accurate to say, "We eat what we are." That is, we use the food we eat to express all kinds of things about ourselves. Whether someone chooses a breakfast of yogurt and granola, lox and bagels, coffee and croissants, or bacon and eggs often has more to do with his or her self-image than it has to do with health. This point is worth making because it easily gets lost when nutrition is discussed. Fears about food and strong commitments to certain types of diet often reflect social beliefs or psychological issues, which are translated into the symbolism of food and nutrition. Food faddism may be a way of dealing with feelings of vulnerability (expressed as resistance to "additives") or discomfort with city living (expressed in a desire for "natural" foods).

Nutrition is undeniably important to health. But the body has a powerful ability to take care of itself, to obtain what it needs from widely differing diets. Recognition of this fact emerged about 150 years ago. The French scientist Claude Bernard was studying the composition of blood. He began to realize that the blood of animals he was studying always contained a particular sugar, glucose, regardless of whether that sugar was present in the animals' diet. Moreover, the level of glucose in the blood was kept within relatively narrow limits, no matter what the animal had been eating. From this observation, a general insight emerged. The body is capable of processing a wide variety of raw materials to supply many of its own specific needs.

In subsequent decades, this observation was confirmed and expanded: The body constructs its own interior environment and has a lot of flexibility in its choice of materials. But there are also certain limits. The general rules go something like this:

- Any of the major components of the diet can be used for energy: carbohydrates, fats, proteins, or even alcohol.
- But the body cannot produce for itself certain structural components; they must be present in the diet. The outstanding items in this list are: about a dozen of the amino acids (the building blocks of protein), calcium and phosphorus (for bones), and, in small quantities, certain fats (which are used to make membranes and some other elements of the cell).

- A host of other substances are needed in minute quantities to help out with chemical reactions that keep the body's engines running smoothly. These include the vitamins and a dozen or more minerals (really chemical elements) such as iron, zinc, iodine, magnesium, copper. The minerals, of course, could not be manufactured by the body because they are chemical elements. Vitamins could, in principle, be produced by our own biochemical machinery (indeed, they all originate from some animal or plant that made them in the first place). But human bodies fail to do so, even though they absolutely require vitamins—usually as catalysts or "cofactors"—for basic chemical reactions. Presumably the major reason vitamins are not made by the body is that they are so prevalent in food. It is, in effect, cheaper to import them than to produce them.

For the better part of a century, nutritionists devoted a great deal of attention to the questions underlying these general rules: What are the necessary inputs for a body? What is the least that can be consumed without hazard? How much can be eaten safely? The answers are now known quite precisely, and, fortunately, they can be rather easily summarized. A diet that is varied enough to include vegetables, fruits, grains, a source of calcium (usually from dairy products in our culture), and protein in modest amounts suffices to keep most people in good health without requiring them to think in much detail about what they are eating. Most traditional diets, if available in adequate quantities, accomplish this goal very successfully. On the other hand, some traditional notions—for example, that we need to eat animal muscles in order to develop big muscles of our own—have been thoroughly undermined; it's perfectly possible to make big muscles from the protein contained in vegetables.

In these terms, contemporary nutrition is a remarkable success. Modern technology may have ruined the tomato, but on the whole it provides an amazing variety of foods, all year round, in easily accessible locations known as supermarkets. This is not to deny the existence of serious nutritional deficiencies. Poverty, even in prosperous countries, is associated with inadequate nourishment. The emerging population of homeless people are clearly at risk of dietary deficiencies along with the other perils they face. People with adequate means occasionally put themselves at risk by choosing an inadequate diet for personal reasons that may have little to do with nutrition but rather are a matter of taste or philosophy. Alcoholism, a prevalent illness, often leads to inadequate food intake. And it seems probable that a good deal of nutritional harm has been done in the pursuit of weight loss through reducing diets. But, on the whole, people living in developed countries are at liberty to eat without giving it much thought.

That doesn't mean, however, that the problem of nutrition has been "solved." Indeed, nutritional progress has led to new questions, which have yet to be answered. The result is a good deal of uncertainty. Unfortunately, many people both in the field of nutrition and outside it feel called upon to express strong opinions one way or another. The result is often controversy, which is a great deal more confusing to the average person than a straightforward admission of ignorance would be.

As in so many other areas of health and medicine, prolongation of life expectancy has changed the nature of concerns about health and well-being. In part—in *large* part—thanks to improved nutrition, people are living longer than ever. But the fact that we are living longer changes the meaning of the term "adequate diet." When life expectancy is 80 years, rather than 40 or 50, previously innocuous habits may become hazardous. For example, gobs of butter and thick red steaks may have been harmless or even beneficial in an era when life was likely to be terminated at an early age by tuberculosis or pneumonia. But now that these infections are highly preventable and treatable, the coronary arteries have become one of the major limiting factors to health and survival in the second half of life. Keeping them clean through diet has become one of the major preoccupations of nutrition in this half century.

Vitamin intake presents a somewhat similar—but even less well understood—problem. The established nutritional requirements for vitamins apply mainly to preventing diseases that emerge after a few weeks to months of total deprivation. The prevailing standards for intake of vitamins, the *recommended daily allowances* or RDAs, are based on the amount required to prevent these deficiency diseases, plus a fairly wide margin of safety. Yet, the RDA may not always be adequate to confer subtle benefits that make a difference later in life. It must be emphasized, though, that this is an area of enormous ignorance. Just because extra doses of vitamins could, in principle, favor a longer life does not mean that they do in fact. And several vitamins are known to be harmful when taken in excess.

Questions such as whether eating less fat or more of a particular vitamin will help us live longer are relatively new, at least partly because most people have only recently been able to contemplate living to older and older ages. Such nutritional questions are also much harder to answer than the more traditional ones, because the time span involved is so long. It was difficult enough to put volunteers on a diet deficient, say, in vitamin B6 and confirm that a deficiency disease would develop in weeks to months. It is vastly more difficult, though not altogether impossible, to conduct dietary experiments that go on for years or decades.

One of the most ambitious such projects ever undertaken is currently in progress. Some 20,000 American doctors have been enrolled in a study that will probably have to last 6 years so that enough information can be collected to show whether a higher than average intake of beta-carotene, a close relative of vitamin A, helps to prevent cancer. Each subject takes a capsule of beta-carotene every other day. In other words, the subjects in this experiment will have consumed a total of 18–22 *million* capsules by the end in order to yield enough information for a clear answer to the question. When evaluating glib statements often made about the role of vitamins or other nutrients in prolonging life, this yardstick should be kept in mind.

Traditionally, the main task of nutrition science has been to assess the body's *need* for a particular substance or class of substances. A newer type of question has to do with how the body responds to materials in the diet, whether or not it actually needs them. That is, foods or nutrients may act on the body in ways that resemble the effect of drugs (but usually more subtly). They may, for example, alter the way the body normally manages its array of chemical reactions. This is now thought to be a very important effect of certain dietary fats. Thus, eating certain types of fat influences the way the body processes all the fats it consumes.

Another set of drug-like effects currently being attributed to food is the ability to alter mood or behavior. Trendy as this area may be, it remains one in which theory vastly exceeds evidence, and popularization has proceeded in advance of knowledge. For example, many behavioral effects have been attributed to sugar—including hyperactivity of children—but most of the evidence points in the opposite direction, that sugar is either quite neutral in its effects or slightly tranquilizing. (Of course, if sweet things are consumed at a birthday party, a good deal of hyperactivity may be observed, but not because of the sugar.)

There is not enough space in this book, let alone in this chapter, for us to provide a complete overview of nutrition. Instead, we'll focus on certain key topics that are currently in the spotlight. By far the most important, and one of the most studied, is the role of fat and cholesterol in the development of atherosclerosis and heart disease.

Fat and the heart

Cholesterol has received enough bad publicity in the last 3 or 4 decades to strike terror into the hearts it threatens to injure. Cholesterol presents the average person with a couple of real challenges. First, it can be a hard subject to understand. Second, it usually comes from tasty foods and thus is a constant temptation. We'll do our best to help with the first; the second is one the reader will have to work on.

Why pick on cholesterol?

The available evidence indicates that high levels of cholesterol in the blood lead to atherosclerosis and heart disease. In human beings this evidence is sometimes circumstantial, but there's so much of it that we would be foolish to disregard it. Here are some of the major items in the indictment:

LONG-TERM STUDIES OF HUMAN POPULATIONS   In groups of people who are followed for long periods of time, those with the highest blood cholesterol levels develop the most coronary heart disease. The Framingham Study, which has followed over 5,000 people since 1948, and the MRFIT (Multiple Risk Factor Intervention Trial) are just a couple of the better known among more than a dozen studies upholding this relationship.

ANIMAL EXPERIMENTS   Animals of many different species develop atherosclerosis when they eat diets that raise their blood cholesterol—and are protected by diets or drugs that lower their cholesterol. Evidence from animals must always be interpreted with caution, but in this case there is so much of it, and it is so consistent, that it provides strong support for the cholesterol hypothesis.

COMPARISONS ACROSS CULTURES   People who shift from the diet of one culture to another tend to acquire the blood cholesterol level associated with their new diet, and the associated risk of heart disease. For example, in their own country Japanese normally consume a low-fat diet, have low levels of blood cholesterol, and experience a low rate of heart attacks. When they move to the United States and shift to an American diet, their cholesterol levels and heart-attack rates go up.

GENETIC DISEASE   There are certain genetic conditions associated with very high cholesterol levels, and these are commonly associated with early development of coronary artery disease.

LABORATORY RESULTS   Cholesterol is found in the atherosclerotic "plaques" that block arteries. Detailed analysis of the way cholesterol gets into artery walls has established that it comes from the blood.

TREATMENT   People who are treated for very high levels of cholesterol lower their risk of dying from coronary artery disease.

Some cholesterol basics

Cholesterol is an essential raw material for a variety of substances required by the body: it is used to stabilize membranes and is the basic substance from which several hormones and bile acids are made. If we ate no cholesterol at all, our bodies would continue to produce the material for these purposes. The basic reason this valuable material can become so harmful has to do with its chemical nature. A white, waxy substance, cholesterol is absolutely insoluble in water, and therefore in blood or body fluids. On the other hand, it very easily penetrates cell membranes, which are composed of oil, protein, and cholesterol, as well as some other chemical odds and ends.

Cholesterol can only be processed by the body if it is linked to carrier molecules—a group of proteins called *lipoproteins*. The lipoproteins are soluble in water, and they have certain specific characteristics which allow them to be recognized as cholesterol carriers. There are, broadly speaking, two major groups of lipoprotein carriers for cholesterol in blood: *low-density* (or LDL) and *high-density* (or HDL).

HDL is the good guy; it acts like a magnet to keep cholesterol from invading the lining surface of the arteries, which is the main area that suffers from exposure to blood cholesterol. To some extent, HDL also serves as a vacuum cleaner, removing excesses of cholesterol deposited in the artery wall. The higher your level of HDL, the less likely it is that you will develop coronary artery disease. Indeed, this is an important reason why women consistently suffer fewer heart attacks than men: they have higher HDL levels.

Low-density lipoprotein (LDL) is the bad guy, because it favors deposition of cholesterol in such tissues as the artery walls. As cholesterol infiltrates the artery, scar tissue forms around the area of penetration. The resulting *plaque* increasingly blocks the channel of the artery, and blood flow is diminished. If the heart muscle requires additional oxygen from the blood during times of exercise or stress, a plaque in the coronary artery may prevent adequate amounts of blood from reaching it. The pain of angina pectoris is a typical result. If the artery becomes totally blocked, a heart attack or sudden death can occur. The higher one's level of LDL-cholesterol, the more likely it is that large plaques will form in the coronary arteries.

There is, as well, a third type of lipoprotein, known as *very-low-density lipoprotein* (VLDL). Packets of VLDL contain little cholesterol but a lot of triglyceride, the basic type of fat used for energy storage. (The fat surrounding, and marbled within, a steak is what triglyceride looks like.) Although blood triglyceride certainly plays some role in the development of plaques, its exact contribution is not yet known. And many experts question whether triglyceride levels in the blood are an important independent predictor of heart-disease risk.

What does an elevated cholesterol mean?

When a laboratory reports your blood test, usually the value given is for *total* cholesterol. This means all the cholesterol in your plasma, regardless of what protein it is attached to. Values may range from 150 milligrams/deciliter (mg/dl) up to 350–400 or higher. Most of this cholesterol, 70–90%, is in the LDL form. Thus, measuring total cholesterol gives a pretty good estimate of the amount that has a potential for harm. But this estimate can be refined by measuring the proportion of HDL cholesterol. The more HDL, the better off you are. This value may be reported simply as an amount, like total cholesterol. Values range from around 40 mg/dl to 65 mg/dl or more. In the case of HDL cholesterol, the more the merrier. In general, having 22% or more of your total cholesterol in the HDL form is desirable; if it's less than 18%, you may want to consider taking measures to raise it. (Sometimes, this information is reported as a ratio of total cholesterol to HDL, in which case, you want a low number, below 4.5, and should be concerned about a ratio above 6.)

There are several ways to evaluate the significance of total cholesterol to coronary health. The simplest is to say that a level of 200 mg/dl is about as high as anyone should want—although the average American value is on the order of 210–220, and traditionally physicians have not been concerned unless the level climbs above 250 or even 300. Obviously, a relatively high total cholesterol is less worrisome if the proportion of HDL is high.

But this doesn't answer a typical question, which goes something like this: "My cholesterol is 235. How much benefit would I get from lowering it to 200?" Recent data from two major studies have provided the same answer to that question: "You will reduce your risk of dying from a heart attack by about 30%." That is, for each 1% you lower your cholesterol, you'll reduce your risk of dying from a heart attack by 2%. (Going from 235 to 200 is a 15% reduction in cholesterol, therefore a 30% reduction in risk.)

Here's another way of looking at the numbers. The risk of having a heart attack goes up considerably after 60% of the coronary arteries are covered by plaque on their inner surface. The age at which that happens depends on the cholesterol level (*see table*). The

• Age at which plaque affects 60% of coronaries, by cholesterol level •	
Blood cholesterol *(mg/dl)*	*Age* *(years)*
150	80
200	70
250	60
300	50
350	40

assumption here is that one's blood cholesterol level doesn't change much in adult life. However, in many people it tends to go up, so the age of high risk is a somewhat moving target. Conversely, lowering blood cholesterol won't instantly change the age of high risk because once plaque appears in the arteries it is quite difficult to remove. Lowering blood cholesterol is more likely to slow progression than to reverse it—although there is some suggestive evidence that reversal may be possible.

Another point to bear in mind is that blood cholesterol acts along with high blood pressure and smoking to raise coronary risk. Someone who smokes or has high blood pressure that is not well controlled by medication can partially offset his or her elevated risk by lowering blood cholesterol. For example, a blood cholesterol of 200 creates a risk for a smoker that is about equivalent to the effect of a blood cholesterol of 275 in a nonsmoker. The biggest benefit to the smoker would come from quitting cigarettes, but, failing that, working for the lowest possible cholesterol level would be a good idea.

In general, someone in middle age with a cholesterol of 250 mg/dl or higher is regarded as having moderately elevated cholesterol and may be a candidate for drug treatment, as well as dietary measures. People with cholesterol levels below about 250 can probably rely on diet alone.

Drug treatment for high cholesterol has been attempted for decades. Success has been mixed at best, and side effects have ranged from the mildly unpleasant to the intolerable. Currently, a new generation of drugs is being tested and introduced to the marketplace. The prototype is *lovastatin,* which interferes with the body's own mechanism for producing cholesterol. It's too early to tell what the long-term experience will be, but lovastatin and its relatives appear to be a real advance. For the time being, use will probably be recommended mainly for people who have very high levels of cholesterol that cannot be lowered by dietary measures alone.

Dietary measures

Most people assume that they should start lowering their blood cholesterol by reducing the amount of cholesterol they eat. Although this measure certainly helps, it is *not* the most important thing you can do. The amount of cholesterol in the diet has a relatively small effect on the levels of cholesterol in the blood. Eggs are the only significant direct source of cholesterol in the American diet. Some seafood, especially shrimp, also contain cholesterol, but recent data suggest the amounts of cholesterol in shrimp are considerably lower than previously thought.

The most important dietary influences on the level of blood cholesterol are (1) the proportion of fat and (2) the types of fat consumed.

The reason that fats other than cholesterol are so important is that they have a much more powerful influence on the LDLs and HDLs—the proteins that are responsible for handling cholesterol. The higher the fat in the diet, and the more of it that is in the form known as "saturated" fat, the more LDL there will be in proportion to HDL. This unfavorable balance between LDL and HDL will result in a net tendency for cholesterol to be deposited in artery walls.

QUANTITY OF FAT   Average Americans get about 35–40% of their calories as fat. LDL cholesterol (and therefore total cholesterol) can be effectively lowered by reducing dietary fat to around 30% of calories—in other words, cutting fat intake by about one-quarter. Going much below that may not be terribly helpful, mainly because diets that are very low in fat seem to reduce HDL as well as LDL cholesterol—with results that are not known.

The main sources of fat in the diet are not necessarily the ones that people recognize immediately. Pats of butter or dollops of mayonnaise are obviously high in fat. But butter or mayonnaise is typically used in relatively small amounts—especially by people who are somewhat conscious of their cholesterol level. The principal source of dietary fat is much more likely to be red meats, those dairy products with a high fat content, and baked goods (especially pies and cakes). The person who decides to use half a pat instead of a whole pat of butter, while ignoring these other sources of fat, may accomplish very little indeed.

TYPE OF FAT   Just lowering total fat intake is not enough for optimum effects on blood cholesterol. It is also important to alter the *type* of fat that is consumed. All the oils we eat are made up of subunits known as fatty acids. It has long been recognized that the proportion of saturated to unsaturated fatty acids in the diet makes a difference to the way the body controls levels of blood fat. *Saturated* (or "fully hydrogenated") fats—the sort that come from animal tissue, but also from coconut oil and from some kinds of processed vegetable oils—have a strong tendency to stimulate production of LDL at the expense of HDL. Two other types of fat, known as *polyunsaturated* and *monounsaturated*, do not have this effect. Indeed, polyunsaturated fats have some ability to *lower* LDL, and in the past a lot of emphasis was placed on consuming high levels of polyunsaturates as a way to protect against heart disease; this occasionally went to the extreme of suggesting that people should actually consume rather large quantities of the substances.

There is little enthusiasm for this approach currently. Concerns have been raised that a high intake of polyunsaturated fats may have adverse effects, including a tendency to promote clotting, to damage the heart muscle, to lower HDL levels, to encourage formation of gallstones, and even to contribute to the risk for cancer. Monounsaturated oil, on the other hand, is not known to have these adverse effects, and it may be about as effective as polyunsaturates in lowering total cholesterol.

The exact proportion of these various oils that would be in the ideal diet is still a matter of debate. One suggestion is that about half the fat in a diet should be monounsaturated, one-third should be saturated, and the remaining sixth polyunsaturated.

TRANSLATING THE MENU   What does this mean in practical terms? Basically, reducing intake of saturated fats from meats such as beef, bacon, and the like, and from those dairy products high in fat, such as ice cream, solid cheeses, and cream cheese, is the first step. Meats and dairy products do not have to be eliminated from the diet—quite the contrary, as milk and milk products are a rich source of calcium. But low-fat versions of many dairy products are available and are preferable. Low-fat meats are being developed, and may prove to be a satisfactory alternative (though this is an industry in its infancy). A second step is to reduce the less well-recognized sources of saturated fat in the typical diet—the butter in a pie crust or a cake frosting, for example.

The richest sources of monounsaturated fats are olive oil, which is 75% unsaturated, and peanut oil, which is 47% unsaturated. Corn, safflower, sunflower, and cottonseed oils are high in polyunsaturated fats. Coconut oil is the most saturated of vegetable oils, and thus no different from butter in its effect on blood cholesterol. It's important to recognize that vegetable oils may be processed to increase their degree of saturation, mainly because polyunsaturated oils go rancid more easily and tend to be liquid at room temperature. (A pie dough won't be flaky if the fat it's made with is not at least semisolid at room temperature; that's why margarine but not corn oil can be used for this purpose.)

Although it's generally a good idea for adults to limit their fat intake, markedly restricting the fat consumption of small children is not a good idea, given the rapid rate of growth during infancy and childhood and the many vital uses to which cholesterol is put during development. Mother's milk contains 40–50% of its calories as fat, and it contains cholesterol—about as much in 6 ounces as in one egg yolk. Presumably, these levels of fat and cholesterol are appropriate for babies and young children.

Fish story

Everything we've said until now about fats and oils in the diet is part of the cholesterol story—which has been unfurling for about 40 years. A brand new wrinkle has been added in the past 2 or 3 years, however. This is the role of oils derived from fish.

Evidence is mounting that fish oil in the diet can help prevent hardening of the arteries (atherosclerosis) and, therefore, heart attacks. This story began in the early 1970s, with a study of the Eskimos living in Greenland. Danish researchers found that about 40% of the calories in the Eskimo diet come from animal fat. This is a high level—comparable to the amount consumed by urban Danes or Americans. Yet, at any given age the Eskimos have a much lower rate of heart attacks than would be expected from such a high fat intake. A reasonable guess would have been that Eskimos simply are genetically resistant to heart attacks. But those few who move to Denmark and shift to the local diet appear to be as prone to heart disease as native Danes, so that's probably not the explanation.

As the research progressed, another trait provided a clue to the mystery of the Eskimos' resistance to arterial disease: a peculiar tendency to bruise easily. The reason for this proved to be that their *platelets* (fragments of cells floating in the blood stream to help with clotting) are less sticky than is typical of Americans or Europeans. This finding suggests that the arteries of Greenland Eskimos are being protected by something that alters the way their platelets function.

And this explanation makes sense. We now know that platelets help to initiate atherosclerosis. The process begins with a bit of microscopic damage to the inner lining of the artery, usually caused by rapid, turbulent flow of blood near a bend or fork in the vessel. Ideally, the injured spot would just repair itself and the problem would go away. But in many people, the damaged inner surface of the artery attracts platelets, which stick to the injured surface and then release chemical signals. These, in turn, stimulate muscle cells in the artery wall to duplicate themselves and also attract circulating white blood cells to collect at the site of injury. The proliferating muscle cells and white blood cells begin to accumulate abnormal deposits of cholesterol and become even bulkier. In this process, a once healthy area of artery wall is turned into a fatty plaque. The artery is narrowed as a result, and blood flow is reduced.

With this background in mind, the researchers surmised that the Eskimos were doing something to protect themselves from their own platelets. That "something" appears to be eating a type of oil that comes mainly from marine sources—fish, seal, walrus, and whale. Fish oils are largely composed of unsaturated fatty acids, like vegetable oils, but they have one major structural difference that influences how the body responds to them.

Blocking cholesterol

Oils taken in the diet find their way into the membranes of many of the body's cells, including platelets. When the content of fish oil in a platelet's membrane becomes high, there is a change in the way the platelet functions.

A platelet draws on the reservoir of fatty acids carried in its membranes to produce chemicals used to signal both other platelets and cells in the artery lining. These chemicals, known as *prostaglandins*, play a crucial role in the clotting of blood. One in particular, *thromboxane*, makes platelets sticky, and it encourages them to aggregate at sites where the cells lining artery walls are damaged. This action of thromboxane is one of the earliest events in the complex sequence known as atherosclerosis.

Our bodies can't make thromboxane "from scratch." We have to get the raw material, *arachidonic acid* (or AA), in our diets. Grains and seeds are, ultimately, the main sources of this substance. Fish oils provide a very similar, but crucially different, material, which cannot be readily converted into thromboxane. Oils known as *n-3*, or ω-3, *fatty acids* are abundant in many fish. The main example is *eicosapentaenoic acid,* or EPA. Essentially by getting in the way of AA, EPA reduces production of thromboxane and thus makes platelets less sticky.

In itself, this effect would probably be sufficient to limit the ability of platelets to initiate a clot. But the EPA of fish oil has yet another effect. It is also accumulated in the cells lining artery walls. These cells normally produce a chemical signal of their own, but one that *inhibits* platelets from clotting. EPA is readily converted into this material, *prostacyclin.* Thus, fish oils work in two ways, tilting the balance of signals so that stickiness of platelets is diminished.

The importance of eating fish oil may be that it acts at such an early stage to inhibit the process of atherosclerosis.

Other benefits

So far, studies with fish oil, or EPA, have indicated that it has a variety of beneficial effects, although the influence on platelets may be one of the most critical. Increasing fish oil in the diet leads to a slight lowering of cholesterol (of the LDL type), and it sometimes reduces blood pressure as well. In people with a hereditary tendency to very high levels of triglyceride in the blood, fish oil leads to a dramatic reduction in the level of this form of blood fat.

In a way, the fish oil story seems almost too good to be true. Not only does this type of oil favor the health of arteries, but it also appears to act against inflammation, and so it may prove useful in a class of diseases, such as arthritis, in which inflammation gets out of hand.

The basis of this effect may be very similar to the action on platelets. Again, the EPA in fish oil, by competing with the AA in vegetable oil, alters production of chemical messengers. In this case, the compounds that are affected are called *leukotrienes,* which promote inflammation and some immune processes. Animal studies suggest that EPA can improve at least some illnesses that result from excessive inflammatory or immune reactions. The success of animal experiments has led to clinical trials of EPA in arthritis, psoriasis, lupus, nephritis (inflammation of the kidneys), and even some cancers in which leukotrienes are thought to play an important role. Because current treatment for these common diseases is generally inadequate, trials of fish oil are generating a lot of interest.

One cautionary note in this story should be borne in mind. Eskimos have a high rate of strokes. Until we have more information about the cause, there is no reason to adopt the Eskimo lifestyle lock, stock, and barrel of fish oil.

Fish oil versus cholesterol

Tempting as it may be to hope that a few servings of fish a week will allow us to eat all the beef and cheesecake we'd like, the reality may not be so favorable. The beneficial effects of fish oil are probably increased by reducing the amount of other fats in the diet. Nevertheless, on the basis of a study conducted in the Netherlands, it seems that eating fish, even just a couple of times a week, can lead to a significant reduction in the risk of heart attack.

But we need to keep this subject in perspective. Our understanding of artery disease is still limited, and the major approach to preventing it is through lowering blood cholesterol levels. Now, however, we are discovering that there are several key points in the process by which arteries become narrowed. We will probably find ways to intervene at each of these points and thus lower the total risk of developing heart disease and strokes. Reducing dietary fat, cutting out cigarettes, and getting adequate exercise are still important; these measures lower cholesterol and shift it into the HDL form. Eating fish oil, which seems to work mainly at an early stage of the process, may well make an independent contribution to the health of the heart and blood vessels. It should be remembered, all the same, that the point of reducing saturated fats and total dietary fats is not only to protect against cardiovascular disease but also to avoid bowel cancers.

The fish to choose

The types of fish that are richest in n-3 fatty acids, including EPA, are those that live in deep, cold waters: salmon, mackerel, bluefish, herring, menhaden. These are also fish that carry fat in their muscles and under the skin. Other fish with a similar habitat, such as cod, tend to have rather dry flesh and store oil in their livers. Thus, cod meat is not a very good source of EPA, but cod liver oil is. However, one must be very careful here. Cod liver oil is also high in vitamins A and D, which can become toxic if taken in large quantities. So it's not a good idea to start taking cod liver oil—at least not in an amount greater than 1–2 tablespoons a day—to obtain EPA; one may get too much vitamin A and D at the same time. It is unlikely that EPA itself will produce serious side effects unless taken in extremely large quantities.

The actual amount of n-3 fatty acids in fish meat varies with the season and with what the fish themselves have been eating. (Unlike beef or chickens, which are raised to tightly controlled standards, fish are wild animals; so estimates of nutrient content for these creatures are less reliable than for domesticated ones.) The table below gives an idea of the range of n-3 fatty acids in some common species. The values in canned products may be somewhat different, but the n-3 fatty acids are not destroyed or removed by the usual canning procedures.

Shellfish also have EPA in them, and the good news is that they are not, as was once believed, high in cholesterol. Mollusks (oysters, clams, scallops, mussels) contain members of the "sterol" family that have been chemically confused with cholesterol, and thus have contributed to an overestimate of the total cholesterol content in these species. Accurate analysis reveals that only about 50% of the sterols in mollusks are cholesterol, and these amounts are very low—comparable to the levels in fish. On the other hand, choles-

• N-3 fatty acids in fish •	
Species	Grams per 4-ounce serving
Chinook salmon	3.6
Albacore tuna	2.6
Sockeye salmon	2.3
Mackerel	1.8–2.6
Herring	1.2–2.7
Rainbow trout	1.0
Whiting	0.9
King crab	0.6
Shrimp	0.5
Cod meat	0.3

• Cholesterol in food •	
Source	Milligrams cholesterol per 4 ounces
Shrimp	181
Crab	113
Lobster	94
Chicken (light meat)	91
Lean fish or mollusk	74

terol is the only sterol in crustaceans (shrimp, lobster, crab, crayfish), but the levels in these species still aren't all that high (*see table, above*).

Supplements

Naturally, with the news of potential benefits from fish oil, EPA supplements became a hot item in health-food and drug stores. No clear benefit of these supplements has been established. It probably would be prudent for people to eat fish instead of red meat a couple of times a week. Taking supplements is premature until it is known how much is needed to achieve benefits and whether EPA can be simply added to a usual Western diet or whether it is necessary to reduce intake of other fats.

In this country, a great deal of fish oil is produced from menhaden—some 100,000 tons. However, it cannot be sold as a food because it is not on the "generally recognized as safe" (GRAS) list. So the menhaden oil is exported to Europe, where it is partially hydrogenated, making it similar to ordinary vegetable oil. Then it is made into margarine and other substances. A certain amount of fish oil is marketed in the U.S. in capsule form. But it exists in a kind of regulatory limbo—not listed as a drug, in that no therapeutic claims are made for it, and not sold as a food.

If fish oil proves to be as beneficial as now appears to be the case, there would be several ways to maintain an adequate supply. Our current production of menhaden oil could be consumed in its natural form instead of being converted into margarine. There may also be other abundant fish species that aren't much favored for cooking but could supply oil.

Ultimately, though, the source of this oil isn't fish but the microscopic plants of the sea, or *plankton*. The Greenland Eskimos don't get their EPA from fish so much as from whale, seal, and other large sea mammals, which have in turn eaten fish, and the fish have obtained their supply from plants. In the long run, the most practical way to develop a supply of this oil may be to short-circuit the process and extract it directly from plankton, or to synthesize it.

Food and cancer

It is now almost an article of faith that diet can be used to control heart disease—and faith is bolstered by the evidence we've discussed. Saturated fat appears to be the main dietary component that can be adjusted to gain some protection from atherosclerosis. The case that cancer can be prevented by dietary changes is, so far, a much softer one. But that hasn't gotten in the way of some major publicity campaigns urging the American public to alter its eating patterns so as to reduce the risk of cancer.

This campaign has three basic strategies: (1) lowering fat intake, (2) raising fiber intake, (3) taking advantage of a couple of vitamins (C and E) and a mineral (selenium) that may be helpful.

Fat (yet again)

For about 20 years, dietary fat has been suspected as a causal factor in two very common cancers: bowel and breast. The suspicion has been based in part on the observation that these cancers are most common in developed countries, where dietary fat intake is very high. Also, in animal experiments high-fat diets have favored the development of these cancers.

Why would eating fat lead to a higher risk of cancer? There are a couple of possibilities. One is that bacteria in the intestine convert undigested fat into chemicals that can either stimulate or promote formation of cancer. This is thought to be a likely mechanism in the case of bowel cancer. With breast cancer the relationship, even in theory, is less clear. Possibly the carcinogens produced by bacteria in the gut are absorbed and stored in the tissues of the breast. The other possibility here is that there are hormonal influences (as high fat intake, and high levels of body fat, tend to be associated with increased production of estrogen).

However, firm evidence supporting the hypothetical association of dietary fat with either cancer has not been obtained. It's just not that easy to keep track of what a group of people may be eating over a long period of time—and presumably diet influences the risk of cancer over a period of decades.

Some of the most persuasive, if circumstantial, evidence associating fat intake with colon cancer comes from the experience of the Japanese and that of their descendants in other parts of the world. As a general rule, colon cancer is more common in developed countries, where dietary fat is usually quite high. But, you could easily argue, there are lots of other differences between developed and less developed countries. Japan, which resembles other highly developed countries in most respects, has been an exception on two counts: it has continued to have low rates of colon cancer and has maintained a very low-fat diet. In the recent past, however, the menu in Japan has been providing progressively more fat—and rates of bowel cancer in that country have begun to rise. Moreover, Japanese who emigrate, for example to Hawaii or California, have the same rate of colon cancer as other Hawaiians or Californians— much higher than in the ancestral home. The case has not been clinched, though. Other research has indicated that consumption of meat rather than fat is most strongly associated with rates of colon cancer. On the whole, it is highly unlikely that dietary fat alone causes colon cancer, and it is quite possible that complicated dietary interactions between two or more nutrients will prove to be the real key to what is going on.

If the relationship of fat intake to colon cancer is debatable, the connection with breast cancer is even less certain. Early in 1987, results were published from a study of nearly 100,000 American nurses who had been given a detailed, and apparently quite accurate, dietary questionnaire. After 4 years, no difference in rates of breast cancer had appeared between those with a relatively high fat intake and those whose intake was low. The methods used in this study, albeit less than perfect, are the best that have been applied to date. Though the results aren't conclusive, they do suggest that modifying fat has little impact on the risk of breast cancer. However, there are other reasons—mainly cardiovascular—to lower intake of fat. So these results should not be seen as *discouraging* efforts to lower fat, but rather as setting some limits to how optimistic we should be about this dietary change as a cure-all for the diseases of developed societies.

Dietary fiber

It's hard to sell *less fat,* but it's fairly easy to sell *more fiber.* So, among the commercial messages beamed out by television these days is one suggesting that fiber of the sort provided in breakfast cereal protects you from cancer.

The manufacturer cites the National Cancer Institute (NCI) as its authority for this claim. The advertiser is trying to sell cereal. The NCI is presumably trying to sell good health. The advertiser may succeed sooner than the NCI. The currently popular, and widely promoted, notion that high-fiber diets protect people against some cancers is still quite controversial.

On the surface, the case looks pretty good. First, the theory that a high-fiber diet helps reduce our exposure to carcinogens makes sense. Cancer-causing substances are essentially unavoidable in any ordinary diet. Some carcinogens are present naturally in foodstuffs. Others are produced by the action of bacteria or yeasts. For example, relatively small amounts of certain molds can introduce carcinogens into food before it is eaten. Microbes naturally and inevitably present in the bowel can act on food after it is eaten to produce carcinogenic chemicals. Some kinds of cooking—notably charcoal broiling—promote formation of carcinogens. In principle, indigestible fiber in the diet could be protective in either of two ways: by hastening removal of fecal matter from the intestine or by chemically binding and removing these substances.

To support the theory, there are various kinds of evidence suggesting that people's environment—including their diet—affects their susceptibility to cancer. For example, when people move from one place to another, the frequency with which they develop colon cancers shifts from that typical of their home country to that of the region where they settle. This observation has stimulated any number of studies comparing the diets and cancer rates in two (or more) groups of people. In most cases, those who eat more fiber and less fat develop fewer colon cancers. To take one example: New Yorkers, who eat little fiber, have been compared with people from Finland, who eat twice as much fiber. The Finns develop about one-quarter as many bowel cancers as the New Yorkers.

Granted, lots of other factors—heredity, for example—may be playing a role in these comparisons between one continent and another. Attempting to pin down the dietary effect a little more precisely, one group of investigators compared the eating habits of

3 groups of people with similar genetic and cultural backgrounds. They were: (1) patients hospitalized for surgery on the colon or rectum, (2) patients in the same hospital, but admitted for other kinds of surgery, and (3) neighbors of the first group of patients who were not in any hospital. The patients with conditions, including cancer, that affect the colon and rectum had a history of eating many fewer vegetables than either of the other two groups. (The greatest difference was in the amount of cabbage consumed.)

Even so, lots of other characteristics that the researchers didn't think to ask about might be the real reason for the difference in rates of bowel disease. Some research results imply that diets high in fat or cholesterol, rather than low in fiber, may be the culprit in colon cancers—although in the case of Finland and New York, fat consumption was about the same. In Japan, on the other hand, people are now getting colon cancer more often than in the past, and the main dietary change has been increasing fat rather than decreasing fiber.

THE RAT PACK Because human behavior is so complex, and people are notoriously so hard to study, researchers have tried to establish the effect of fiber on rats—which have a reputation for providing tidier results than humans do. In this case, though, the rats haven't exactly cooperated. Sometimes, rats fed a diet of fiber and carcinogens get fewer cancers than controls receiving only carcinogens, without the fiber. But sometimes they get cancer at the same or even a higher rate. It appears that the type of fiber fed to the rats, as well as the type of carcinogen, affects the outcome of these experiments.

Which brings us to a crucial point: all fiber isn't created equal. The word "fiber" is used to describe a variety of vegetable substances that are digested partially or not at all by human beings (or rats). The human digestive system doesn't make a dent on *cellulose*, which is the principal component of bran from grains and beans, and is also present in virtually all vegetables. But digestive juices can partially break down other fibers such as *gums* (derived from stems or seeds of tropical plants, often purified and used as additives in food), *pectins* (in apple pulp and cabbage), *lignins* (in alfalfa stems), *cutins* (in tomato skins and berry seeds), or *hemicelluloses* (in corn bran and wheat bran). Many foods contain a mixture of these fiber types, of course.

Most fibers have one property in common: they help to make the stool soft and bulky (thus, those fiber-consuming Finns with a low rate of bowel cancer were found to produce stools with more than 3 times the volume of the New Yorkers'). Some of this bulk is the undigested fiber, but much of it is contributed by water, which the fiber attracts and holds. A bulky stool is more rapidly evacuated, so the time during which the intestine is exposed to foreign substances is reduced.

There, however, similarities between the various types of fiber end. Too infrequently discussed are the differences between fiber types, and how they may affect the way fiber interacts with other nutrients. These differences could well mean that one type of fiber gives more protection from cancer than another. Some, for example, bind bile acids—which are secreted by the gallbladder to aid digestion of fats but may also have irritating effects on the intestinal lining. Others sweep up chemicals related to steroid hormones and carry them out of the intestine.

By now the reader can imagine most of the ways that fiber could, in principle at least, help reduce the risk of bowel cancer.

- Because fiber seems to shorten the time that fecal material spends in the bowel, it may help to minimize contact between the bowel and any carcinogen.
- Fiber may encourage the growth of some natural bacteria in the intestine and discourage others in a way that alters the production of carcinogens.
- Simply increasing stool bulk may be enough to dilute carcinogens in the bowel.
- Fiber could have other effects on the body that might reduce the production of potential carcinogens, such as bile acids.
- Some forms of fiber actively bind carcinogens, at least when they are studied outside of the body, so perhaps these kinds of fiber bind harmful chemicals within the intestine, and thus keep them from doing mischief.

DRAWBACKS This might seem like enough theory to persuade any consumer that it's better to err on the side of eating too much fiber rather than too little. Here again, though, the rats have made trouble. Rats in fiber-feeding experiments live longer, but fiber may not be the real reason for this effect. Rats are not all that fond of diets that are very high in fiber; they eat less than normal of these experimental diets. As it happens, underfed rats live longer than usual, at least partly because they have lower rates of cancer. So in some experiments the effect of fiber may simply be to discourage the animals from eating. (People aren't necessarily like rats, at least not physiologically. Nobody has proved that human beings who shift to a high-fiber diet will permanently reduce their food intake, or live longer if they do eat less—but popular books have made both claims.)

The confusion doesn't end there. When a group of rats were exposed to chemical carcinogens, then fed wheat bran as 20% of their diet, their intestinal cells showed *more* precancerous changes than did those of rats that ate no added fiber. And the evidence from humans is at least as equivocal. Studies of people living in Puerto Rico and Hong Kong have found that those who ate more fiber had more, not fewer, colon cancers than those with low-fiber diets.

Quite apart from any effect on cancer risk, increasing dietary fiber can have other consequences that are not fully understood. Some kinds of fiber are capable of binding trace minerals and removing them from the bowel. A diet very high in fiber might thus interfere with absorption of needed minerals. Even if no real damage is being done, however, sudden increases in fiber intake will probably lead to gas and intestinal discomfort—a problem that should diminish with time.

Not only do various studies on dietary fiber disagree with one another—a common problem when research is conducted in different settings—but some authorities feel that even the data showing fiber's beneficial effects could be explained in other ways. For example, people with diets high in fiber usually also eat less fat. The statistical association between fat content of the diet and rates of colon cancer has often been very high. Fiber isn't the only dietary component thought to reduce the risk of bowel cancer. High calcium intake may do so as well. Why this should be so is uncertain, but one suggestion is that harmful fatty acids and bile acids become bound to the calcium and are thus deactivated (much as they would be deactivated by attaching to dietary fiber). So it may be worth observing that the Finns with so much less bowel cancer than the New Yorkers also consume lots of high-calcium dairy products. Other components of the diet that may, or may not, protect from cancer include various vitamins, minerals, and even certain food additives.

OTHER AILMENTS Like most health practices that have a season of popularity, high-fiber diets have been recommended as "good for what ails you"—virtually from tooth decay to ingrown toenails. At a more serious level, fiber has been tested as a treatment for at least four major conditions associated with "refined" diets: constipation, diverticulosis, type-2 (adult-onset) diabetes, and obesity. The original rationale for using fiber to treat these conditions was based on a historical speculation. After 1880, it was reasoned, when roller-milling of flour began, these diseases became more prevalent. Perhaps the high-fiber elements of the pre-1880 diet were protective.

Fiber is a perfectly sensible and suitable treatment for constipation because of the changes it causes in fecal matter. It also appears that bulkier, faster-moving stools reduce pressure within the colon, and this effect helps to prevent or alleviate diverticular disease—a condition in which small portions of the bowel are forced into outpouchings, presumably as a result of high internal pressure. (For at least a decade it has been known that the older practice of reducing fiber intake for diverticular disease was counterproductive.) In one test, 85% of a group of people with diverticular disease obtained relief by eating a diet high in fiber.

The role of fiber in diabetes is somewhat less clear. Fiber, particularly of the sort found in beans, peas, and other legumes, appears to be helpful in the control of blood sugar. Fiber seems to slow digestion and delay the absorption of sugar, thus lowering the peak demand for insulin immediately after a meal. However, when high-fiber intake has been tested with diabetics, it has been in conjunction with a diet high in complex carbohydrates, which are now known to be an important element favoring good control. Results have not been equally good with other types of high-fiber diet that have been tried. So the relative importance of fiber versus high-carbohydrate intake has not yet been fully established.

Some high-fiber diets have been heavily promoted for the treatment of obesity, but here the evidence is poor. The old idea that pure bulk in their stomachs makes people less hungry has long been disproven. Right after a meal, people report feeling more satisfied by meals that are relatively high in fiber. But over the long haul, both people and rats tend to compensate by eating enough to maintain their weight. However, there is one report that a few women lost a few pounds while eating food prepared with guar gum as an additive. Cellulose, by contrast, not only hasn't helped rats to lose weight; it has caused their cholesterol levels to go up (and also reduced absorption of certain nutrients).

FIBER MORAL   Something about eating high-fiber foods seems to be beneficial, although this cannot be said with the same assurance for fiber supplements. Many foods high in fiber also contain calcium and vitamin A, both of which have an aura of virtue clinging to them. But even if fiber turns out not to be as protective as some studies indicate, enough other benefits come from cabbage, broccoli, carrots, grains, and legumes to warrant regularly including them in one's diet. The only exception to this rule may be certain people with intestinal disorders that interfere with absorption of nutrients.

A standard recommendation is to aim for a total of 30 grams (an ounce) of dietary fiber a day. However, it's difficult to estimate one's fiber intake with any accuracy, so gauging it by the bulk and frequency of bowel movements may be somewhat more practical.

Vitamins and other nutrients

Reducing fat and elevating fiber intake have a similar goal: to minimize the body's exposure to carcinogens—by not eating a potential raw material, in the case of fat, and by hastening removal from the bowel, in the case of fiber. Raising intake of certain vitamins or minerals is now often recommended as yet another defense against cancer. In this case the hope is that these nutrients can bolster the body's defenses against carcinogens. Vitamins A, C, and E have received the most press in this regard. Selenium and calcium are the minerals with a reputation for anti-cancer activity. Frankly, the evidence for any of them isn't all that solid.

VITAMIN A   The strongest case has been made for vitamin A and its relatives—collectively known as the carotenoids. These substances are found in dark green and yellow vegetables, such as broccoli, romaine lettuce, squash, and carrots, as well as fruits such as apricots and cantaloupe. A good deal of laboratory research has shown that animals deficient in carotenoids are more susceptible to cancer, whereas those with a high level are protected. The evidence for a similar effect in human beings is much less clear. Various case-control and epidemiologic studies, the mainstay of this type of research, have come out on both sides of the question. Recently, it has been popular in health books to suggest that carotenoids will protect smokers from lung cancer. This is an exceedingly dubious proposition, based on current evidence, and no one who smokes should kid himself or herself that the potential for protection comes close to offsetting the higher risk.

We can hope for a definitive answer on vitamin A from the doctors' study mentioned at the beginning of this section. But the 20,000 doctors will have to take another 5 or 6 million capsules of beta-carotene over the next couple of years before the results can be known.

There is no very good guess as to *why* carotenoids might be protective against cancer. This class of substances seems to help cells reach their differentiated (or adult) form, and it may be that they counteract the tendency of cancer to take cells back toward a more "primitive" stage of development.

Readers should bear in mind that overdosing on vitamin A is fairly easy to do—and that the resulting toxicity is very unpleasant. The safest, and quite possibly most effective, way to get this vitamin is from vegetables. Supplementation with vitamin A should be avoided. Beta-carotene is not toxic; whether supplements make a difference is not yet known, as we have said.

CALCIUM As we mentioned in discussing fiber, there is now some evidence that calcium prevents cells in the large intestine from beginning the series of changes that seem to lead to formation of cancers. The study demonstrating this effect was quite elegantly designed and carried out, but it still requires confirmation. The reason why calcium might be protective is not known, but a plausible inference is that it binds to potentially carcinogenic substances and prevents them from having an effect before they are eliminated.

THE "ANTIOXIDANT" NUTRIENTS The basic reason given for taking vitamins C and E, as well as selenium, to protect against cancer is that they all perform similar functions (though in different locations within the body). These substances protect against the destructive effects of chemicals known as *free radicals,* which are formed all the time simply as a result of the fact that we live in, and breathe, an atmosphere of oxygen. Life-giving though it is, oxygen is potentially very toxic to tissues—not directly, but because it permits the formation of highly reactive compounds that have the capability of damaging DNA and thus of triggering the process that leads to abnormal cell growth and cancer.

Our bodies have evolved with several protective mechanisms to minimize the subversive potential of free radicals. Not only are vitamins C and E, as well as selenium, used in reactions that detoxify these chemicals, but there are special enzymes within cells that maintain a constant search-and-destroy mission. The outlines of the way these substances work are well known. What is not known is whether the protective activity inside cells can be increased by taking extra amounts of vitamins C and E and selenium.

There are indications from research that, in humans, once there is a sufficient level of these nutrients coming in (and they're all fairly easy to obtain from any balanced, varied diet), consuming extra amounts doesn't enhance their effect. However, vitamin C has been the object of vigorous promotion, not only for cancer protection but several other potential benefits, so we'll take a little more time to look at the claims made on its behalf.

Vitamin C: when is enough enough?

It is now 17 years since Linus Pauling's book *Vitamin C and the Common Cold* appeared. This very successful little volume converted ascorbic acid from a deservedly popular vitamin into one of the nutritional superstars of our time. In 1970 Dr. Pauling opined that the average person needs 1–2 grams a day of vitamin C for "optimum health. " By 1986 Pauling was advocating a routine daily intake of 6–18 grams, as a way not only to prevent colds but to treat cancer and prolong life.

That's a lot of vitamin C. The average American diet supplies 60–70 milligrams a day, or about one fifteenth of a gram; 25% of the population consumes a good deal more, but even at that the amount ranges between 130 and a little over 200 milligrams. In the United States, the recommended dietary allowance (RDA) has been set at 60 milligrams—very near the typical intake. Someone who regularly consumes this amount of vitamin C is well protected from scurvy.

And the reason everyone *must* take in at least some vitamin C is to prevent scurvy. Unlike all but a few other animal species, human beings are incapable of producing ascorbic acid from sugar (which the vitamin chemically resembles). As a result, connective tissue breaks down, because collagen, a crucial structural protein, can't be manufactured. Easy bruising or bleeding, loosening of teeth, failure of wound healing, and feeling thoroughly miserable are among the major signs of this nasty deficiency disease. Unless vitamin C comes to the rescue, sudden death from uncontrollable bleeding follows. However, 10 milligrams a day is all it takes to cure or prevent scurvy. By consuming 60 milligrams a day, the average American maintains body stores adequate to stave off the illness for a month or two if suddenly switched to a diet with no vitamin C whatever.

Nobody is really arguing that point. The live controversy is whether vitamin C has some benefit other than preventing scurvy, and whether a larger intake than average is needed to obtain it. Yes, says Dr. Pauling, who has received one Nobel prize for his work in basic chemistry and another for his efforts to reduce the risk of nuclear warfare. An effective writer and skilled debater, Dr. Pauling has won many converts to his point of view. Where does the evidence now stand?

Colds

Dr. Pauling's 1970 book presented the case that taking large amounts of vitamin C would reduce the number of colds people get, or make the symptoms milder when a cold managed to break through defenses presumably enhanced by the vitamin. In the next 10 years several tests of his hypothesis were conducted. The results of these trials have been quite consistent. There is no measurable reduction in the frequency of colds when people take vitamin C at these levels, and specific symptoms, such as sneezing or runny nose, are not affected. On the other hand, people who take extra vitamin C do seem to feel better during the cold and are likely to take less time off work. According to the Canadian investigator Terence W. Anderson, who conducted three studies on more than 5,000 adults, the sense of well-being that comes from taking additional vitamin C is probably achieved with a daily dose of 200 milligrams or less. People who don't regularly take extra vitamin C may get some benefit if they take as much as 1 gram a day for up to 4 days at the beginning of a cold.

Dr. Pauling criticized most of the studies conducted to test his hypothesis on the grounds that not enough vitamin C was given. (This is, of course, a conveniently elastic criticism.) In general, much larger doses of the vitamin were given than anyone normally receives in the diet. The design of the research projects was not airtight, but on the whole these studies were carefully executed on enough subjects to warrant the conclusion that vitamin C does not have the dramatic effect predicted in the 1970 book. On the other hand, it's fair to say that a modest increase of vitamin C taken during a cold often makes people feel better, even when they don't know they are taking vitamin C. The effect is enhanced if subjects know or guess that they are taking the vitamin.

Cancer

Dr. Pauling and some colleagues subsequently put forth a more startling claim for vitamin C: that it could improve survival rates in people with cancer—particularly cancer of the colon, which has been highly resistant to chemotherapy. The basis for this claim was the reported experience of terminal cancer patients at a Glasgow hospital. These patients were given 10 grams a day of vitamin C. Their length of survival was then compared with that of other patients who had not been so treated. An important flaw in this study was that the investigators picked their control cases (10 for every patient given vitamin C) from hospital records. This procedure is notoriously unreliable. If the people selecting control cases unconsciously chose records of patients with more advanced disease, the effect attributed to vitamin C could have been completely spurious.

Two careful investigations at the Mayo Clinic have attempted to test vitamin C as an anti-cancer agent. Patients with incurable bowel cancer were selected and randomly assigned to vitamin C or a placebo. Neither the patients nor the investigators knew who was getting what. Vitamin C was given as long as the patient could take oral medication or until the disease had progressed, as measured by a 50% growth in the diameter of the tumor, a weight loss of at least 10%, or marked worsening of symptoms. Neither study showed any benefit to the patients receiving vitamin C.

The first Mayo investigation was conducted on patients who had received prior treatment, such as chemotherapy. Dr. Pauling objected that chemotherapy weakens the immune system and thus had probably undermined the potential effectiveness of vitamin C, so the second study was conducted on patients who had received no previous chemotherapy for their disease. Dr. Pauling criticized this study on the grounds that it did not exactly reproduce his procedure, which was to give vitamin C in very high doses until the patient died. Dr. Pauling speculated that the Mayo result came about because withdrawal of the vitamin led to a kind of "rebound" in which the patient was made worse. There was, however, no evidence for such a rebound in the Mayo subjects, whose experience after withdrawal of the vitamin was no different from that of the control patients after the placebo was withdrawn.

On the basis of evidence currently available, vitamin C seems highly unlikely to be effective at controlling cancers that resist other forms of therapy. On the other hand, vitamin C may play a useful role in *preventing* some kinds of cancer.

The reason for thinking so is based partly on laboratory results, which indicate that vitamin C prevents formation of nitrosamines (potent carcinogens) in the digestive tract. Many foods, especially cured and charcoal-broiled meats, contain nitrates and nitrites, which can be converted by bacteria to nitrosamines. Vitamin C inhibits this process. Vitamin C also has been found to inhibit formation of a carcinogenic substance in the bladders of female mice. In several recent epidemiologic studies from Australia, southern Louisiana, and Hawaii, people with diets relatively high in vitamin C appeared to be protected from bowel, stomach, or bladder cancer, respectively. These results are only suggestive, though; they are not conclusive.

Longevity

In his latest book, *How to Live Longer and Feel Better* (1986), Dr. Pauling advocates taking 6–18 grams of vitamin C supplements a day as the keystone of a program to prolong life by 25–35 years. Readers must decide for themselves whether this premise is credible or extravagant. There is hardly any evidence on which to base a discussion.

Minimum, optimum, maximum

The human body is remarkably adaptable. It seems capable of getting by on relatively small amounts of vitamin C, and it protects itself quite well from overdoses of this vitamin. On the other hand, in some people large doses could be something between a nuisance and a health hazard.

The main nuisance from very large doses is diarrhea, but many people seem capable of adapting to high intake of the vitamin with-

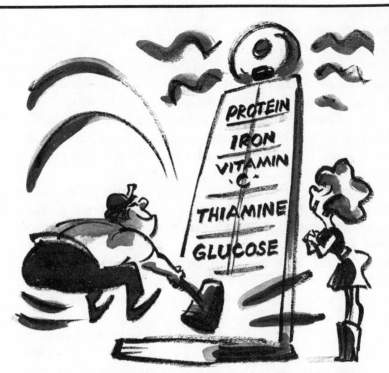

Protein is another of those things, like vitamins, of which it can be said, "Enough is enough." Once you've met your daily requirement—3 or 4 ounces of pure protein at most—you've received all the benefit there is to get from it. The rest is broken down by the body, and substances are released that must be excreted by the kidneys. There is some indication that modest intake of protein may actually be better for the kidneys in the long run.

out much difficulty. There's a theoretical possibility that people whose bodies have grown accustomed to eliminating excess vitamin C would develop scurvy if for any reason the high doses were abruptly stopped. This doesn't seem to be a common occurrence. Pregnant women are advised not to take large quantities of the vitamin to avoid inducing such a rebound in their babies after birth. High intake of vitamin C may slightly increase the risk of forming kidney stones in some people. Because vitamin C favors the absorption of iron, people who suffer from an excess of iron storage in their bodies would be harmed by taking large doses. On the other hand, people who need iron probably are helped by this effect.

Taking high doses of vitamin C can interfere with certain standard laboratory tests, including those that check for blood in the stool (which will be falsely negative) and tests for urine sugar (results on Tes-Tape and Chemstrip can be falsely lowered, whereas Clinitest gives a falsely high result).

Skepticism about vitamin C should be tempered by the recognition that standard recommendations for intake (such as the RDA) may not be high enough to account for all the potential benefit that vitamin C could offer. By and large, these recommendations are based on the quantity known to prevent scurvy and provide a margin of safety. The useful amount beyond that is anybody's guess. Ours is that the range is somewhere between the current RDA of 60 milligrams and, at the very most, 250 milligrams a day. The main reason for choosing the higher figure is that this is around the dose that will saturate the body's ability to store vitamin C. Amounts in excess of 250 milligrams daily do not produce significantly higher tissue levels; most of the dose is lost in the urine. On the whole, people probably would do better to get their vitamin C from food than from supplements, because the foods that are high in vitamin C have other good things as well.

Though most people taking supplements of up to 1 gram or so a day probably won't be harmed, the long-term consequences of taking this amount of vitamin C really aren't known. And anyone who is taking medications or needs regular medical testing should check with a physician to make sure that the excess vitamin won't interfere with his or her care.

Sweet stuff

As we said at the beginning of this section, there's no way to compress a complete discussion of nutrition into the space we have available. We've tried to hit the high spots of controversy and promise in the late 1980s. Another 10 years, we suspect, and the story may look quite different. But even if we haven't been able to provide a full "meal" in this section, we'll end with dessert: some remarks on sugar and sweeteners.

Sugar is one of the great paradoxes of modern life. All told, people seem to be consuming more sugar, in all its forms, than ever before—around 120 pounds a year. At the same time, sugar is routinely disparaged as a nutritional no-good, with nothing to offer but calories. The reality, as always, is more complicated.

The word *sugar* usually brings to mind the white granules of sucrose that used to come in sugar bowls and now appear in paper packets. Most of this stuff is derived from sugar cane or sugar beets. The juice of the plant is separated into *raw sugar* (sticky crystals) and molasses syrup. Raw sugar is banned in this country because it carries a lot of impurities, such as insect parts and bacteria. So the raw sugar is dissolved in water, filtered, and recrystallized into virtually pure sucrose. *White sugar* has long been favored by consumers simply because it comes in a tidy, crystalline form that is easy to handle and store. *Brown sugar,* which gives a richer taste to baked goods, sauces, and some other foods, can be prepared in a couple of ways, but it is basically white sugar with a thin coating of molasses.

An increasing proportion of our national sugar intake now comes from *corn sweeteners,* a mix of sugars derived from corn starch. Corn sweeteners cannot always be substituted for sucrose, because they have a distinct flavor, or because they don't work the same way in cooking. But they are economical for use in candies (which are less likely to crystallize when made with corn sweetener) and soft drinks. Enzymes can be used to increase the fructose content of sugar derived from cornstarch, and thus make it sweeter. The resulting product, *high-fructose corn syrup,* is gaining a larger share of the market.

The differences between one form of sugar and another are not fundamental. Some sugars are associated with a flavor other than sweetness (maple or honey, for example). These flavors sometimes limit the appeal of one or another sweetener; at other times they are exploited to give a distinctive taste to foods. There is no particular reason, however, to claim that "natural" sweeteners are healthier than "refined" or "processed" sweeteners.

Sources

Sugar turns up in the most unexpected places. Here are some examples: crackers (Ritz crackers, 11.8% sugar), ketchup (Heinz, 29%), Russian dressing (Wishbone, 30%), artificial lightener for coffee

(Coffeemate, 65.4%). But let's keep these figures in perspective. Few people consume enough ketchup or coffee lightener to get significant amounts of sugar from them. Much more important sources are soft drinks, fruit juices, candy, baked goods, and other desserts.

Even the distinction that is commonly made between sugar and "complex carbohydrates"—meaning starches such as potatoes, rice, pasta, breads, and so on—is not as crucial as the impression sometimes given in dietary recommendations. All carbohydrates are broken down to sugar before they can be digested and used by the body. There is some difference in the rate at which absorption occurs, but it is often surprisingly small and is not easy to predict. A food identified as sweet, such as ice cream, may yield its sugar more slowly than, say, a plain potato (because the fat in ice cream delays emptying of the stomach). Other foods eaten at the same time will also have their effect. In other words, popular impressions that blood sugar levels swing up and down in relation to the sugar content of a meal are not well founded in fact.

An important feature of most "sweets," other than soft drinks, is not their sweetness, but their high fat content. Sweetness as such is not a very popular flavor. Relatively few people eat teaspoons of plain sugar, which bears a faint resemblance to cardboard. What people with a "sweet tooth" tend to like is sugar in combination with butter or cream. To that extent, the sugar becomes something of a trap, because it entices them to eat foods with a high content of saturated fat. But the sugar itself is a relatively innocuous component of food.

Sugar and health

The clearest hazard of sugar intake is tooth decay. But, in this connection, the source of the sugar is also very important. Between raisins or dried fruits, which are often seen as more "natural" and healthful than candy, and a chocolate bar, the latter is much less damaging to teeth. The reason is that components of dried fruit tend to cling to the teeth and provide a growing surface for bacteria. By contrast, the fat in a chocolate bar, which coats the enamel, seems to make it more difficult for bacteria to adhere to the tooth.

Other health hazards often attributed to sugar seem not to exist. It is quite clear that a high sugar intake has nothing to do with causing diabetes, and there is no demonstrated connection with heart disease, cancer, or other illnesses. (But again, a diet high in sweets may be high in fats, and these are not harmless.) Likewise, obesity cannot be attributed purely to sugar consumption. The leaner you are, the higher your sugar intake is likely to be. The reason seems to be that leaner people tend to be more active, and to use sugar for a fuel.

On the other hand, sugary foods or beverages may be criticized for what they *don't* have. Sodas, for example, are sometimes fortified with vitamin C, but on the whole they provide nothing but calories. There's nothing wrong with pure calories, provided one's intake of other nutrients is adequate. To the extent that a person is attracted to sugary foods that don't have much in the way of calcium, iron, fiber, vitamins, or minerals, he or she may well be consuming an inadequate diet.

Substitutes

Artificial sweeteners promise to give us the sweetness of sugar without the calories. Surprisingly enough, there is remarkably little scientific evidence as to whether people who use artificial sweeteners actually reduce their intake of calories. Under laboratory conditions, with short-term observation, there may be a slight effect, but even that cannot be said with confidence. On the whole, artificial sweeteners appear to be added on top of what people would eat anyway, rather than helping to subtract calories.

The reason is probably fairly straightforward. The tongue is the only part of the body that is fooled by these substances. The rest of the body in some sense "knows" that it's being cheated. Hunger is not appeased—even the craving for something sweet may not be satisfied but stimulated.

However, artificial sweeteners do not cause tooth decay and, in chewing gum, may actually help to retard caries. At least this can be said in their favor.

SACCHARIN   Saccharin, the oldest of the artificial sweeteners in general use, is a completely artificial chemical, about 500 times sweeter than sucrose. It has been associated with bladder cancer in experimental animals, and for that reason there was a move in the late 1960s to have it banned from use in the United States. But several epidemiologic studies have been unable to confirm that there is an increased risk in people; in one of these, no overall increase in cancer risk was found in a survey of more than 9,000 people. In any event, special legislation has specifically exempted saccharin from the general ban on sale of substances that cause cancer in any species (the Delaney clause).

Two cautions should be considered, however. Saccharin may act as a weak carcinogen in heavy smokers. And there is simply no information on the long-range effects of ingesting saccharin from early childhood through old age. There is generally no reason for pregnant women or small children to consume artificially sweetened substances, and it may not be a good idea.

ASPARTAME   By now, this relatively new sweetener, marketed as Nutra-sweet or Equal, and included in soft drinks and dietetic foods, has become one of the major sugar substitutes in the United States. Aspartame is a relatively simple molecule, about 180 times sweeter than sucrose, that strongly resembles natural compounds because it is composed of two naturally occurring amino acids, one with a slight chemical modification. On the whole, one would expect it to be quite safe, and testing has not revealed serious problems. Aspartame should not, however, be consumed by anyone with phenylketonuria (PKU), because it breaks down to phenylalanine, a substance that people with this hereditary disorder must avoid.

Some controversy about the safety of aspartame for normal people continues, despite its generally encouraging record, in the main because of a theoretical worry that the substance could produce behavioral or neurological effects, at least in people who consume very large amounts or are quite sensitive to the substance. Children *may* be especially vulnerable to the effects of aspartame for several reasons: (1) Their smaller body size means that the relative dose from a can of soda, say, is higher; (2) their nervous systems are potentially more vulnerable; and (3) they will be exposed to aspartame for much longer than adults who have begun consuming this recently introduced product.

CYCLAMATE   At one time, cyclamate (marketed in Sucaryl and other products) was popular in the United States. In combination with saccharin, this sweetener provided quite a "natural" sweetness. But laboratory findings of increased cancer in animals led to the banning of cyclamate from sale here. That decision has been criticized, but never rescinded. Cyclamate is still used in many other countries, however.

SORBITOL   Sorbitol is a slightly sweet substance, a complex alcohol, that cannot be absorbed or digested. It is used to sweeten candies and gums, as a rule. Sorbitol serves as a noncaloric sweetener simply because it's indigestible. However, bacteria in the intestine can metabolize this material, and the products that result can lead to explosive diarrhea. Whether diarrhea occurs depends pretty much on the amount of sorbitol that is consumed, but relatively small amounts can produce distress—particularly in children.

2 | Reducing the Risks: Cigarettes, Alcohol, and Other Drugs

After 20 years or so of liberalized attitudes toward the use of recreational drugs, the United States is returning to an anti-drug outlook. On the whole, this swing of the pendulum is in the right direction. There is little evidence that recreational drugs offer any real benefit to health—although many people claim simply to enjoy them as a feature of the "good life."

Where to draw the line between drugs that can be legitimately regarded as consumer items and those that should be banned from civilized society is not always as clear as it may seem. All of the substances considered in this chapter—coffee, alcohol, marijuana, tobacco, and cocaine—are potentially addictive, although true addiction seems to be exceedingly rare with marijuana. All of them alter mental function to at least some degree. All of them also have effects on the body. All are the objects of intensive promotional campaigns—some of them open, others covert—and all, in varying degrees, have been decried as a menace to health.

Consumerist tolerance of drugs is most widespread when it comes to coffee, tobacco, and alcohol. All three are legal and universally available, although sale of tobacco and alcohol to minors is everywhere restricted, and coffee is not commonly thought suitable for children in the United States. Use of all three of these drugs—and of marijuana—usually becomes established in adolescence. Cocaine typically gets a somewhat later start.

Advertising creates attractive images of the legal drugs: sex-stereotyped glamor for tobacco; comfort and homeyness for coffee; relaxation and companionship for beer; success for whiskey. Marijuana and cocaine have also become associated with "images" in the public eye: youthfulness and unconventionality for marijuana, stardom for cocaine.

National programs to discourage drug abuse appear periodically. Whether they have much effect is difficult to ascertain. And two of the most devastating substances in current use—alcohol and tobacco—retain a powerful, and legal, hold on the public. Marijuana has not emerged from its status as a counter-culture drug with a reputation for ill effects that are sometimes overstated. The bad press for this drug, whether or not it has been completely accurate, has probably had a favorable effect. Fewer young people are using marijuana than just a few years ago, and regular use seems to taper off sooner than it used to. This change in use patterns appears to have very little to do with government efforts to prevent importation and sale of marijuana. Rather, it reflects a general shift in attitudes that is progressively more approving of drug-free living.

Cocaine is the current exception. A drug that once was a distinct curiosity in the marketplace of illicit substances, cocaine has become *the* fashionable stimulant—occupying a position not unlike that of the amphetamines in the 1950s and 1960s. This is particularly sad, because cocaine is one of the most addictive and most destructive of all drugs. Eradicating it will not be easy, and may be impossible. The substance is compact and therefore easy to transport. The market is sufficiently lucrative to provide dealers with incentives to evade detection and capture—or to run the risks. Many experts now say the major hope is that educational campaigns can induce a much higher level of sales resistance to cocaine.

Cigarettes

Contrary to the impression given by the cigarette industry, there is no uncertainty among reputable scientists that cigarette smoking is eminently "dangerous to your health." A few questions about the details remain, but the main point has been proven: Cigarette smokers die younger than nonsmokers, and in large numbers.

The magnitude of the effect is hard for most people to grasp. In the United States, cigarettes cause about 300,000 deaths a year. Since 1964, the date the Surgeon General of the United States issued the first report on smoking and health, cigarettes have been responsible for an astounding 6 million deaths. In the same period, military operations have killed no more than 60,000 people.

War kills young people, you could argue, whereas cigarettes take a few years off the end of one's life. Is the comparison valid? Even if you count years of life lost, cigarettes have taken a much greater toll (well over 30 million years) than the 3 million years of life consumed by war in the last couple of decades. No matter how you estimate it, cigarettes have been responsible for greater loss of life than any effort by our military enemies in the 20-plus years since the danger was first officially recognized. However, the victims of cigarettes die one-by-one in hospital beds—not on battlefields. Thus, the cigarette crisis is not "news" and is often neglected by newspapers and magazines, many of which are dependent on cigarette advertising for revenue. However, this source of income may be starting to dry up. In 1985 consumer magazines lost 13% of their revenue from tobacco advertising (and 10% from alcohol advertising).

The toll

Cigarettes attack the heart and lungs primarily. Smoking is responsible for one-third of all deaths from coronary disease and one-third of *all* cancer deaths—not only from lung cancer but from a variety of other tumors as well. About three-quarters of all deaths from chronic lung disease (bronchitis, emphysema) are attributed to smoking.

Although men bore the brunt of illness from cigarettes for many decades, women, who have been increasing the amount they smoke for 30 or 40 years, are now shouldering an equivalent burden of disease. Fifteen years ago, lung cancer caused only half as many deaths among women as breast cancer; now it slightly exceeds breast cancer as a killer of women. Cigarette smoking is also responsible for two-thirds of the heart attacks afflicting women under the age of 50. A woman with a 1½-pack habit in this age bracket runs a 5-fold greater risk of having a heart attack than a nonsmoker.

The baby of a cigarette-smoking woman is likely to have a low birth weight and possibly to suffer other developmental failures. In the first years of life, the child, if exposed to its parents' smoke, will have more bronchitis, tracheitis, bronchiolitis, colds, and other respiratory illnesses than a nonsmoker's baby. The children of smokers are also more likely to take up the habit.

And nonsmoking adults who breathe high levels of second-hand smoke are also injured by their exposure. At least 14 epidemiologic studies have asked whether "passive smokers" are more likely to develop lung cancer than people who live in a smoke-free environment. Thirteen of these studies have said yes. More recently, similar studies have been looking at the rate of heart attacks in passive smokers—chiefly the wives of smoking men. These investigations indicate that being married to a current smoker triples the risk of having a heart attack.

Not incidentally, smoking endangers the lives not only of smokers but of nonsmokers by way of the fires that result from the habit. According to an estimate based on a 3-year survey of house fires in the city of Baltimore, cigarettes ignite house fires that kill almost 2,000 nonsmokers in the United States every year. This represents 40% of all deaths resulting from house fires.

Thus, in many ways, smoking may be regarded as a "contagious" disease. It is also an addiction, much like heroin dependence or alcoholism.

Harder than heroin

By some estimates, nicotine (in the form of cigarette smoke) is several times more addictive than alcohol and at least as addictive as heroin. The cigarette habit is almost always acquired during childhood or adolescence. Virtually all regular cigarette smokers become addicted between the ages of 12 and 18.

Whatever psychological reasons people may have for smoking, the fact is that as many as 95% of smokers are physically dependent, at least to some degree, on the nicotine they inhale. This drug seems to produce addiction in *at least* three ways: (1) by providing an active sensation of pleasure, (2) by leading to fairly severe discomfort during withdrawal, and (3) by leaving the smoker susceptible to craving long after obvious withdrawal symptoms have passed. Nicotine appears to be most addictive when it is absorbed from the lungs, and less so when absorbed from the lining of the nose and mouth—the main route for nicotine obtained from cigar and pipe smoke, chewing tobacco, snuff, or the newest form of oral nicotine, therapeutic chewing gum.

With each puff of cigarette smoke, blood passing through the lungs is loaded with a high concentration of nicotine, which reaches the brain 7 seconds later. (Heroin shot into a vein in the forearm takes 14 seconds and in the process of reaching the brain is also diluted by blood returning from other parts of the body. Some authorities speculate that the addictive potential of cigarettes is partly the result of this ability to receive a very prompt and intense reward for a simple behavior.) Cigar and pipe smokers, plug chewers, and snuff dippers get their nicotine in lower concentrations, delivered more gradually.

After months to years, tobacco users appear to require some nicotine in their blood in order to feel comfortable. The addiction of cigarette smokers may have a second component—not only a need for a fairly constant level of blood nicotine, but a yearning for a series of nicotine "jolts" of the sort delivered by each inhalation of smoke. The sense of gratification is sometimes difficult for the smoker to describe: it may be characterized as a slight "rush," a distinct sense of pleasure coming from the whole body.

Nicotine also produces unpleasant symptoms, such as nausea and wooziness, when blood levels get too high. Smokers thus have a balancing act to perform. They seek the sensation provided by a rush of nicotine, either because it is pleasant or because it helps prevent the discomfort of withdrawal, but they don't want to overdose and get sick. After a period of exposure, the majority of smokers can tolerate quite high levels of nicotine in the blood, but all of them have their limits. Most smokers take 200–300 puffs a day and, with that much practice, become adept at regulating nicotine intake.

The most powerful incentive to smoke, for someone who has been at it a few years, is preventing withdrawal. Indeed, smokers find a cigarette "relaxing" largely because it reverses the tension that signals the beginning of withdrawal. When a smoker goes without cigarettes for very long, he or she begins to complain of irritability, anxiety, and craving. Nausea, constipation, or diarrhea may follow. The heart rate regularly slows, brain-wave patterns may change, levels of certain hormones fall, and blood pressure tends to go down. Weight gain (with or without eating more than before) may also occur.

Most confirmed smokers also report difficulty in concentrating when they try to abstain; this may, indeed, be one of the most disabling symptoms of nicotine withdrawal. It can persist for weeks or months. Not only does the abstaining smoker *feel* unable to concentrate, but psychological tests give objective support to this bit of self-observation. If a recent quitter is given tasks that require vigilance or tracking, he or she performs less well than when smoking.

Although the major symptoms of withdrawal often abate during the first 7–10 days of not smoking, some (such as drowsiness, difficulty with concentration, and craving) may become worse about 2 weeks after quitting. And at least slight craving may persist for very long periods. According to the long-term study of British doctors who quit smoking, about one-fifth of them continued craving for as long as 5–9 years. The fact that some craving persists over such a long period helps to explain why smokers who quit are extremely vulnerable to relapse.

Research on other forms of addiction suggests that the sheer availability of cigarettes is a major reason why people resume smoking. In Vietnam, for example, heroin was easy to get, and a significant number of American servicemen became addicted. After they returned to the United States, where the drug is not so easily obtained, 70% of these veterans readily dropped their habit without entering a treatment program. No quit-smoking program has reported such a high rate of recovery lasting more than a brief period of time. Because access to a drug—whether alcohol, a narcotic, or tobacco—is such an important factor in maintaining the addiction, and because cigarettes are about the easiest lethal drug to obtain, it is no surprise that tobacco is such a hard habit to kick.

Safer forms of tobacco?

Low-tar cigarettes

In the past 20–30 years, cigarette companies have vigorously marketed low-tar, low-nicotine cigarettes. The unstated implication of this enormous campaign is that lowering the tar and nicotine delivery of cigarettes makes them safer. Certain federal and state regulations have favored this trend. And the public has bought the message. In the late 1970s and early 1980s, American smokers made a massive shift to smoking the low-tar type of cigarette.

It is not clear, however, that this shift in buying and smoking habits has made much of a contribution to smokers' health. Several studies of people who switched to filter-tips from the high-tar brands smoked during the 1940s and 1950s did report that filter smokers ran a slightly smaller risk of lung cancer (and probably of heart disease) than those stubborn (or thoroughly addicted) devotees of the older smokes. However, the two groups of smokers may have differed in other ways that were more important than the type of cigarette they bought. Those who voluntarily switched to filters may have been puffing or inhaling less to begin with. They may have been trying to quit as a result of increasing health-consciousness. So these studies cannot be taken as conclusive proof that switching to a filtered brand was what made the difference. More recent studies have indicated that low-tar cigarettes offer little health advantage to those who smoke them. According to one well-designed investigation, male smokers between the ages of 30 and 54 suffer heart attacks at the same higher-than-average rate, regardless of whether they smoke low-tars. Another investigation, sponsored by the National Research Council, has questioned whether there is any reduction in the risk of lung cancer as a result of smoking low-tars.

People who actually inhale less tar and nicotine should suffer fewer ill effects than those who take in a full dose of these substances. But there are several reasons for thinking that merely switching type of cigarette does not guarantee a lowered exposure to tar and nicotine. In the first place, the official rating for tar or nicotine delivery may have little to do with the actual amounts a given brand yields to a human smoker. The ratings come from machine measurements, and the method has not been completely standardized. So different types of cigarettes may not be accurately represented in the tar and nicotine ratings published by the Federal Trade Commission.

What an individual smoker is capable of extracting from a cigarette may also be very different from what the machines measure. There is good reason to believe that most smokers automatically adjust their intake of smoke to maintain "comfortable" levels of nicotine. Those who switch to low-delivery brands compensate by smoking more cigarettes, inhaling more deeply, or puffing more often. Even if less "tar" is inhaled, the substances given off by newer brands are not necessarily the same as those yielded by standard brands. The treatments used to produce low-tar tobacco may raise the proportion of the most dangerous components. Data on this point are hard to obtain and, once available, will probably be even harder to interpret.

How to smoke them (if you must)

Someone who smokes low-tar cigarettes may hold them in such a way as to prevent the cigarette from doing the good it was designed to do. One of the main ways low-tar cigarettes reduce smoke delivery (and therefore delivery of tar and nicotine) is by mixing smoke-free air into the stream. Tiny ventilation holes placed around the edge of the filter admit the air (*see illustration*). Depending on the brand, as much as 80% of a puff can be air. Usually you can see the holes if you examine a filter, but some brands (such as Merit) make them invisible. Obviously, if your lips or fingers block the holes (which may be necessary in order to light this type of cigarette), you increase the amount of smoke, as well as nicotine and carbon monoxide) in each puff. With most low-tar brands, you can tell whether you have blocked the holes of your cigarette (and thus converted it from low- to medium- or high-delivery) by looking at its filter tip after you have smoked it. If you see a brown bull's eye surrounded by a white halo, you have smoked the cigarette correctly. But if the tar stain has spread over the entire filter, you have been blocking the holes. (This test does not work for some brands, which have a different filter design.)

So if you want to protect yourself from cigarette smoke, the only

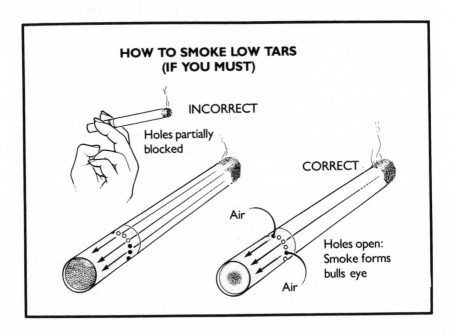

HOW TO SMOKE LOW TARS (IF YOU MUST)

INCORRECT

Holes partially blocked

CORRECT

Air

Air

Holes open: Smoke forms bulls eye

way is to inhale less of the stuff. Switching to low-tar cigarettes will not automatically accomplish this goal. But, theoretically, they could help reduce the hazard to a smoker who conscientiously goes on a tobacco "diet." The Addiction Research Foundation has published some rules for those smokers who want to reduce their intake of cigarette smoke. We quote, with permission, from the ARF's pamphlet, "Tar and Nicotine Ratings May be Hazardous to Your Health: Information for Smokers Who Are Not Ready to Stop."

- Smoke as few cigarettes as possible, no matter what their yield. (Studies show that people who were smoking 40–50 cigarettes a day have been able to cut back successfully to 10 per day.)
- Smoke the lowest-yield cigarettes that you find acceptable, realizing that it may take weeks to get used to the lower-yield cigarettes. The greater the decrease in yields, the better: differences of only 2 milligrams of tar and 0.1 milligrams of nicotine are too small to be important.
- Do not block vent holes on filters.
- Take fewer puffs per cigarette.
- Leave longer butts (the last part of a cigarette delivers the highest yields).
- Avoid inhaling; if you do inhale, take more shallow puffs.
- Do not hold the cigarette in your mouth between puffs.

What about pipes?

Many a former cigarette smoker has switched to a pipe in the hopes of reducing his risk of diseases caused by cigarette smoking. However, some studies—and casual observation—indicate that these "secondary" pipe smokers may continue to inhale the even more irritating smoke of pipe tobacco. Those who can switch to a pipe without continuing to inhale significant amounts of smoke are, nevertheless, at less risk than cigarette users.

   In one study, blood nicotine levels (a good indicator of the amount of smoke that is inhaled) were measured right after each subject smoked one pipe-bowl of tobacco. Before they lit up, with one exception, the group of 8 secondary pipe smokers had nicotine levels as low as the primary pipe smokers—those who had never used cigarettes. After finishing the experimental bowl, however, the secondary pipe smokers had much higher nicotine levels than the primary pipe smokers—meaning that they were now inhaling pipe smoke.

To the degree that former cigarette smokers switch to pipes, and desist from inhaling, their new habit will indeed produce less lung disease and probably less heart disease. Certainly primary smokers of pipes and cigars, though not as healthy as nonsmokers, are at much less risk than cigarette smokers. However, users of "oral only" forms of tobacco—pipes, cigars, snuff, and plug (or chewing tobacco)—are still at higher risk of developing mouth and throat problems, including cancer.

Smokeless tobacco

Television has given us the opportunity to watch baseball players close-up as they work away at a wad of tobacco jammed into their cheek. In addition to this unpaid publicity, manufacturers of "smokeless tobacco"—snuff and plug—have engaged in a vigorous advertising campaign. High school and college athletes have responded, exactly as you would expect, by taking up the habit in droves.

Although the chewing and snuff-dipping habits do not appear to be as lethal as cigarette smoking, very definite hazards are associated with smokeless tobaccos. Evidence comes from a study conducted in North Carolina by the National Cancer Institute. In rural areas of the state, snuff dipping (inserting powdered tobacco between the gum and the cheek) is an old tradition that is still common enough to make possible the gathering of adequate statistics. Cancer of the mouth and upper throat proved to be much more frequent in snuff dippers—as much as 50 times more common in those who had made a lifetime practice of keeping tobacco in their cheek.

Switching to snuff or chewing tobacco might reduce the risks for cigarette smokers, but young people who take up these habits have nothing to gain from them except addiction to nicotine, bad breath, discolored saliva and teeth, gum disease, missing teeth, and, eventually, cancer of the mouth or throat.

Clove cigarettes

Yet another potential hazard for young smokers is the growing popularity of flavored cigarettes. Sweeteners have long been tossed into tobacco. Now cloves are being added to the recipe. Cigarettes containing cloves are an increasingly popular alternative to the traditional variety. In 1984, for example, 150 million clove cigarettes were imported from Indonesia and sold in the U.S. Most consumers are teenagers and young adults.

Clove cigarettes typically contain roughly two-thirds tobacco and one-third cloves. Although many people believe their lower tobacco content renders them less harmful than regular cigarettes, this is not necessarily the case. Recent reports from the Center for Disease Control (CDC) suggest that people who smoke clove-containing cigarettes could be at risk for serious lung injury. These reports make a suggestive case that when a mild upper-respiratory illness is already present, smoking clove cigarettes may lead to severe breathing difficulty. The main concern, however, is that these cigarettes are likely to serve as yet another way youngsters become exposed and addicted to tobacco.

One of the reasons that clove-containing cigarettes may be more noxious than conventional cigarettes could be that puff-for-puff they deliver twice as much nicotine, tar, and carbon monoxide as moderate-tar American brands. Another reason may be the clove component itself. Eugenol, the active ingredient in cloves (which dentists have used as a topical anesthetic for years), deadens sensation in the throat and allows smokers both to inhale more deeply and to hold the smoke in their lungs for a longer time. As yet there is no proof of any long-term health hazard due to clove cigarettes (beyond the disastrous effects of smoking tobacco), but it is known that close chemical relatives of eugenol produce the kind of damage to cells that may eventually lead to cancer.

Quitting

The value of giving up cigarettes has been well publicized. People who quit smoking cigarettes get almost instant benefit to their health (even though they may not *feel* better at first). In particular, the risk of having a heart attack diminishes rapidly within the first year. There are probably several reasons. Heart rate and blood pressure go down. Blood cholesterol shifts from the unfavorable LDL form to the protective HDL form. The amount of oxygen the blood can carry increases, because carbon monoxide is no longer being inhaled. Moreover, the ability of the lungs to clear themselves of foreign matter and bacteria is also rapidly restored. Risk of lung cancer goes down more gradually, but it does go down, along with the risk of other cancers caused by cigarette smoke.

So why don't more people give up cigarettes? About one-third of American adults continue to smoke. There seem to be two major reasons: (1) many people don't *really* try, and (2) those who do try and, at first, succeed often then relapse.

The reasons that people don't try are complex. Some don't believe what they're told about the damage cigarettes cause; these people are simply misinformed. Others don't believe they are as vulnerable as other people to the illnesses caused by cigarettes. This is a matter not so much of being misinformed as of retaining the childhood belief in one's own immortality. Perhaps a few smokers believe that they are making an informed choice.

Most smokers, however, do want to quit. Every year, according to national surveys, a very high percentage of them try to kick the habit. What makes the difference between success and failure?

The chief characteristics of people who eventually succeed are (1) they do it on their own, (2) they do it cold turkey, and (3) they have tried to quit at least once before. Indeed, the probability of success seems to *increase* with each successive attempt. Thus, people who see themselves as hopeless failures after breaking down and smoking a cigarette are probably succumbing to a self-fulfilling prophecy. Although the attitude that it's okay to smoke a cigarette now and then almost certainly undermines efforts to quit, the other extreme—thinking that quitting is an all-or-none process—is probably equally unhelpful. Smoking an occasional cigarette, or trying to "taper," seems to prolong the process of withdrawal and make complete quitting more difficult. But despairing of the effort after the first relapse would make it impossible ever to quit.

How valuable are the various programs to help people stop smoking? The answer is remarkably unclear. Most of the people who respond to a community- or clinic-based effort, or who sign up for a commercial program, will quit smoking for a while. But after a year or two, the rates look much less impressive. At least one very intensive program (associated with the MRFIT research) has reported that nearly half of its graduates remained nonsmokers after 4 years. This is an extraordinarily good statistic compared with the more typical 10–15% figure from most programs. But the people who enter formal programs for smoking cessation may be those who have special difficulty giving up. Thus, even a modest success rate may be more meaningful than it appears. On the other hand, success measured 4 years after a program is over may not reflect any particular value of that intervention but rather the dogged determination of the people who tried it—and subsequently went on to try other methods.

What a quit-smoking program usually has to offer is psychological and social support combined with a variety of techniques, loosely termed *behavior modification,* that have been devised to help people get control over habits and change them. These techniques may involve self-monitoring (such as keeping a record of every cigarette smoked and of the reason for wanting it); stimulus control (avoiding the situations in which craving is stimulated); substitution (putting something besides a cigarette in the mouth); and rewards (depositing a sum of money that is refunded when a certain criterion of success is met).

Aversion therapy has also been tried. The idea is to associate smoking with unpleasant experiences, such that the very thought of a cigarette brings on nausea. Probably the most common form of aversion therapy involves requiring the subject to smoke so much that he or she becomes physically ill from the overdose, and then to repeat this tactic whenever the desire for a cigarette comes back. This routine may be combined with sessions in which every unpleasant aspect of the cigarette habit is discussed. Although very high rates of quitting with this aversion technique have been reported in the short run, it does not appear to have a much better record than other techniques over the long haul.

Gumming up the cigarette habit

A new twist in treatment of the cigarette habit came with the introduction in 1984 of nicotine chewing gum, marketed in the United States as Nicorette. Each Chiclet-sized pellet of this peppery-tasting gum delivers approximately the equivalent of a cigarette's nicotine, which is absorbed gradually through the mucous membrane of the mouth. Delivered this way, the nicotine doesn't produce the same "rush" that comes from a deeply-inhaled puff of smoke. Yet it is capable of diminishing withdrawal symptoms by maintaining a blood level of nicotine.

The theoretical hope for using oral nicotine to help people stop smoking was that it would allow a kind of 2-stage withdrawal. Smokers could deal with the various forms of psychological dependency first—the habits associated with smoking, the anxiety-provoking situations that customarily led them to reach for a light. Then, when these patterns had been broken, they could be more easily weaned from the drug itself.

Several years' experience with the gum have now been reported in the medical literature. The consensus is that the gum improves rates of quitting; but as with all other techniques, results are better in the short run and look less significant as time passes. Nicotine gum probably is most helpful to the subset of smokers who are most heavily dependent on nicotine and most clearly smoke for relief of withdrawal symptoms. These are also, as a rule, heavy smokers.

The best results with nicotine gum appear to be achieved when it is used as part of a program involving intense counseling and group support. When dispensed in a general-practice setting and with a minimum of advice, the gum produces a negligible improvement in the rates of quitting. On the other hand, *quitting* may not be the only criterion to consider. If the gum helps some smokers to reduce their intake to relatively low levels, even if they continue to smoke a little, there is probably a net benefit to health.

Side effects of the gum are fairly minor: belching, jaw fatigue, air swallowing, nausea, soreness of the mouth, heartburn. Such complaints are reported in 5–25% of users. Because the consistency of Nicorette is heavier than that of normal chewing gum, it has reportedly loosened fillings and caused difficulties with dentures. This is a problem that the manufacturers are seeking to correct.

No matter what form it is supplied in, nicotine has some undesirable properties that are not really side effects because they are part of its main action on the body. Nicotine stimulates the heart and thus causes disturbances of the heart rate (palpitations), but these have been reported by fewer than 1% of persons using oral nicotine—and they presumably get a similar effect from smoking. Oral nicotine also appears, at least in monkeys, to cause a shift of cholesterol to the unfavorable LDL form. People who have to give up smoking because they have uncontrolled angina, serious disturbances of heart rhythm, or a recent heart attack probably should give up cold-turkey; nicotine in any form is bad for them. Nicotine is also bad for the developing fetus and should be strictly avoided during pregnancy.

Finally, because nicotine is addicting, nicotine gum is potentially addicting. Some people transfer their dependence to the gum and continue to use it beyond the recommended period. When they are given a placebo gum, they go through physical withdrawal symptoms similar to those that abstaining smokers feel. And a Nicorette habit could be more expensive than a cigarette habit, as a month's supply costs roughly $120.

Blaming the victim

Until recently, most programs directed against the cigarette habit have been aimed at helping the individual smoker to quit. Logical as this approach may seem, it has several drawbacks as an overall strategy. It puts pressure on the individual, through education and strength of will, to overcome an addiction that gives pleasure and is painful to abandon. But it leaves intact the very circumstances that help to make cigarette smoke so powerfully addicting—including the very easy availability of cigarettes. It could even be argued that our national emphasis on quit-smoking programs is a form of "blaming the victim," in that it puts all of the pressure on people who unwittingly became addicted as minors.

We shouldn't underestimate the value of educational programs, which do appear to be gradually reducing the number of smokers in this country. However, education has been most effective only with one group of smokers: relatively affluent and well-educated white males. As one authority has expressed it, the people who have benefited most from the current educational efforts are those "who wear neckties to work."

If our goal is to reduce the toll that cigarettes take, ultimately the most important population to focus on is young adolescents. Any effort that reduces their vulnerability to the cigarette habit will have a high yield in the long run. Such measures might include a ban on cigarette sales through vending machines, confining the sale of cigarettes to liquor stores, and more rigid enforcement of penalties for sale to minors.

Limiting the opportunities for people to smoke cigarettes will also have an effect. The harder it is for a smoker to find an acceptable place to smoke, the less likely it is that he or she will do so. (In effect, restricting opportunities to smoke is equivalent to limiting availability of cigarettes.) The current emphasis on "nonsmokers' rights" is thus likely to have two important consequences: (1) It will protect nonsmokers from a health hazard that is coming more and more to be recognized as real. (2) As a by-product, it will almost certainly reduce consumption of cigarettes by smokers.

Raising the cost of cigarettes by heavily taxing them seems like an obvious way to deter purchase, and there is evidence that consumption goes down if the price of cigarettes goes high enough. Historically, however, in many countries, including our own, cigarette taxes have been a significant source of tax revenue, and this fact may have discouraged governments from pursuing more vigorous anti-smoking efforts. In effect, the government becomes addicted to its tobacco tax revenues.

Restrictions on cigarette advertising could be introduced as a way to reduce the attractiveness and credibility of the product. Advertising does not have quite the same claim to First Amendment protection that other forms of speech have. Other democratic countries, such as Norway, have enacted total bans on cigarette advertising—and have seen smoking rates go down as a consequence. Given the enormous amounts of money spent on cigarette advertising in this country, however, such a move would have important economic implications, not only for the embattled cigarette industry but for the publications that continue to accept cigarette money.

Finally, many politicians feel that the only realistic approach to the "tobacco problem" in this country is to plan—over at least a 20-year period—a replacement economy for tobacco production and distribution. Until recently it wasn't obvious that such a plan would be necessary. Although the cigarette industry was no longer growing, it wasn't shrinking and it remained highly profitable. (Granted, cigarette exports to the Third World were compensating for some loss of domestic revenue.) However, increasing awareness of the deleterious effect of second-hand smoke may well lead to legal restrictions that will ultimately undermine cigarette sales in this country. Planning for the demise of the industry seems more appropriate than ever.

Alcohol

Alcohol has been a social lubricant for most of human history. The ancient Egyptians brewed alcoholic drinks; the ancient Chinese wrote poems about being inebriated. Until the relatively recent past, fermented beverages served perhaps a more important function than making people feel friendly, relaxed, giddy, sleepy, or just plain drunk. Making alcohol from fruit or grain was a way to store calories in an era when food preservation was much more difficult, and much less successful, than it is now. By turning the grape harvest into wine, and some of their grain into beer, our ancestors could take advantage of not only the psychological but the preservative qualities of alcohol.

Until just about 300 years ago, various forms of wine and beer were the main alcoholic drinks. The alcohol content was relatively low (and remains so, at 5% in beer and 12–13% in table wine). By 1700, though, the progress of technology made distillation possible on a large scale, and the liquor produced with this method was 40–50% alcohol. Cheap gin—followed by whiskey, brandy, and other forms of hard liquor—became available to large numbers of people, who had no previous experience with such potent stuff. For about a century thereafter, drunkenness became epidemic in countries where distilled alcohol was consumed. (This chapter of European history was repeated when "firewater" was introduced to native Americans.) Currently, alcohol in all its forms is widely available in the United States, and per capita consumption is very high.

In this country, the amount of pure alcohol sold per person is currently about 2.6 gallons a year. Since many people are nondrinkers—either taking a rare drink on special occasions or never drinking at all—the intake of the rest of the population must be correspondingly higher than this deceptive "average" figure. About 20 million people in the United States drink so much that they are classed as "alcoholics"—a term that describes not only how much someone drinks but how he or she reacts to it.

Dividing people into three categories of alcohol consumption—nondrinkers, social or "controlled" drinkers, and alcoholics—has some descriptive value, but these terms can also be deceptive. It is not, for example, absolutely clear that most alcoholics are different in some fundamental way from other people—more vulnerable to addiction because of genes or personality. To be sure, there is increasing evidence that a subgroup of alcoholics—mostly young men who begin drinking early and go through a severe course—are biologically destined to have special trouble with keeping their drinking under control. But there isn't much support for the notion that the majority of alcoholics, at least when they begin, are inherently more prone to develop the condition.

Most alcoholics give no advance indication that they will become drug dependent. Simply living in an environment where alcohol is abundant—and where drinking to get drunk is common—may be sufficient to turn many people into alcoholics (those who don't react by becoming teetotalers). The societies with the fewest alcoholics are those that undertake programs to restrict the amount of alcohol sold, make it harder to obtain (with short hours and few outlets), or otherwise impose limits on consumption (for example, through strong cultural norms about when and where drinking is appropriate). In other words, the major risk factor for becoming an alcoholic is exposure to lots of alcohol. Drinking beer or wine instead of "hard" liquor is not protective—what counts is quantity, not kind.

In the body

Because alcohol is a small molecule that dissolves in both blood and fat, it can travel rapidly throughout the body, crossing barriers that block other substances. Small amounts appear in the blood stream within a few minutes after a drink is taken. When blood levels reach a peak depends on many factors, such as how much food there is in the stomach when drinking begins. From the blood, alcohol rapidly diffuses into the brain (where it interferes with normal function), the lungs (from which it enters the breath), and kidneys (which excrete it). Alcohol easily crosses the placenta to reach the developing fetus, and it enters breast milk.

The liver is the main organ responsible for metabolizing alcohol. As a rule, it takes about an hour for the liver to completely process a single drink. In the first step, a chemical known as acetaldehyde is produced. This compound is highly toxic and is partly responsible for the ill effects felt after drinking. Some drugs interfere with the body's mechanism for removing acetaldehyde. Metronidazole (Flagyl), which is used to treat certain infections, is one of them. Larger than normal amounts of acetaldehyde accumulate, so even a single drink may result in extreme discomfort. Another drug with this effect is disulfiram (Antabuse), which is sometimes prescribed for those alcoholics who are sufficiently motivated to take it regularly. Knowing that a drink will make them sick helps deter people on Antabuse from giving into temptation, but only if they resist the temptation to stop taking the drug.

After acetaldehyde, the next product of alcohol metabolism is acetate (the principle component of vinegar). The body also obtains acetate from fat and sugar. Acetate is then used as the main material from which energy is extracted. Water and carbon dioxide are the end products.

A gram of pure alcohol yields 7 calories' worth of energy. By comparison, a gram of fat yields 9 calories and a gram of carbohydrate (say sugar) or protein, when used as an energy source, yields 4 calories. Most ordinary, unmixed drinks, beers, or wines contain somewhere between 75 and 120 calories a drink. Mixed drinks, with juice or a sweetened soda, have still more calories, and a real extravaganza—say half a cup of holiday eggnog—can be worth 225 calories, give or take. It doesn't take much computation to recognize that someone who drinks at all heavily—say 5 beers a day, at 8 ounces each—may be getting one-fifth to one-quarter of his or her calories from alcohol.

Excess

This person is probably also getting sick from alcohol. Above an intake of about 3 standard drinks a day, the body's disposal system begins to show signs of stress from overwork. After only a few weeks of taking 4 or 5 drinks a day, liver cells begin to accumulate fat. This situation quickly returns to normal when drinking is stopped. But if it continues, the chance increases that the drinker will develop *alcoholic hepatitis*—inflammation and destruction of liver cells. About 15% of people who continue drinking beyond this stage go on to develop *cirrhosis*, an irreversible, and often progressive, condition in which there is scarring and destruction of liver tissue.

The liver is hardly the only organ that suffers from alcohol exposure, although it is probably the most vulnerable. Nor is cirrhosis the only disease caused by excess intake.

CANCER   After cigarettes, alcohol is probably one of the most important environmental influences on cancer—a fact that is not sufficiently understood. Excessive alcohol intake clearly raises the risk of developing cancer in the liver, mouth, and esophagus. Many other cancers—in the lung, pancreas, intestines, prostate, and, recently, breast—have also been related to alcohol intake.

BLOOD DISORDERS Alcohol diminishes the production of both red and white blood cells. By itself, heavy intake of alcohol can lead to anemia and lowered resistance to infection. The diseases and dietary deficiencies that often accompany alcoholism make the situation worse.

PNEUMONIA A variety of unusual pneumonias affect alcoholics—probably because the drug makes people less able to protect themselves from inhaling saliva, and also because it impairs immunity.

GASTROINTESTINAL DISORDERS Alcoholics have a much higher incidence of peptic ulcers and pancreatitis (inflammation of the pancreas) than nonalcoholics. In addition, many suffer from repeated episodes of nausea, vomiting, and abdominal distress—most often due to superficial gastritis (inflammation of the lining of the stomach).

NERVOUS SYSTEM DAMAGE Well-known are the acute problems of intoxication and (in the physically addicted person) withdrawal—including delirium tremens (DTs) which leads to death in about 10% of cases. Alcoholism also contributes to permanent damage to the brain and peripheral nerves. Among such chronic effects are Wernicke's disease (rapid mental deterioration, paralysis of eye movements, stumbling gait); polyneuropathy (loss of sensation and strength due to nerve damage); and cerebellar degeneration (deterioration of the part of the brain controlling stance and balance). A report from Denmark has suggested that intellectual impairment may be a serious problem for the younger alcoholic. The Danish study involved measurements of intellectual functions and liver damage in 37 alcoholic men under age 35 in whom no other explanation for possible brain damage could be found. Nineteen percent of the group turned out to have cirrhosis, but 59% showed signs of intellectual impairment on standard testing (memory, concentration, comprehension), with 11 of the 37 showing enough impairment to be described as "occupationally disabled." The researchers concluded their report with this chilling statement:

"Disabling intellectual impairment may be the earliest complication of chronic alcoholism and may arise early in the alcoholic career."

HEART DISEASE Despite recent information suggesting a possible beneficial effect of small amounts of alcohol on coronary artery circulation, there is little doubt that large amounts of alcohol can damage heart muscle directly—a disease described as alcoholic cardiomyopathy.

SUGAR AND FAT METABOLISM When liver supplies of glycogen (a storage form of sugar) are depleted—as occurs in malnourished alcoholics—alcohol ingestion can lead to hypoglycemia (low blood sugar). Alcohol also produces elevated levels of blood fats—especially triglycerides and very low density lipoproteins. These elevated fats contribute to the "fatty liver" described earlier.

SEX AND REPRODUCTION Alcohol interferes particularly with sexual performance in the male. As Shakespeare's character observed, it "provokes the desire, but it takes away the performance." With even moderate amounts of alcohol on board, many men find themselves unable to achieve an erection or maintain it. The sexual function of women may not be as noticeably affected by alcohol intake, but reproduction is disastrously impaired. Approximately one-third of the infants born to women who imbibe 6 or more drinks a day during pregnancy are born with devastating abnormalities: mental retardation, stunted growth, and facial deformities. This condition has come to be known as the *fetal alcohol syndrome*. The risk drops to about 10% at an intake of 3 drinks a day. The real question for many pregnant women, however, is whether increased risk of birth defects occurs at *all* levels of alcohol intake down to an occasional drink. In a controversial decision, the Surgeon General of the United States has taken the position that pregnant women should avoid all alcohol, because there is no certainty about the "safe" level.

BLOOD PRESSURE Increasing evidence indicates that alcohol raises blood pressure. There may actually be two different mechanisms. Alcohol itself may cause blood pressure to rise. But withdrawal from alcohol also seems to raise blood pressure. In other words, it can get you coming and going. People with mild high blood pressure who want to minimize their need for antihypertensive drugs would be smart to go on the wagon—or reduce their intake of alcohol to very low levels.

OTHER DRUGS   The two prime "targets" for alcohol—the brain and the liver—are also affected by many other drugs. The combination with alcohol can range from the merely unpleasant to the downright lethal.

In some cases, mixing alcohol and another drug enhances the effect of both. Tranquilizers and antihistamines are notorious for their ability to impair alertness and judgment when mixed with alcohol. Alcohol also enhances the anti-clotting effects of aspirin, and the combination of these two drugs can lead to severe bleeding. Many drugs given to lower blood pressure may have an enhanced effect if taken with alcohol (somewhat paradoxically). Thus, combining one of these drugs with a drink can lead to a sudden drop in blood pressure, and possibly loss of consciousness.

Sometimes, however, alcohol reduces the effect of a drug. The reason is that alcohol stimulates the liver before destroying it. A major function of this organ is to convert biologically active compounds—such as drugs or certain poisons—to harmless ones. The liver has a whole collection of enzymes that it can use to inactivate substances that it "perceives" as potential poisons. Alcohol is among the substances recognized by liver tissue as potentially dangerous; like many such chemicals, alcohol induces the liver to increase its level of protective enzyme activity. These enzymes work to remove not only alcohol from the system but other drugs as well. Thus, a dose of drug that is adequate for most people may become insufficient to affect the person whose alcohol intake is high.

The aspirin substitute acetaminophen (Tylenol, Datril, and Panadol) is an interesting variation on this story. As the first step in inactivating acetaminophen, the liver converts the drug to a highly toxic substance. Ordinarily, the very next step is to combine the toxic substance with a small, protein-like substance known as glutathione, which renders it harmless. In an alcoholic, however, the first process may go on faster than usual, whereas the second step may be very slow because many alcoholics do not always have an adequate supply of glutathione. Thus, the toxic breakdown product of acetaminophen may accumulate in excess. Severe, even lethal, liver damage can result.

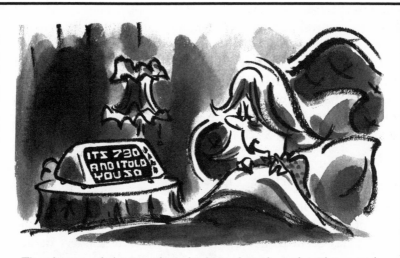

The danger of driving after drinking doesn't end with a good night's sleep. Driving performance can still be seriously impaired the "morning after" even if no alcohol remains in your blood. And whether you feel hung over is not a reliable indication of your ability to drive well.

ACCIDENTS Long before alcohol erodes the liver or permanently injures the brain, it may kill by a swifter mechanism: accidents. The danger of drinking and driving is too well known to require discussion here. What is less well recognized is that alcohol may impair driving even after blood alcohol levels have returned to zero. A study conducted in Sweden involved 22 volunteers who got drunk and then took a driving test the next day, when no alcohol could be detected. The investigators found a 20% decline in driving ability the "morning after." Behind-the-wheel performance did *not* correlate with how the person felt. On average, skill deteriorated as much for those who felt fine as for those who acknowledged having a hangover.

Walking under the influence can be quite as dangerous as drunk driving (but with less likelihood of injuring innocent bystanders). In Belfast, Northern Ireland, a study of the alcohol levels of 50 pedestrians injured in traffic accidents revealed that intoxicated pedestrians were 3.5 times more likely to be injured than sober pedestrians in the same place at the same hour. The severity of the injury also correlated with the amount of alcohol the pedestrian had consumed.

Alcohol plays an important role in causing other kinds of violent death. The risk of suicide may be as much as 80 times higher in alcoholics than in nonalcoholics. Alcohol has been consumed by a majority of the victims of such mishaps as choking (70%), drowning (70%), assaults (65%), burns (70%), and falls (50%).

The confusing mortality curves

Having said so little that is good about alcohol, we come to an apparent paradox: the finding that people who take a couple of drinks a day seem to live longer than either teetotalers or heavy drinkers. Since 1974 several different studies have come up with this same conclusion. The low mortality of light drinkers, as reported by these studies, has generally been attributed to a lower rate of coronary artery disease.

The explanation most commonly offered for this apparent benefit of alcohol to the heart has been that it raises the "good" or HDL form of cholesterol—the type that seems to prevent damage to artery walls. One group of researchers has even gone so far as to suggest that 3 beers a day may be just as effective at raising HDL levels as regular jogging—and, by implication, equally effective at forestalling heart disease.

Dr. Edward Eichner of the Department of Medicine at the University of Oklahoma, who has conducted a thorough analysis of the studies on alcohol, HDL, and coronary artery disease, has picked enough holes in the theory that alcohol helps the heart to make it seem, at best, unproven.

Statistical problems

Several factors could have created a statistical illusion that teetotalers have a higher rate of coronary artery disease than light drinkers. First is a problem of definition. The groups identified as "teetotalers" and "light drinkers" are not homogeneous. For example, in virtually all studies the teetotaling group contains both lifelong nondrinkers and those who have given up alcohol in the fairly recent past. The so-called light drinkers are also an extremely diverse lot, including a lot of people who drink very little as well as others who drink more regularly. It appears possible that the way various types of drinkers and former drinkers are distributed between these two groups could be responsible for creating a false impression that the use of alcohol "in moderation" somehow contributes to better cardiac health.

There are some other problems that may be clouding the picture. "Light drinking" is statistically associated with higher social status in the United States; both teetotaling and heavy drinking are somewhat more common in lower income groups. So "light drinking" might simply be a proxy for "high income" and "more education," which in our society lead to better health and lower mortality from heart disease.

Finally, results from various studies cited as showing the protective effect of light drinking are not all that consistent; particularly, the effect is less likely to appear in nonsmokers than in smokers, which suggests that some interaction of smoking habits and drinking habits might be obscuring the real relationships.

Theoretical problems

The data that were produced to "explain" the statistical finding that alcohol protects the heart also appear to have a serious flaw. Although drinking does seem to raise levels of HDL cholesterol, it turns out that the "wrong" kind of HDL is involved. There are two important kinds of HDL cholesterol, and one of them is better than the other. (Sorry about that; we know it's confusing. Everybody who isn't an expert in this area gets confused by it. HDL cholesterol is "good" and LDL is "bad," but HDL comes in several types. Among these is a type 2, which is what does the work, and a type 3, which is not particularly useful.) Measurements of HDL that don't discriminate between the two types may thus be misleading.

When this distinction is made, and the effects of alcohol and exercise are evaluated, it turns out that alcohol raises the amount of ineffective HDL_3 and exercise raises the amount of active HDL_2. Thus, the theoretical reason for thinking that alcohol might help protect against coronary disease is also relatively weak.

Finally, it is becoming clear that drinking alcohol can make both high blood pressure and diabetes worse, and these are two very common risk factors for coronary artery disease. Exercise, on the other hand, probably helps to prevent these two diseases, and it appears to be an effective component of treatment programs for both type-2 diabetes and mild high blood pressure.

On the whole, then, it is unlikely that 3 beers a day is an adequate substitute for a pleasant workout. Indeed, this level of intake is probably the highest that is really compatible with reasonable health and adequate performance. More than 3–4 drinks a day clearly begins to shorten life and reduce its quality.

The way back

People who drink too much are clearly better off not drinking at all than continuing an excessive intake. But this alternative is not appealing to many people, who would like to continue so-called social drinking without succumbing to alcoholism. There has been an active, and often acrimonious, controversy as to whether alcoholics can really return to controlled drinking.

The controversy about such a basic question as this has come about because honorable investigators have obtained different answers, depending on how they asked the research question. The debate has been passionate because the subject is extremely important and because both sides of the debate are defending political and social viewpoints as well as attempting to solve a complex medical and psychological problem.

In brief: Between 1973 and 1978, there appeared reports of two major studies on the subject of controlled social drinking. One of them was conducted by a group at the Rand Corporation; the other was carried out by Mark and Linda Sobell, then at Patton State Hospital in California. Both reports indicated that certain alcoholics had successfully returned to asymptomatic (that is, controlled or social) drinking after treatment with behavioral methods.

At the time this research was begun, there were several reasons for thinking that social drinking could be achieved by at least some alcoholics. Laboratory studies, for example, had shown that even people who seemed to be strongly dependent on alcohol could modify their drinking patterns in response to learning or to a change in their social environment. At least, this seemed to be the case in laboratory or inpatient environments. Questionnaire results from studies in the community also identified people who claimed to have recovered control after a period of abusing alcohol.

Both the Rand investigators and the Sobells alleged that, after treatment, many of the study subjects were able to control their drinking for months to years. Moreover, the Sobells found that the subjects who attempted social drinking were more successful at avoiding relapse into alcoholism than those who were trying to remain wholly abstinent, at least in the year or so after treatment.

There were serious flaws in the design of the Rand study, however. Its standard of "control" over alcohol use seemed unrealistically relaxed. More to the point, long-term follow-up has shown that the Sobells' subjects ultimately did not fare well. Within 1 to 5 years after treatment, all but one lost control over their drinking.

Drinking behavior has also been studied in two large groups of men who were followed for more than 30 years, from youth through middle age. As reported in *The Natural History of Alcoholism* by Dr. George Vaillant, all of these men were psychologically "normal" to begin with, but some of them lost control over drinking for a period of time. Some became severely alcoholic. To be sure, there were men in this study who lost and then regained control over their drinking without having to give up alcohol altogether. These were people who had developed relatively few alcohol-related problems (such as illness, blackouts, difficulty with employment), and their alcohol problem had not brought them to the attention of a professional, or garnered them a formal diagnosis of alcoholism.

By contrast, those men who had ever developed more than a few alcohol-related problems, or who had been diagnosed alcoholic by a clinician, evidently had progressed too far in their illness to manage a return to asymptomatic drinking. They either became abstinent or they continued to suffer from alcoholism.

We must believe reports from the community studies showing that some alcoholics have been able to return to controlled drinking. But we also must recognize that virtually nobody who has gone so far as to require admission to an alcohol-treatment program will be able to go back to symptom-free drinking for very long.

This finding does not imply, however, that there are two distinct classes of people—"problem drinkers" and "alcoholics"—with two basically different capacities for handling their drinking. This is a common error in interpreting the research findings. There is no real difference, except in degree. Those who recognize the early warnings of lost control and who respond by taking measures to limit their use of alcohol may succeed in achieving some stability in their drinking patterns. The process of becoming dependent on alcohol begins with the first drink. Whether we avoid alcoholism is determined, in part, by the way we learn to control how we use alcohol.

Thus, it is probably not a good idea to assert categorically to an alcoholic that he or she can never drink again. The statement is not helpful, and it may not be true. The principle that Alcoholics Anonymous uses *is* helpful: to advise abstinence one day at a time. Alcoholics are extremely reluctant to give up the hope of taking another drink, as many nonalcoholics would be.

When someone with a clear alcohol problem hopes to manage the shift to social drinking, the following strategy, as outlined by Dr. Vaillant in an interview with the *Harvard Medical School Health Letter,* may be used. The person is told: "Drink any day you like, but never have more than 3 drinks in a 24-hour period." A drink is (somewhat generously) defined as one shot (1.5 ounces) of whiskey, one 12-ounce can of beer, or one 6-ounce glass of wine.

As Dr. Vaillant says, "My experience is that nobody to whom I have given this prescription has been able to stay within it. At that point, both the patient and I get the message. He or she has lost the ability to control consumption of alcohol. Abstinence—one day at a time—becomes the treatment goal." The exercise serves as a structured experiment from which the alcoholic can learn about herself or himself. It helps to define the task and cut through the denial that is a universal feature of alcoholic thinking. It also reinforces the point that alcoholism is a life-long disease, like diabetes or high blood pressure.

It is the structure of denial that makes alcoholism so difficult for not only the victims but families and friends to cope with. One of the greatest problems with relatives or close friends is that they protect the alcoholic's drinking. Like the alcoholic, they tend to deny what they know is really happening. That is the worst thing they can do. The earlier this disease is detected, the better one's chances of halting its progression.

If your own life is made painful because someone close to you has an alcohol problem, *you* have an alcohol problem as well. The first step is to recognize that simple fact. The second step is to go to Al-Anon, an organization of relatives of alcoholics, to learn what other people have done to get comfort for themselves and help for their relatives. The third step is to find a professional, through Al-Anon or an alcohol treatment clinic, and think through how to confront the alcoholic relative or friend and begin the treatment process. There is time. Alcoholism is never a problem of the moment. It puts a person at risk for a lifetime and must be approached as a lifetime disease.

Alcoholics Anonymous

Treatment may have to begin with a professional (alcoholism counselor, psychologist, social worker, psychiatrist, or other), but such help is by its nature hard to find and expensive. It may also be somewhat counterproductive because it is likely to undermine the alcoholic's already poor sense of self-esteem. Sooner or later, and preferably sooner, the alcoholic should be induced to attend meetings of Alcoholics Anonymous (AA).

There is nothing magic about Alcoholics Anonymous. And the view of alcoholism that it presents is probably not altogether correct, from a scientific standpoint. But that is beside the point. AA is available; it is free; and it offers a behavior modification program that even its psychologist-critics have to respect. It provides contact with people who have succeeded in staying sober. And it offers a variety of ways to restore the alcoholic's hope and self-esteem.

At least as important as all these features, AA provides a community of caring people whom the alcoholic has not injured in the past. One of the greatest burdens in any alcoholic's life is knowing that he or she has hurt everyone that he or she loves. The people at an AA meeting are not angry at the newly arriving alcoholic; and the alcoholic does not come into the room feeling guilty for inflicting past injuries on these people.

Telephone numbers for Alcoholics Anonymous, Al-Anon, and other sources of information and help can be found in the Yellow Pages under "Alcoholism Information and Treatment Centers."

Coffee

Coffee is the most widely consumed drug in North America and northern Europe. Although the beverage has an ancient heritage in the Middle East, it took hold in European cultures only about 250 years ago. Since then, it has become an important feature of daily life for very many people. The appeal of coffee as an agent to enhance alertness, more or less on demand, is augmented by positive associations from advertising—cozy evenings by a fire or heart-to-heart talks with an old friend.

The arousal effects of coffee are usually attributed to caffeine, though other substances may also play a role. In any event, the presumptive benefits—a sense of wakefulness or increased energy on one hand and relaxation on the other—all have their down side. It's surprisingly easy to overdo one's coffee consumption. Anxiety and sleeplessness are among the better documented results of doing so. The paradoxical sense of relaxation that coffee can bring is probably due to the fact that caffeine is fairly addicting. Abstaining from caffeine often produces a well-defined withdrawal syndrome, including lethargy, irritability, and headache. A cup of coffee becomes relaxing indeed when it is undoing these effects of withdrawal.

The behavioral drawbacks of coffee drinking, once recognized, can usually be controlled by regulating the amount that is consumed. More worrisome to many people is the thought that a lifetime of moderate coffee consumption could be injurious. For example, does coffee cause cancer, heart disease, or other serious illness?

Getting an early start

Many of us were first exposed to coffee before we were born. But pregnant women nowadays commonly avoid coffee for fear that the beverage might cause birth defects. This concern arose primarily because pregnant animals given large quantities of caffeine sometimes produce offspring with low birth weight or limb deformities.

However, studies of human mothers and their babies have been reassuring. One report has suggested that the mothers of children with birth defects consumed more coffee than a matched group of women whose babies were normal, but the design of the research was open to question. More rigorous investigations on larger groups have not confirmed the association. In one large study, even heavy coffee consumption carried no increased risk of low birth weight or birth defects. In another, the investigators specifically looked for an association with such common and major birth defects as cleft palate, heart malformations, or spina bifida. They did not find any.

After birth, however, a baby's behavior can be affected by caffeine in breast milk. The drug finds its way from the caffeine-containing products that a mother consumes into her milk, though at relatively low levels. It is unlikely that a cup or two of coffee would much affect a nursing infant, but nursing mothers with a very high intake may find that their infants are sleepless or irritable.

One lump or two—or none at all?

In the past 8 years or so, more attention has been paid to the breast itself than to breast milk as a target for caffeine. Ever since a group of doctors asserted that women with cysts of the breast could become nearly cyst-free when they eliminated coffee and other caffeine-containing products from their diets, much has been made of this claim. Although some small and poorly controlled studies have suggested that caffeine in the diet encourages cysts to form—and that abstaining increases the likelihood that they will disappear—the weight of the evidence indicates that coffee consumption has no consistent relationship to lumpy breasts, or so-called fibrocystic breast disease (*see Chapter 5*). This is not to deny that some women with cysts experience some relief when they reduce or eliminate caffeine intake, but this measure doesn't seem to help the majority.

Along the same lines, it is often claimed that caffeine worsens the so-called premenstrual syndrome or contributes to dysmenorrhea (excessive discomfort associated with menstruation). Again, no solid research supports these claims, though many women maintain that they have been helped by giving up caffeine. Little harm, other than the pangs of withdrawal, can come from giving up coffee, so abstention may be worth a nondogmatic try.

Coffee, caffeine, and cancer

While there is still some doubt about the relationship between caffeine consumption and lumpiness of the breasts, there is absolutely no evidence that coffee drinking leads to breast cancer. On the other hand, in the past 10 years articles appearing here and there have linked coffee to a variety of other cancers—bladder, pancreas, and colon most conspicuously. The best-publicized came out in 1981, when a group of researchers from the Harvard School of Public Health reported finding a connection with cancer of the pancreas. Careful analysis of the study, however, showed flaws. Since then, the original investigators and others have failed to find a clear relationship. Some researchers continue to suspect that *decaffeinated* coffee puts people at risk of developing pancreatic cancer, but this connection has not been established.

The connection to bladder cancer is more problematic. A weak relationship between coffee drinking and bladder cancer has appeared in many reports published in the past 10 or 15 years. But the studies have differed in significant ways, so interpretation is difficult. Some investigators have found increased rates only in male coffee drinkers and others only in females, for example. In no case has there been any evidence that the risk increases with the amount of coffee consumed. So it's reasonable to speculate that coffee is only incidentally associated with bladder cancer. Perhaps some other habit, one that goes along with coffee drinking, is the real cause of the cancer.

Isolated or occasional reports linking coffee to cancer of the ovary, colon, or kidney, among others, have peppered the medical literature. But support for these claims is not widespread. It seems unlikely that coffee plays an appreciable role in causing any of them.

Unfortunately, epidemiology is not a highly exact science. Failure to demonstrate a connection between a particular substance and cancer in humans, though somewhat reassuring, is usually far from air-tight. Thus a judgment about the potential of a substance to cause cancer should be based on as wide a variety of information as possible, including chemical and biological tests.

In the laboratory, brewed coffee flunks one of the standard screening tests used to determine cancer-causing potential. When bacteria are dunked into coffee (in the so-called Ames assay; *see Chapter 7*), some of them undergo genetic mutation. On the other hand, laboratory animals put on a life-long coffee break do not develop any more cancer than they would otherwise. Caffeine itself is probably not a cause of cancer, and some studies even suggest that it may be protective. Others, however, suggest that caffeine may be a co-carcinogen, a chemical that brings out the potential of other dietary or environmental substances (such as tobacco) to cause cancer. Caffeine is known to have a faint chemical resemblance to some carcinogens.

Coffee, cholesterol, and coronaries

The last 20 years have seen a lot of debate on whether coffee contributes to coronary heart disease. Four main areas of controversy persist: (1) Does coffee raise cholesterol levels? (2) Does it raise blood pressure? (3) Does it disturb the heart's rhythm? (4) Whether or not it does any of these things, is coffee consumption statistically associated with a higher death rate from heart attacks?

The cholesterol quarrel was stirred up by a report in 1985 which indicated that men who drink more than 2 or 3 cups of coffee a day have higher cholesterol levels than those who drink less. This research has to be interpreted with caution because only a small number of men were enrolled in the study. A major investigation in Norway, where some of the world's heaviest coffee drinkers live, has also found an association with elevated cholesterol. Their conclusions, reported in 1983 as the Tromsø Heart Study, were based on findings in over 14,000 people. In the Tromsø sample, those consuming the most coffee had the highest cholesterol levels. But almost two-thirds of the people in the Tromsø group drank more than 5 cups of coffee a day. (Some critics have suggested that the results could reflect higher cream intake from the extra cups of coffee. But Norwegians happen to like their coffee black.) A more recent release from the Tromsø investigators reports that when habitual coffee drinkers with high cholesterol abstain from coffee, their cholesterol levels fall an average of 13%.

However, other research reports on blood cholesterol have not incriminated coffee. The disparity between these various research results fuels controversy and also suggests that if there is a relationship between coffee drinking and elevated cholesterol, it may depend on some factor that isn't well understood. Among the possibilities are choice of brewing method and bean, temperature of the water, or even the water itself. Drip-brewed coffee on average contains more caffeine than either percolated or instant coffee, for example, and the levels of other ingredients may also be affected by brewing technique.

There is no question that a cup of coffee can increase blood pressure. But the increase is usually mild, and there is no clear evidence that regular coffee drinking causes high blood pressure in an otherwise healthy person or aggravates it significantly in someone with hypertension. Coffee also has a reputation for causing arrhythmias, or irregularities in the heartbeat, and this reputation, too, is by and large overstated. However, coffee can trigger serious disturbances of the heartbeat in some people, especially those with preexisting heart conditions or those who are taking certain medications. Here the culprit appears to be caffeine, so that decaffeinated brews probably pose less of a threat.

If coffee increases such risk factors for heart disease as blood cholesterol levels or blood pressure, that fact should be reflected in a higher cardiovascular mortality of coffee drinkers when other factors, such as cigarette smoking, are controlled.

Late in 1986, a widely publicized study from the Johns Hopkins Medical School reported that there is a connection between coffee intake and cardiovascular disease or death. The results of this 25-year follow-up of 1,000 white male physicians indicated that 3–4 cups of coffee a day were associated with twice the average risk for coronary events, and drinking more than 5 cups brought the risk to nearly 3 times average.

Although this study had some real strengths, it also had weaknesses—mainly the fact that very few coronary deaths were recorded, so that it became necessary to lump together some conditions, such as chest pain, that are harder to document. Also, the only potentially associated aspect of "lifestyle" that the investigators controlled for was cigarette smoking. No effort was made to evaluate diet, obesity, level of exercise, stress, or other variables that might have contributed to the coronary outcome. In short, the new report is not powerful enough to offset the results from the great majority of studies, in which no significant relationship could be detected between death from heart disease and coffee consumption.

The scoop

Whether coffee has any adverse effects on health is still very much debated. Many factors complicate research. The mere fact that people have trouble accurately recalling and reporting the amount of coffee they drink makes data collection difficult. And coffee tends to keep some tough company, such as cigarettes. Weeding out the effect of this variable can be very difficult. Another problem may be that one person's heavenly brew is another one's poison, so to speak. The ingredients and the exact composition of a cup can vary considerably.

Since no one is entirely certain what components of coffee are

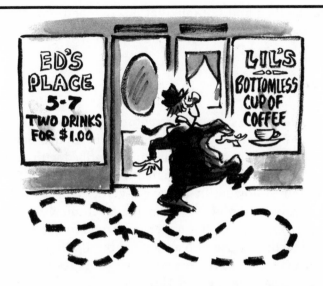

Contrary to myth, coffee is no antidote to alcohol. You can be just as drunk after several cups of coffee as you were before. You may be a drunk with "coffee nerves," but not a safer driver or otherwise better off.

biologically active, it has been hard to conduct detailed laboratory studies on the beverage. Caffeine, which is the most familiar and best studied, may not be the ingredient that has greatest impact on health. A nice illustration of this fact is that decaffeinated coffee provokes the stomach to secrete acid just as effectively as does regular coffee. Thus, the once-common recommendation that people with ulcers drink decaffeinated coffee in preference to the real thing proved not to be particularly sensible advice. (There is no clear evidence that coffee actually causes ulcers, even in people who are prone to develop them. But people with an ulcer are probably well advised to limit their coffee intake.)

What, then, can be concluded about coffee and health? The best that can be said at present is that there is no definitive evidence that coffee contributes to disease. While there is some suggestion that in certain populations heavy coffee drinking may predispose to coronary heart disease, not even this relationship has been borne out for Americans. Almost certainly, other aspects of our lifestyle (such as cigarette smoking and saturated fat intake) contribute far more to such illnesses as heart disease and cancer than does coffee.

Marijuana

Marijuana has been around for centuries—as both a recreational drug and a medication. Around 1900 in the United States, recreational use of marijuana was primarily identified with urban black culture. It then came to be associated with jazz music, and the drug had a certain following in the avant-garde, bohemian fringes of American culture. An active campaign to criminalize the drug as both dangerous in itself and a stepping stone to harder drugs was conducted by the Bureau of Narcotics in the 1930s and 1940s. This campaign appears to have been effective in suppressing the popularity of marijuana until the mid 1960s.

Then something remarkable happened. Within a decade, marijuana became a truly common recreational drug—not by any means the equal of tobacco or alcohol, but sufficiently popular that one-fifth of the population had at least tried it and somewhat less than 10% were identified as regular users. Marijuana use became particularly prevalent among adolescents and young adults, and if the trends to ever-increasing use in this age group had continued, marijuana might well have rivaled alcohol, if not tobacco, in popularity. But by the mid 1980s, this did not appear to be the probable outcome. The marijuana wave crested around 1978, and popularity of the drug now appears to be waning.

The reasons for this change are not altogether clear. Government programs to prevent importation and sale may have played some role in reducing the supply, but most people, especially teenagers, respond to surveys by saying that they think marijuana is easy to get, and lack of supply isn't what prevents them from using the drug. It seems more likely that demand has declined. The reason for a shrinking demand is not known. To the extent that fashion played a role, marijuana may simply lack the glamor it once had. And, as laws affecting possession and use have relaxed, it may have become harder for youngsters to make a "statement" by smoking a joint.

Whatever else is going on, the decline in use of marijuana is associated with an increasing perception that the drug is harmful. The reason for this shift in attitude is not known. On the whole, medical research on the drug has not turned up a "smoking gun." As drugs go, marijuana appears to be intermediate in risk—certainly nowhere near as dangerous to the average occasional user as regular consumption of cigarettes or alcohol. This is not to say that marijuana is a problem-free drug. Long-term consequences of heavy use are not really known; 25 years is a relatively brief period in the life of a drug. It took over 50 years for the hazards of widespread tobacco use to be generally recognized.

Animal experiments can give us some clue as to possible risks, but they cannot be trusted to predict the actual outcome in human users. Experiments with people are possible, but ethical considerations and time limitations restrict their utility. Even observations made on heavy marijuana smokers elsewhere (Jamaica, Costa Rica, Egypt, Greece) have limited applicability to Americans because of differences in environment and pattern of use.

Highs and lows

People using marijuana for the first time are commonly motivated by curiosity about its effect and by the urging of friends. Those who return to using marijuana usually do so for the mild euphoria, loosening of inhibitions, and alterations in the quality of perceptions and sensations without true hallucinations. Other aspects of the marijuana "high" vary widely from person to person and from time to time in the same person. The drug's subjective effects usually last for 2 or 3 hours.

Objective changes also occur. While high, marijuana users often become somewhat clumsy (though they may feel graceful). They react more slowly than normal, perceive the passage of time less accurately, pay attention less well, and make more errors in performing arithmetic tests. They also show defects in short-term memory during the high. Impaired driving can pose a serious threat to health. Marijuana can interfere with driving skills, although it does not appear to stimulate aggressiveness behind the wheel the way alcohol does. Moreover, the effect on driving skills lasts several hours beyond the period when a person feels high; even someone who feels "normal" drives worse than usual. It is foolish and dangerous to drive while under the influence of marijuana.

A few individuals may react to the marijuana high by becoming extremely anxious. Their minor "bad trip" is best handled by reassuring them and helping them wait out the period of intoxication. There is no solid evidence that other, more serious or lasting psychological effects are likely to result from marijuana use. A marijuana high may trigger prolonged symptoms in unstable people, but does not itself appear to be responsible for mental illness.

Marijuana users typically claim that the drug does not produce addiction. This both is and is not true. Two of the hallmarks of addiction are *tolerance* and *withdrawal symptoms*. As tolerance develops, people require more of a drug to produce its usual or desired effect. Withdrawal is manifested by irritability, craving, and various physical symptoms occurring when the drug is no longer taken. Marijuana appears capable of producing both tolerance and withdrawal, but neither is seen in people who use the drug occasionally. Much heavier exposure to marijuana is required to elicit either feature of drug dependence. Indeed, both tolerance and withdrawal have only really been observed in experimental settings with prolonged administration of high doses of the active component of marijuana, THC (tetrahydrocannabinol). True addiction to marijuana—of the sort produced by nicotine or heroin—seems to be rare or nonexistent outside a laboratory.

On the other hand, an effect sometimes claimed for marijuana, "reverse tolerance" has not been observed in experimental settings. The notion that people become more sensitive to effects of the drug as they gain more experience with it was once popular among counter-culture users of the drug. It seems likely that placebo effects were involved, and that users "trained" themselves to achieve these effects more rapidly.

Another effect that has been attributed to marijuana proves not to be as important as once thought. The claim that chemicals from marijuana accumulate in the body is true. But this does not mean that the drug remains active in the body. THC quite rapidly leaves the blood stream and enters tissue with a high fat content. However, it is either inactivated in these tissues or released so slowly and in such small quantities that it appears to have no further effect.

Marijuana has been blamed for producing apathy, loss of motivation, and narrowing of interests in people who use it heavily. There is no clear evidence that the drug does indeed produce such an "amotivational syndrome," although clinical observation certainly indicates that young people who become heavy marijuana users may lose interest in achieving well at school or work. However, carefully designed studies of both unskilled workers and college students have failed to support the notion that routine use of marijuana commonly impairs overall performance. Heavy use of the drug may really be a *symptom* of depression and low self-esteem, rather than a cause. Young people who are depressed and have low expectations for themselves—and whose parents expect little of them—are more likely than others to make heavy use of marijuana.

Physical consequences

No convincing report has yet been published to show that marijuana permanently damages the brain. In the early 1970s, an x-ray study published in the *Lancet* reported that atrophy of the brain had been observed in 10 young men who used marijuana regularly. The method for measuring brain size was not particularly accurate, however, and two more recent studies using computed tomography, a very reliable method, showed no evidence of atrophy. It would not be particularly surprising if there were some effect on the nervous system from heavy, prolonged use, but the weight of the evidence, at the moment, suggests that there is none.

Marijuana is usually smoked—a method of administration that is about as efficient as injecting a drug intravenously. Smoking anything damages the lungs. Paradoxically, THC, the active ingredient, opens air passages of the lungs. For this reason smoking marijuana during an asthma attack was sometimes recommended in the last century, when medicinal use of the drug was still legal. But heavy smoking of marijuana clearly has the opposite effect. Smoking about 5 cigarettes a day narrows the air passages and inflames their lining. Sufficiently heavy, long-term marijuana smoking probably leads to chronic bronchitis, just as tobacco smoking does. Marijuana smoke contains more than 400 chemicals besides THC and some of them are quite similar to tobacco "tars," including those that contribute to lung cancer. It is likely that smoking marijuana can lead to cancer of the lung, but, even if the risk is fairly high, another 15 to 20 years must pass before enough evidence accumulates in this country to show how much marijuana smoking is necessary to create a significant risk. On the other hand, to keep a perspective, the typical tobacco smoker inhales 20–30 cigarettes' worth of smoke a day; the occasional or social user of marijuana probably has a far lower exposure to lung-damaging smoke.

Marijuana stimulates the heart to beat faster and work harder. Although this effect is insignificant in healthy people, it may be a hazard for anyone with heart disease.

Early studies indicated that marijuana reduces levels of the male hormone testosterone and also impairs sperm production. It now appears that there is little or no effect on testosterone levels of adults, but that sperm production may be reduced. However, there has been no clear evidence of infertility in males who smoke marijuana, and the effect on sperm production appears to be temporary and reversible when the smoker abstains. In boys entering puberty, marijuana may have a more important hormonal effect. There is some evidence suggesting that cannabis stimulates the body to convert testosterone to estrogen, the female hormone, and that this action of the drug has resulted in delayed puberty.

Effects of marijuana on female sexual and reproductive functions are even less well known. It appears that marijuana is capable of disturbing the menstrual cycle and increasing the number of infertile cycles. During pregnancy, THC can pass into the placenta (where it tends to be stored) and enter the fetus. A nursing mother concentrates THC in her milk and passes it to her baby. Milk production itself can be reduced by exposure to THC.

Whether typical marijuana use causes genetic damage that is passed on to a fetus is not known, but appears doubtful. The subject has been controversial for over 15 years, and it remains so. Also not known is whether marijuana is capable of causing miscarriages or developmental defects in a fetus, but the results of one large study suggests that it is. Given the general sensitivity of fetal development to drug exposure, it is prudent to recommend that women who are pregnant, or likely to get pregnant, should add marijuana to the list of drugs that have a potential to harm their fetuses.

Much has been made of marijuana's ability to suppress immunity. There are clear indications from laboratory studies that exposing immune cells to THC inhibits certain functions. Studies of whole animals also show an impairment of immune functions tested experimentally. However, there is no clear evidence that regular human smokers of marijuana have a defective immune response. There are not enough data to indicate whether marijuana smoking increases susceptibility to the development of AIDS.

Keeping off the grass

Little is known about marijuana's long-term effects on health or behavior. Like tobacco smokers at the beginning of this century, current marijuana users are engaged in a massive and uncontrolled "experiment." Yet, the "volunteers" for this experiment can hardly be thought to have given their *informed* consent, particularly not the adolescents and young adults who represent the majority of marijuana users. Even if marijuana proves to have few or no adverse effects on the health of young people, the time they spend "high" is time that could be spent in normal learning and physical activity. It is difficult to imagine that recreational drugs make any positive contribution to growth and development.

It seems appropriate to take measures that will diminish marijuana use by young boys and girls, but how to do so is not very clear. Research conducted in the past 10 years has some tentative implications for parents who wish to discourage their children's use of marijuana:

- Limit access to the drug.
- Encourage friendships with nonusing companions.
- Attempt to delay a child's first experience with marijuana.
- Take stock of parental attitudes about alcohol, marijuana, and other drugs.

Parents protect children from drug use by being close to them, remaining actively involved with them and their friends, supporting their self-esteem, and expressing high expectations for achievement in and out of school. Once heavy involvement with drugs is established, however, parents are often no longer able to help their children.

It is probably not productive to let marijuana become ammunition in the war between the generations or to treat experimentation with the drug as a catastrophe. Just because tobacco and alcohol are more familiar drugs does not mean that they are safer than marijuana. They are a very real threat to health at every age.

One tactic to reduce marijuana use cannot be condoned: spraying of defoliants such as paraquat to limit production of the drug. Contamination of marijuana with this substance has been the most clearly defined health hazard presented by the drug. The amount of paraquat-contaminated marijuana in this country is not large—

perhaps 10%. Unfortunately, inhaling this material can lead to severe lung damage. Paraquat on marijuana can be detected with an ultraviolet light, which reveals a red fluorescence on the leaves, as well as on the lips of someone who has been smoking material contaminated with herbicide.

Cocaine

Ten years ago we would not have included cocaine in this book—except perhaps for a passing historical mention. Few people needed medical or psychiatric help for cocaine problems. Now cocaine is in the news every day—the second most popular illicit drug in the United States, a 30-billion-dollar-a-year business, a favorite subject of crime dramas and tales of disaster among entertainment celebrities. Once an exotic pleasure of outlaws and the very rich, it can now be found in homes, college dormitories, offices, and factories all over the country.

The coca plant has been cultivated for thousands of years in the Andes and Amazon regions of South America. There, Indians still chew the leaf daily to prevent fatigue, chill, and hunger, and they use it medicinally as a local anesthetic and stimulant. There is little evidence that cocaine ingested this way—by mouth, slowly, in a dilute form, mixed with other chemicals in the leaf—creates any serious health hazards or social problems.

Pure cocaine was first extracted in 1860 and introduced into medicine in the 1870s and 1880s as a treatment for a wide variety of illnesses. Abuse and dependence soon became problems, and by the early 20th century cocaine had been subjected to the same laws as the opiate narcotics, such as morphine and codeine. Medical interest in its stimulant powers declined, and it is now used in medicine only as one of many local anesthetics. Eventually new synthetic stimulants, the amphetamines, replaced cocaine both in doctors' offices and on the streets.

When new legal restrictions were imposed on amphetamines in the 1970s, the market for cocaine began to recover. The new enthusiasm for recreational drugs of all kinds then led to a revival of the cocaine traffic. Because of its expense, cocaine became known as the champagne of drugs; but now the price has fallen, availability has increased, and use has spread to all social classes and income levels. In one survey of cocaine users calling a telephone information hot line, 50% of the callers earned less than $25,000 a year, the mean family income in the United States.

Crack

The highly publicized emergence of "crack," a form of cocaine that is smoked, has certainly increased the hazards associated with cocaine use. Although cocaine is active when swallowed (unlike nicotine), it is rarely used that way, because the effect is not immediate or strong enough. The three common methods of ingestion are snorting (snuffing), freebasing (smoking), and injection, usually intravenous. Any of these can produce serious ill effects, but freebasing and intravenous injection are particularly dangerous and particularly common among severe cocaine abusers. Injection and snorting have been practiced for more than a hundred years, but freebasing was not discovered until the early 1970s.

Illicit cocaine is usually sold in the form of hydrochloride salt, which is soluble in water and convenient for injection or snorting. It tends to decompose on heating, but is easily converted to cocaine proper (the free base) by the addition of baking soda or another alkaline substance. "Crack" is just a term for the cocaine base when it is sold as such, rather than converted by the consumer. Cocaine base is more volatile than cocaine hydrochloride and can be smoked in a glass water pipe. According to surveys available a couple of years ago, more than a million people—perhaps 10% of cocaine users—had at least experimented with freebasing. The marketing of crack has no doubt greatly enlarged that number.

Effects of cocaine

The immediate effect of cocaine is a mood of exhilaration, alertness, confidence, and high energy that lasts 20 minutes to an hour. The main physical effects are dilation of the pupils, constriction of peripheral blood vessels, increased heart rate and blood pressure, and loss of appetite. (Snorted cocaine also produces a sensation of numbness in the nose.) The elation is sometimes followed by mild irritability and lethargy. High doses or repeated use can produce a state resembling mania, with impaired judgment, incessant rambling talk, hyperactivity, and paranoia that may lead to violence or accidents. There is also an acute anxiety reaction, sometimes severe enough to be called panic, which can be treated with injections of diazepam (Valium) or other anti-anxiety drugs.

Serious acute physical reactions are also possible. By constricting blood vessels and increasing the heart rate, cocaine can produce cardiac symptoms, including irregular heartbeat, angina, and myocardial infarction. High doses may also cause nausea, headache, cold sweat, tremors, and fast, irregular, shallow breathing. People who have high blood pressure or damaged arteries may suffer strokes. Death usually results from convulsions followed by paralysis of the brain centers controlling respiration, leading to cardiac arrest. In serious cases, acute overdose must be treated with oxygen and anticonvulsant drugs. Any method of ingestion can kill, but intravenous injection and freebasing are especially dangerous. A common cause of death is intravenous injection of a speedball—a combination of heroin and cocaine. The reported number of deaths involving cocaine has risen from fewer than a dozen to several hundred a year over the last decade.

Habitual use

Animal experiments and studies of coca chewing indicate that as long as only a limited quantity is consumed, cocaine can be taken daily for years with no apparent ill effects. But it is one of the most powerfully addicting of drugs. When laboratory animals are connected to an apparatus that supplies unlimited intravenous cocaine, they eventually kill themselves by repeated injections. Human users often become aware of the insidiously seductive quality of cocaine and may find the appetite for it hard to control.

A damaging habit usually develops over a period of several months to several years. It begins with a need for another snort after the first to counteract the mild let-down feeling and proceeds to all-night parties on weekends, taking cocaine for energy in the afternoon at work, needing it early in the morning, and then perhaps concealing the habit, freebasing or intravenous injection, and an increasing preoccupation with cocaine to the exclusion of most other things. Compulsive users cannot turn the drug down. They think about it constantly, dream about it, spend all their savings on it and borrow, steal, or deal to pay for it.

Short-term tolerance develops very fast with repeated doses during a single session; users often say that they never quite recapture the euphoria of the first snort. After months of use, long-term tolerance may also arise, although this happens less strikingly and consistently. Experiments have shown that tolerance to amphetamines also develops as the user becomes tolerant to cocaine. There is some evidence, though, that users become more, not less, sensitive to the seizure-inducing effect of cocaine.

Whether cocaine can be said to produce a withdrawal reaction depends partly on definitions. It does not cause physiological addiction of the kind associated with alcohol, sedatives, and opiates, in which the central nervous system becomes hyperexcitable when deprived of the drug. Therefore abstinence does not usually result in acute physical discomfort. A common pattern of cocaine abuse, observed in laboratory animals as well as human beings, consists of binges or runs followed by crashes. A week-long run produces acute tolerance as well as exhaustion from lack of food and sleep. The user becomes agitated and depressed, then falls into several days of severe depression, excessive sleep, and heavy eating. Sometimes chills, tremors, or muscle pains are felt.

The crash is more like a hangover than an alcohol or opiate withdrawal reaction; during the acute phase there is no desire for cocaine. Afterward the abuser may go through a period of unhappiness and lethargy that stimulates further craving. Even many months or years later, a passing but intense craving can reemerge, especially when certain moods or situations have come to evoke a conditioned response.

Alcohol, sedatives, and narcotics are often used to calm cocaine-induced agitation, and this practice may create a dual dependency that is particularly hard to treat. Since long-term heavy use of cocaine is physically hard to sustain, many abusers eventually switch to alcohol or opiates. When heroin addicts in methadone maintenance clinics start using cocaine, they are likely to be on the way back to heroin.

Chronic cocaine abuse resembles amphetamine abuse in its effects on health. Some physical effects are exhaustion, headaches, tremors, blurred vision, nausea, seizures or loss of consciousness, and malnutrition resulting from loss of appetite. At first cocaine is often sexually stimulating, but chronic abusers tend to lose interest in sex, and men may become impotent. Cocaine dependence interferes seriously with work, family life, and friendships. Suicide attempts are common. Intensive and compulsive users become jittery, irritable, and sometimes subtly cool, distant, and self-absorbed. They suffer from loss of concentration and perceptual and thinking disturbances. Often they become hypersensitive to sound, light, and touch. Resulting symptoms are snow lights (flashes in the peripheral visual field), animated shadows, and hallucinations of objects touching the skin, especially the feeling that insects are crawling under the skin.

Another typical symptom is absorption in apparently meaningless repetitive activities—scribbling, counting, pacing, sorting and ordering, taking apart and reassembling mechanical objects. Exaggerated interest in detail together with anxiety and hypersensitivity to peripheral sensory cues may result in paranoid thinking. Cocaine abusers have been known to sit before the door of a room for hours, holding a revolver and awaiting an imaginary intruder. A paranoid psychosis may occur; it is usually transient but may last several days. Because consciousness is clear, the hallucinations and delusions of a cocaine psychosis are hard to distinguish from an acute paranoid psychosis not produced by drugs.

Each method of ingestion also has its own special dangers. Snorting causes sinusitis, runny and clogged noses, cracked, bleeding, or ulcerated nasal membranes, and once in a while a perforated nasal septum that requires surgery. Intravenous injection with contaminated equipment can lead to skin infections, hepatitis, internal fungus infections, endocarditis (infection of the lining of the heart), polyarteritis nodosa (inflamed and broken arteries), and acquired immune deficiency syndrome (AIDS). Freebasing causes bronchitis and lung damage that reduces the capacity to exchange oxygen and carbon dioxide. Death from pulmonary edema (fluid collection in the lungs) has been reported.

The proportion of experimental and recreational cocaine users who develop a serious problem is not known. There is no evidence that cocaine abusers necessarily have any particular personality type. Certain people may be more susceptible—especially those who suffer from depression, manic-depressive disorder, or attention deficit disorder of the residual (adult) type. But many cocaine abusers have not been suffering from any psychiatric disorder. The drug has a powerful attraction that is enhanced by certain features of Western culture—its emphasis on activity, efficiency, speed, self-sufficiency, and aggressiveness. Cocaine abusers are sometimes caricatures of the society in which they live.

Treatment for chronic abuse

Treatment suggestions and treatment centers for cocaine abuse and dependence are proliferating—information hotlines, cocaine clinics, public and private hospital wards, psychotherapy, counseling services, and mutual aid groups. Although there are no adequate controlled experiments or follow-up studies, it appears that some cocaine abusers succeed in solving their problem either by themselves or with professional help.

The abuser must first become convinced that treatment is necessary. As in all types of drug and alcohol abuse, more or less subtle forms of denial are common; for example, abusers may want relief for some of the side effects without giving up the habit itself. Sometimes they are induced to come in for treatment only by pressure from families, employers, or the law. People seek treatment at different stages of dependency, and the severity of the symptoms varies greatly.

Sometimes cocaine abusers can help themselves. One device that has been advocated is a form of aversive conditioning. The user makes a promise to himself or herself not to use cocaine at certain times and places, with explicit self-imposed penalties if the promise is broken.

A variant of this technique is so-called contingency contracting, which requires the cooperation of a professional. The cocaine abuser deposits a letter with a counselor. If the urine turns up positive for cocaine or a sample is not produced for inspection, the letter is to be mailed. It contains an admission likely to be embarrassing or damaging professionally or financially. Since the penalty is severe and public, motivation to fulfill the contract is presumably strong. This method has been reported to be highly successful, at least among well-educated and well-motivated cocaine abusers who have a great deal to lose. Even so, many who are offered contingency contracts turn down the proposal, and almost all of these eventually drop out of treatment or resume cocaine abuse. Possibly abusers who refuse contingency contracts have more serious problems, or many who sign such contracts are already prepared to give up the drug anyway.

Psychotherapy alone rarely solves any drug problem, but it can be an important part of treatment. Supportive psychotherapy is a relationship with a sympathetic professional who provides comfort and encouragement to help the abuser stay away from the sources of cocaine and manage impulsive behavior in general. Interpretive or exploratory psychotherapy can help abusers to understand what functions cocaine has been fulfilling in their lives and find other ways to cope.

Many cocaine abusers have also joined mutual help groups—Alcoholics Anonymous, Cocaine Anonymous, and Narcotics Anonymous. All these programs have more or less the same approach: confiding in others who have the same problem, sharing feelings, making a resolution to overcome the dependency, and getting the support of the group to confirm that resolution. Members admit their powerlessness over the drug and seek help from a higher power, while taking a "moral inventory" of themselves and pledging abstinence one day at a time.

In severe cases, detoxification in a hospital may be necessary. Some authorities favor hospitalization whenever there is chronic freebasing or intravenous cocaine use, dependence on other drugs, or severe psychological and social impairment. Others would hospitalize only when other treatments have repeatedly failed or when severe depressive or psychotic symptoms have lasted more than a few days. They believe that hospitalization only delays the necessary encounter with the stresses and temptations that originally led to cocaine abuse.

Withdrawal procedure

Cocaine can be withdrawn suddenly, since removal of the drug does not produce a physically dangerous syndrome. The severe depressive symptoms of a crash will usually go away by themselves in a few days. Withdrawal in a hospital can be followed by further treatment including psychotherapy and group therapy, and then a discharge plan that includes job placement, guidelines for the family, and further psychotherapy.

An intensive or compulsive user who is being rehabilitated must do everything possible to avoid situations and people that may tempt him or her to return to cocaine use. It is important to destroy cocaine paraphernalia and avoid dealers and friends who use the drug. Sometimes an abuser must find a new place to live and get a new job to avoid familiar drug scenes. Usually it is necessary to give up alcohol, marijuana, and other drugs as well, because they excite the desire for cocaine while reducing the capacity to resist it.

Several drug treatments for cocaine abuse have been proposed, but it is doubtful whether any of them will prove entirely effective. Some researchers believe that the amphetamine-related stimulant methylphenidate (Ritalin), often prescribed for children with hyperactivity or attention deficit disorder, is also effective for cocaine abusers who have been medicating themselves for the adult variant of that disorder. Other drugs may also be tried, particularly when the treating physician believes that another disorder, such as depression, underlies the tendency to abuse cocaine. But right now there is no known drug that eliminates the desire for cocaine or supplies a safe substitute for most users.

Probably no single treatment will turn out to be effective for most cocaine problems or even for any particular group of cocaine abusers that can be identified in advance. Cocaine abuse presents the same kinds of difficulties as amphetamine or alcohol abuse. Despite the uncertainty about methods, reports from clinics have been fairly hopeful. To determine whether optimism is justified or illusory will require more clinical experience and controlled studies.

3 Living with Progress: Environmental Hazards of Modern Life

Is progress killing us? Many people, perhaps especially those who read or watch the daily news, go around thinking so. The feeling that modern life is fraught with lethal hazards is actually rather an old one. For about the last 150 years it has been a major theme for commentators living in societies undergoing industrialization. The worry that the most fundamental elements of life—air, food, water—will be irrevocably poisoned is a persisting one. In many ways, the worry is both symbolic and real. It is symbolic when the pressure of living and working in a highly industrialized, time-conscious society is expressed not as emotional discontent but as anxiety about being poisoned. It is also very real. We are all aware that toxic gas *can* leak from a chemical plant to kill or injure thousands, that leakage of radiation from a nuclear power plant *can* make a whole region of the earth uninhabitable for decades, that workers *can* develop terminal disease from handling hazardous products without adequate protection or information.

On the whole, though, technological advance appears to have improved life expectancy rather than shortened it. People in industrialized countries live much longer than those in developing countries, and this is no longer a result solely of reductions in infant mortality. A person of 40 living in the United States can now expect to live longer than one who reached the same age a couple of decades ago. So, overall, technology appears to have succeeded in prolonging most people's lives.

By the same token, the lives of some people are shortened by modern ways. One of the central problems of technology is how to provide benefits to the majority without exposing a minority to undue hazard. Workers in certain industries may be exposed to high concentrations of hazardous chemicals, to radiation, or to accidents that they might not have suffered if we were all living a simple life. People who live near airports must put up with—and

143

perhaps suffer from—high levels of noise in order for passengers to enjoy the convenience of rapid transportation. In some instances the person at risk is the consumer who purchases a product that has been inadequately tested and proves to be hazardous. The only way to prevent this type of mishap is with an adequate early-warning system alerting consumers and manufacturers to the health hazards involved.

In this chapter, we focus on certain important and recurring themes arising from the effect of modern living on health—chiefly problems of the workplace, but also problems of the environment and of housing.

Noise Pollution

We *expect* cities to have a noisy soundtrack: honks, crashes, rumbles, and plunks of cars, construction sites, delivery trucks, and portable stereos. But noise can also follow those who flee from modern life. After building a dream-house retreat near Altamont Pass, a California family lost a lot of sleep when a windmill farm was built next door. Another windmill, in a northeastern vacation community, drove its neighbors crazy (first) and into court (second), where they succeeded in getting an order to have it turned off. The roar of passing automobiles or low-flying airplanes is a pretty standard feature of all but the most remote areas. There's no doubt that noise is an almost universal irritant—but is it a health hazard?

Sound versus noise

Webster's definition of noise has a nice ring to it—"any loud, discordant, or disagreeable sound." Of course, a sound does not have to be loud to be annoying or bothersome. Noise is unwanted sound; the experience has both a psychological and a physical component. One person's music may be another's noise.

Sound begins as the movement of air molecules. A vibrating object (like the sound box of a guitar) sets up alternating bands of compression and expansion in the surrounding air. When these vibrations strike the ear drum, they are transmitted to delicate cells, known as *hair cells,* in the inner ear. Hair cells, responding to the pattern of vibrations, convert them to another code, which is transmitted to the temporal lobe of the brain. Here begins the process of decoding the sound to extract information, pleasure, or annoyance.

Sound carries both energy and information, which are really just different aspects of the same process of wave formation. Waves have two main properties: the speed at which they vibrate, and the intensity of each vibration. (If you think of the ocean's surface, you can imagine these properties as, respectively, the rate at which waves hit the shore and the average height of their crests.) With sound, it is chiefly the intensity (essentially, how tightly air molecules pack together with each vibration) that creates the sense of loudness, though frequency also makes a contribution, with higher sounds perceived as louder.

Thus, there is more than one way to describe the volume of a sound. The actual amount of energy it is carrying can be measured; this is usually expressed in *decibels,* abbreviated *dB*. For many purposes, though, a modified form of the decibel scale is used. Called the "A-scale," this system of measurement compensates for the effect of frequency and corresponds very closely to the way people actually hear sound. When the A-scale is used, decibels are abbreviated *dbA*.

Although the decibel scale is based on physical measurement of sound pressure, what most people are really interested in knowing is the quantity we call "loudness," which has to be evaluated by having people listen to sounds and rate them. When loudness is measured this way, an increase of 10 decibels generally makes a given sound twice as loud, and an increase of 20 decibels is heard as a fourfold increase. (Thus, the decibel scale is not a linear scale, like a ruler marked in inches, but logarithmic.) The rustling of leaves measures about 10 dbA; human conversations average 50, and a ringing telephone commonly reaches 60. Household appliances, such as vacuum cleaners, measure around 90; and subway trains, jack hammers, and disco music may exceed 100. Depending somewhat on the circumstances, sounds over 60 are perceived as intrusive, those over 80 are annoying, and those exceeding 100 decibels are extremely bothersome. (Obviously, the audience at a rock concert assigns a somewhat different value to these measurements.)

Because sound is a form of energy, it has the potential to damage human tissue. Most vulnerable to injury are the sound-sensing hair cells themselves. Thus, hearing impairment is the major physical consequence of loud sound. A single, explosive noise is capable of

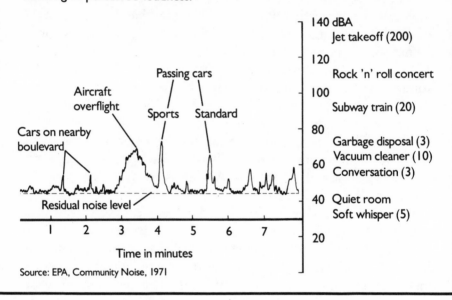

NOISE POLLUTION

The graph below shows 8 minutes of noise sampled on a city street in the early afternoon. The volume ranges from about 45 dBA to a peak of more than 70 when a sports car drives by.

The volume of some familiar sounds, as measured by the decibel "A" scale, is indicated on the graph at the right. Distance, in feet, from the source is given in parentheses. An increase of 10 dBA indicates an approximate doubling in perceived loudness.

140 dBA
Jet takeoff (200)

120
Rock 'n' roll concert

100
Subway train (20)

80
Garbage disposal (3)
Vacuum cleaner (10)
60
Conversation (3)

40 Quiet room
Soft whisper (5)

20

Passing cars

Aircraft overflight
Sports   Standard

Cars on nearby boulevard

Residual noise level

Time in minutes

Source: EPA, Community Noise, 1971

damaging hair cells, but hearing loss is usually the result of continual exposure to volumes over 80–85 decibels. Current estimates are that 8 million production workers in the United States are exposed to noise at this level, and about 1 million of them have detectable hearing loss as a result. To prevent this type of hearing loss, several steps have to be taken. Equipment can be engineered to make it run more quietly. Workers who wear ear plugs or earmuff-type shields can reduce their noise exposure by 7–20 dBA, and this precaution is recommended to anyone who is routinely exposed to noise from industrial machinery or aircraft at levels above 80–85 dBA. Rock musicians, whose sound exposure during a work night may be roughly comparable to a steelworker's exposure during a work shift, have not routinely protected themselves and are now often proving to suffer occupational hearing loss.

The hair cells are the only parts of the adult body that have been shown to suffer physically from exposure to audible sound, but the possibility has been raised that intense noise can harm the fetuses of pregnant women exposed in the workplace. This concern was raised by studies of babies born to women living near large airports. A higher rate of low birth weight and such defects as cleft palate or cleft lip was reported. The National Research Council investigated these reports and concluded there was not sufficient evidence to prove that exposure to noise of high intensity is harmful to fetuses. However, it is theoretically possible that loud sounds could be directly noxious to the fetus, or could produce changes in the mother's physiology that lead to damage. So, even though there is no solid proof that such damage occurs, the Council did recommend that pregnant women avoid exposure of long duration to very loud sounds.

Someone else's drummer

Physical reactions to noise can occur, even when the volume itself is not loud enough to produce tissue damage. Unwanted, uncontrollable, and unpredictable noise well below 85 decibels may have physiological effects. Your neighbor's stereo does not have to be loud to prevent you from falling asleep. The fact that you have no control over it and cannot turn it off may be sufficiently upsetting. Noises from passing trucks or trains have that same quality; they intrude on an activity—or rest—and cannot be controlled. When the source of the noise is particularly disliked, then the sound may be even more irritating than it otherwise would be.

A typical response to this sort of intrusive lower-level noise is the complex of physiological responses known as *stress* or *arousal*. These reactions may take the form of a change in heart rate or rhythm, an increase in blood pressure, a temporary rise in the level of blood cholesterol, or excessive secretion of certain hormones. Stress reactions are more common, and usually more severe, when the unpleasant stimulus is combined with a sense that there is no getting away from it and nothing to be done about it.

Whether people who live in noisy environments actually suffer such ill effects is not firmly established. Several European studies have reported that people living near noisy airports have more evidence of cardiovascular and circulatory problems than those living out of earshot. Higher-than-average blood pressures have been reported for children living near the Los Angeles airport. These community studies certainly suggest that noisy environments are a health hazard, but further research with more rigorous methods is needed to confirm or refute the relationship.

Noise may have a less direct, but nonetheless real, effect on health by disturbing sleep. Even people who believe that they have adapted to the sound of passing elevated trains or overhead jets often have disordered sleep patterns. Frequent shifts in the course of the night from deep to lighter sleep may lead to an ongoing sense of fatigue. The associated lapses of attention or concentration could become a safety hazard.

Bad vibes

Whether or not physical health is affected by noise, mental health does seem to be affected. The heads as well as the hearts of people living near noisy airports have been studied, and it has been found that these people are admitted to hospitals for mental health reasons with higher than average frequency. But this kind of correlation has many pitfalls of method and must be interpreted with caution.

Social behavior may be impaired in noisy environments. There's an abundance of anecdotal evidence—such as accounts of fights breaking out because someone is playing a radio too loudly—supporting this notion. One field study has demonstrated that people are less helpful, if not more hostile, in a noisy place. The experimenter dropped a load of books in an area where there were many passersby. People were much less likely to stop and help when a loud lawn mower was running nearby than when the area was quiet. This effect has been confirmed by other research showing that people who ask for help or for directions get less help in a noisy than in a quiet environment.

A good deal of psychological research on the effects of noise has been conducted in the area of learning. Noise begins to take its toll on learning at a fairly early age. Young children acquire language skills more slowly and are less likely to explore their environments when they live in a noisy home. Part of the reason may be that children have less opportunity to interact with adults when the environment is noisy.

Studies of children in day care and at school have indicated that learning is slowed in a noisy environment. Preschoolers attending a day care center near one of New York City's elevated trains scored below normal in certain psychomotor tasks. Also in New York, children living near the two airports or a noisy highway were found to have lower reading scores than average for the city. In schools near the Los Angeles airports, children scored low on measures of problem solving.

One particularly interesting test of the noise hypothesis was conducted in a classroom adjacent to elevated train tracks in New York. The reading ability of sixth-graders in this room was found to be a year behind that of sixth-graders on the quiet side of the building. Pressure was then placed on the transit authority to install rubber pads on the tracks near the school. The Board of Education also installed acoustic ceilings in the rooms facing the tracks. The result was a somewhat quieter learning environment. After these changes were made, the children's reading scores were found to be the same on the two sides of the building. In the light of these results, the city is now planning to use noise-reduction methods in schools under flight paths to the airports—in the hope that reading scores will go up.

Noise and progress

A lot of changes associated with modernization of life lead to noisier environments. Large, spacious offices in which workers are separated only by partial dividers are plagued by the cacophony of typewriters, copying machines, calculators, telephones, and electric pencil sharpeners. Household appliances—dishwashers, hair dryers, vacuum cleaners, and garbage disposals—contribute their share of noise to the environment. Sometimes increased noise is the result of compromise, as when the New York Transit authority ordered shiny, smooth-riding subway cars that were also very loud owing to the type of motor installed. Sometimes the noise is intentional, as when a penetrating beeper is installed on a truck to warn when it is backing up.

Most of these noise problems can be solved with available engineering methods. The solution may sometimes be expensive, of course. On the other hand, living with a noisy environment has its own invisible costs. The employer who invests in sound-damping walls and ceilings, or in quieter equipment, may realize gains in productivity. At least, this possibility is suggested by studies of the adverse effects of noise on problem-solving ability.

Sometimes, noise reduction is not so much a matter of equipment as planning. A school can be noisy (in the sense of having sounds where they aren't wanted) simply as a result of putting classrooms or libraries, which should be quiet, near gymnasiums, where loud sounds are expected and perhaps even desirable. Other typical problems in school buildings include noisy heating or ventilating equipment, vibrating ductwork, poorly sealed doors, and just plain overcrowding.

As a direct hazard to health, noise takes a relatively limited toll. Damage to hearing, which can be permanent, is the outstanding risk of prolonged exposure to loud sound. Less easily measured, but quite possibly significant, are the indirect effects on both emotions and cognitive processes. This is an area where such terms as "health," "comfort," and "ability" become blurry. Although not conclusive, the available studies indicate that there are real losses in learning ability, social interaction, and productivity in noisy environments.

Indoor Air Pollution

People who live in the North try to keep the winter cold out of their homes by spending at least 5 months enclosed in what they hope is a highly insulated, air-tight space. People who live in the South turn on their air conditioners, close all their windows, and try to keep the coolness from escaping. In both cases, the quality of indoor air is treated mainly as a matter of temperature control. But researchers are now learning that some of our efforts to control indoor air temperature and to conserve energy, admirable though they may be, can lead to a very serious threat to health in the form of air pollution. The exact scope of the problem in the U.S. has yet to be determined, but we do know that the average American is indoors 90% of the day. So even low levels of indoor pollution can have adverse effects, simply because we are exposed to it so much of the time.

When, in the effort to save money on heating and cooling costs, buildings are constructed so that they drastically reduce the exchange of air with the outside, the saving in energy may actually lead to added costs in health problems. Sometimes a building meets the required ventilation standards for air flow and exchange, but because of design defects, occupants actually breathe relatively stagnant air. For example, in large work spaces broken up with low partitions, virtually all of the air circulation may be overhead, with little of it reaching inside the cubicles themselves. Substances that vaporize from the building materials, or pollutants that are added by the inhabitants themselves—primarily cigarette smoke—may contaminate the air.

Common sources

Contaminants enter indoor air in a number of ways. In both commercial and residential structures, newer types of building materials (including urea-formaldehyde insulation) or carpets and furnishings may give off formaldehyde gas over a period of months or years. Certain pesticides used to saturate building foundations may be picked up in the heating system and spread through the interior. Asbestos insulation, if it starts to break down, can scatter high levels of hazardous fiber into the indoor environment. Microbes such as bacteria and molds can grow in the water of air-conditioning or humidifying systems, as the emergence of Legionnaires' disease has taught us.

Tobacco smoke

One of the major indoor air pollutants is cigarette smoke. Cigarette smoke inhaled "passively" is made up of the fumes given off by idling cigarettes (sidestream smoke) and the residue exhaled by smokers. Although sidestream smoke is diluted in a large volume of room air, to begin with it contains a higher concentration of ammonia, benzene, carbon monoxide, nicotine, and certain carcinogenic tars than mainstream smoke. So it may be proportionately more hazardous.

Environmental tobacco smoke is a health hazard to both adults and children who are exposed to it.

The children of smoking parents have more respiratory infections than those of nonsmokers, and their lungs do not develop at the normal rate. Although a minority of adults smoke, a majority of children live in homes with at least one cigarette smoker. Thus, the problem of smoke exposure in childhood is a fairly large one.

Nonsmoking adults exposed to the smoke of others over a long period of time have slight but measurable abnormalities of lung function, and they are more likely to develop lung cancer than people with low exposure to tobacco smoke in their environment. The increased risk of lung cancer in passive smokers has not been precisely measured yet, because collecting the necessary data is extremely difficult. But the fact of an increased risk is no longer regarded as doubtful.

Late in 1986, the surgeon general of the United States released conclusions on "The Health Consequences of Involuntary Smoking." In summarizing the evidence, this report not only concluded that the health of nonsmokers suffers as a result of exposure to second-hand smoke, but also: "The simple separation of smokers and nonsmokers within the same air space may reduce, but does not eliminate, the exposure of nonsmokers to environmental tobacco smoke."

In public and commercial buildings, the presence of smokers considerably increases the need for circulation of fresh air. According to careful research conducted at Yale University, permitting cigarette smoking in such buildings increases the fresh air requirements by 5 to 10-fold, in order to satisfy 80% of the occupants that the air is not unpleasant to breathe. In a large building, this requirement translates into millions of dollars a year in heating and cooling costs, which could be sharply reduced if smoking were curtailed or confined to separately ventilated areas. It is not yet clear what standards should be established for air contaminated with cigarette smoke.

An approach that might seem plausible on the surface would be to keep the concentration of smoke particles at the same level that is acceptable for particles in outdoor air, but such a standard would almost certainly be too lenient. The freshly produced particles of cigarette smoke are chemically more reactive than particles that have been floating in the air for a while. In addition, if one lives or works near a smoker, exposure to cigarette smoke is likely to go on for longer each day than exposure to street fumes, for example.

Carbon monoxide

Tobacco smoke adds carbon monoxide to the air, but in many homes it is not the only source of this pollutant. Carbon monoxide is likely to come from kerosene heaters, unvented gas heaters, or poorly designed wood heating systems, and it can build up to dangerous levels, especially in a tight structure. (If doors and windows are tightly sealed, a supplemental wood stove may have to draw its air for combustion through the flue of the regular furnace. In doing so, it may pull carbon monoxide from the furnace into the house.) Although relatively few cases of carbon monoxide poisoning are reported in the U.S., the potential is there. In Korea, the use of unvented burners for room heating leads to some 2,000 carbon monoxide deaths a year.

Nitrogen oxides

The use of natural gas or propane stoves in poorly ventilated kitchens leads to very high levels of nitrogen dioxide and may be associated with respiratory illnesses. Some 40–50% of residential gas burned in this country goes through pilot lights, which are a steady source of nitrogen dioxide. A relatively easy way to reduce exposure is to convert from pilot lights to spark ignition.

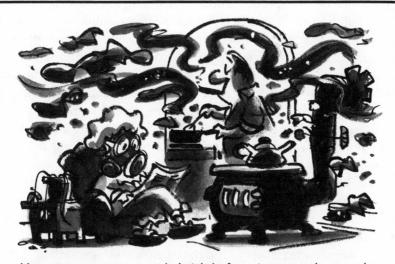

Houses or apartments sealed tightly for winter may have problems with indoor air pollution. Among the pullutants to watch for are cigarette smoke, nitrogen dioxide (from gas stoves and their pilot lights), and carbon monoxide (from kerosene heaters, unvented gas heaters, or furnace exhaust pulled back into the house by a supplemental wood stove).

Unexpected hazards

It's always possible to introduce unusual poisons into the home environment. A poignant example comes from a low-income family that burned wood treated with copper-chrome-arsenate (CCA) as a preservative (so-called pressure-treated wood). For several years this Wisconsin family used plywood remnants from a construction site as the principal fuel for their wood-burning stove. The ash and fumes from the burned plywood permeated their home, and especially the warm area around the stove, where the mother and smallest children spent most of their time in winter. Hair loss, respiratory difficulties, skin rashes, and abnormalities of blood clotting, among other problems, plagued the family as their arsenic levels built up in late winter and spring. Then the problems would improve until cold weather returned.

The "sick-building syndrome"

When the design of buildings deals with thermal comfort at the expense of other aspects of indoor air quality, in extreme cases the "sick-building syndrome" may develop. This condition is diagnosed when an unusual number of people in a building begin to complain of discomfort in their eyes, upper airways, or chest. Although many of the explanations listed above have been proposed for the sick-building syndrome, so far no one can be certain whether any of them is the real reason for the symptoms. For that matter, no one really knows how many buildings are sick. But a report from Great Britain suggests that there may be many more than had been suspected. The investigators gave detailed questionnaires to workers in 9 office buildings. A couple of these buildings were studied because the workers were complaining of symptoms. Other buildings were selected for study without any advance knowledge that there might be a problem.

The British researchers found that people who spend their days in an air-conditioned environment are much more likely to have health complaints than those in buildings with natural ventilation. Discomfort in the nose and eyes, dry skin, headache (usually mild), and lethargy are prominent complaints. Whether or not air is humidified seems to make no difference in these complaints, although people working in buildings with a humidification system often add a sense of tightness in the chest to this list. Headache and lethargy become increasingly prominent as the day wears on.

The reason for the problems encountered is not immediately apparent. Urea-formaldehyde insulation was not present in the buildings studied, so the symptoms cannot be attributed to formaldehyde in the atmosphere. Neither humidification nor recirculation of air seemed to be the critical factors: most symptoms occurred in air-conditioned buildings whether or not these systems were present.

Although the number of buildings studied was small, they were chosen without bias, and the difference in symptoms were strikingly large and consistent. The study results thus suggest that air conditioning may assure a comfortable temperature but at the price of other kinds of discomfort.

Radon in houses

In the past couple of years, a form of indoor air pollution that was previously unsuspected has emerged as a major health concern. It is caused by the radioactive gas radon, which is released by the uranium naturally contained in rock and soil. When it is present, radon seeps through cracks in the basement or floor and enters the air of a house. The gas rapidly decays to certain radioactive solids, and these become attached to dust particles. Like any dust, the radioactive motes can be inhaled; once in the lungs, they will decay further. The radiation released in this process contributes to an increased risk of lung cancer. The radon problem is not a new one; it has probably been around as long as people have lived in heated houses. Nevertheless, for most of us, household radon appears to be our largest source of radiation exposure.

The danger

Estimates of the actual amount of lung cancer resulting from this process vary from 5,000 to 30,000 new cases a year (out of a total of 149,000) in the United States. In as many as a million homes in the United States, according to Anthony Nero, a physicist at the Lawrence Berkeley Laboratory, radon levels are high enough (at 8 picocuries per liter) to warrant efforts at reduction. For an American, the average cancer risk from radon is estimated as being in the range of 0.1–0.9%, which is low compared with the lifetime risk of death from smoking, judged to be about 25%, or driving a car, 1–2%. But it is very high compared with many risks that are regulated by the Environmental Protection Agency. Nero gives, as examples, benzene, vinyl chloride, and certain pesticides, with lifetime risks of 0.001% for the average person and approximately 0.01% for people with high levels of exposure.

These estimates depend on certain assumptions about the potential of low-level radiation to cause cancer. Attempts to confirm them with epidemiologic studies have yielded mixed results. One survey of lung cancer rates in Maine has indicated that the higher rates are to be found in areas with high radon levels. But surveys conducted in Italy and China have not found a clear association.

The actual magnitude of household exposure to radon is not known with any accuracy. The levels of radon in any home are affected by a host of factors, not all of which have been clearly defined. The most important influence, clearly, is the nature of the ground on which a house is built. Certain kinds of rock (notably granite) with a high content of uranium are apt to release radon.

Some areas of high radon exposure are known. They include parts of Maryland and eastern Pennsylvania, as well as communities in Montana, North Dakota, Colorado, and Washington. But because there has not been a systematic survey, other areas with high radon levels have yet to be identified. Even in a given region, though, dwellings may vary considerably in their radon levels, for reasons that really aren't known. A group of Canadian investigators surveyed the row houses in an Ontario development and found that houses with the lowest radon levels were located side by side with others that had the highest levels.

A major challenge, at the moment, is to find houses with high radon levels. Some research programs are now under way. In the meantime, people who want a measurement of radon in their own dwellings can arrange to have one made through a private company or a few nonprofit concerns. The Environmental Protection Agency has published a study of companies and organizations that offer to measure levels of household radon; 75 groups met the agency's standards. Interested readers may request a copy of the results by writing Radon Testing Proficiency Report, Environmental Protection Agency, Press Office, Washington, D.C. 20460.

What to do?

Although modern construction methods, leading to tighter houses, seem to have increased the level of radon in dwellings, even this is not a hard-and-fast rule. Some very tight houses have quite low levels of radon, and other, draftier structures may still have relatively high levels. The reason for this situation is fairly complex, and not fully understood. But basically what happens is that houses seem to suck radon out of the soil into themselves. Two very simple features of a building are responsible for this effect. (1) A house sticks up from the ground, thus causing wind flow to create areas of high and low pressure. (2) It is heated, and the rising column of heat, in effect, creates a suction on the basement.

Most attempts to seal the basement or create more ventilation in a house proves to be either ineffectual or impractical. Caulking doesn't work unless every conceivable crack is caulked. Ventilation may simply make a house unbearably drafty without appreciably lowering the radon levels. Thus, other solutions are often needed. Finding the right one, though, may not be easy. Construction companies that specialize in control of radon levels are appearing. A call to the state agency that specializes in radiation protection is probably the best way to locate one that is nearby, competent, and reasonably priced. But many states have little experience with household radon, and officials may not be able to give firm recommendations.

An approach that has worked well in some houses with finished basements is the following: two or more pipes are driven through the concrete floor into the gravel below (*see illustration*). These vertical pipes are then connected to another, which leads to an exhaust fan. This system is tightly sealed at all joints. What it does is create a slight suction underneath the basement floor. The pipes draw radon-loaded air to the fan, but more importantly, the lowered pressure under the basement floor offsets the house's tendency to draw air from the basement into the rooms above.

Unfinished basements and crawlspaces can often simply be vented with one or more small fans. The fans create a low-pressure area near the soil surface and draw radon-contaminated air away from the house. More elaborate and more expensive solutions may be required in special situations.

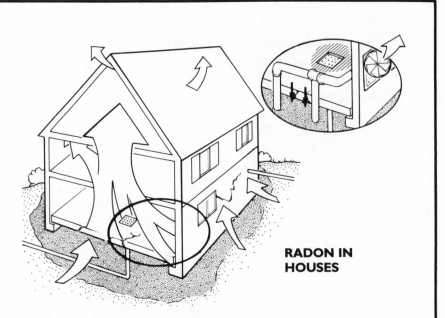

RADON IN HOUSES

Radon seeps into this basement through cracks in the floor and walls, as well as around pipes that enter and leave the basement. The radioactive gas is drawn upward by lower pressure near the roof. Diagrammed in the circle is a relatively simple system for lowering pressure beneath the basement floor and drawing exhaust air to the outside. Pipes sunk through the floor are connected to a horizontal pipe that in turn is vented to an exhaust fan.

Although the radon problem appears to be a significant one in some areas, there is no cause for general panic. Most of us will not much affect our life expectancy by taking steps to lower the radon levels in our dwellings. A rational, and nation-wide, program of detection and control, however, could eventually have a salutary effect. In many ways, this new discovery of an old health hazard is an optimistic one, as it provides an opportunity to reduce a cancer risk that otherwise would have been regarded as just part of the inevitable "background."

Asbestos

Asbestos is a kind of soft rock made of compressed fibers. Since ancient times, people have recognized that asbestos has the useful property of not burning. In fact, lamp wicks, theater curtains, fabrics, and many other things have been made of asbestos because it is both fire-resistant and one of the best insulators known. It protects what it covers from heat, corrosion, or electrical damage. Asbestos is also strong and durable. The mineral fibers can be spun, woven, made into felt, or bonded with other materials to form durable products for construction, heating insulation, fire protection, and more.

Over 3,000 uses have been made of asbestos. Buildings have been insulated with it. Huge amounts have been used to insulate boilers and pipes in ships. Automobile brake linings and clutch plates have been made of asbestos since the early 1900s. Asbestos has been incorporated into cement to strengthen it for use in concrete pipes and other formed objects. Asbestos filters are used in the manufacture of some imported wines. For many years, hair dryers were insulated with the material. Until recently, asbestos was commonly incorporated into the spackling and taping compounds used for dry wall construction. From 1946 to 1973, asbestos was added to coatings that could be sprayed onto walls or other structures to avoid the need for plastering them.

In all, some 30 million tons of asbestos have been used in the United States since the beginning of this century. By the end of the twentieth century, however, despite the many valuable properties of the material, an estimated half a million people will have died as a result of their exposure to asbestos.

The problem

Asbestos produces disease mainly when it is inhaled. Minuscule fibers of the material (some too small to be seen with a standard microscope) are drawn into the lungs. There the fibers are taken up by cells responsible for cleaning the air passages. These cells ordinarily do a good job of cleaning the lungs. But the cells cannot easily break down the fibers of asbestos to remove them from the lungs. Instead, the asbestos fibers remain in place or slowly migrate toward the outer parts of the lungs. Some tiny particles may even travel across the diaphragm into the abdominal cavity (peritoneum).

The desirable properties of asbestos as an insulating material are also the ones that make it dangerous. It appears that asbestos creates problems solely because of its physical properties, not because of its chemical nature. The tiny size of asbestos particles is important. If they were larger, the inhaled fragments would settle out in the large airways, which are better equipped to remove foreign substances than the very small ones. The shape of the asbestos particles also matters. The needle-like dimensions typical of the asbestos crystal appear to increase its ability to cause disease.

Thirty years or so after asbestos dust is inhaled, but sometimes much sooner (depending on dose), it begins to cause several types of detectable disease:

ASBESTOSIS   This potentially fatal condition hardly ever occurs except in people who have worked with asbestos or with products containing it. It is the most common disease produced by exposure to the material, though not the most common cause of death, which is lung cancer. Asbestosis is a kind of scarring process that takes place within the lung or on its outer surface. As a result of this scarring, the air spaces within the lungs become smaller or obstructed, and the lung itself becomes more rigid. Breathing is difficult, oxygen and carbon dioxide are poorly exchanged, and lung infections are easily acquired. There is no effective treatment to prevent or reverse the scarring. Asbestosis or its complications can progress, even without further exposure to asbestos.

LUNG CANCER   Lung cancer is extremely common among people who have worked with asbestos, many of whom smoke. For some unknown reason, the combination of cigarette smoke and asbestos is much worse than would be predicted by adding together the risks from each. Anyone who has been exposed to even small quantities of asbestos dust should do everything he or she can to avoid cigarette smoke. The outlook for those who stop smoking is much better than for those who continue. As is the case with all forms of lung cancer, by the time symptoms occur, it is usually too late for curative treatment, and no good tests for earlier detection are available.

MESOTHELIOMA   Mesothelioma, another type of cancer, occurs almost entirely in people exposed to asbestos dust. These tumors arise from the membrane that lines the chest or abdominal cavity, and they are highly malignant. Although they are rare, mesotheliomas can occur even after a limited exposure to asbestos dust and may affect people who were not directly involved in handling the material, such as relatives of asbestos workers. A very long time—40 years or more—can elapse between exposure and the appearance of mesothelioma, although many cases appear earlier.

Some other types of cancer, occurring outside the lungs, also appear to be somewhat more common in people exposed to asbestos dust.

What to do?

The asbestos situation raises two questions: What can individuals do to protect themselves and their families? What should we do as a nation to prevent further injury from exposure to asbestos?

The answer to the first question is reasonably straightforward for people who do not work with the material. Asbestos is only dangerous when it produces dust. Left undisturbed or bonded into durable slates, tiles, or other materials, it presents virtually no risk. But asbestos-containing insulation around pipes or boilers and in walls, wall coverings, or spackling compounds that are sawed, cut, sanded, or exposed to damage from routine use may give off considerable quantities of asbestos dust.

People who work with such materials should be adequately trained and fully protected from inhaling the dust. Face masks and respirators are not as effective as ventilation control or improved handling methods, such as "wet processing."

Deteriorating asbestos materials should be removed, covered with an effective sealant, or enclosed under another covering. Expert advice is needed both to determine whether there is an asbestos problem in a given area and to choose the proper method for dealing with the hazard.

Spray-on wall coverings that contain asbestos present a special problem. This inexpensive technique was rarely used in homes but quite frequently in school construction. Water damage, heavy use, and occasionally vandalism have caused the coatings to start disintegrating in some schools, and several states have initiated programs to detect and correct the problem. Unfortunately, such efforts are expensive and, all too often, underfunded.

People who work with asbestos and its products, including those who repair existing objects that contain the material or are covered with it—such as plumbers, shipyard workers, brake and clutch workers, construction workers—are entitled to protection from asbestos and the diseases it causes. They should be fully aware of the amount of asbestos dust that they breathe while they earn a living.

Unfortunately, employers in both private industries and the government have often been negligent, failing to inform employees about asbestos exposure or to protect them from it. Workers at risk of exposure should insist that the air they breathe be sampled frequently and analyzed by an appropriate method. Employees and workers should cooperate in bringing fiber counts in the air well below the current legal standard (2 million fibers per cubic meter), which is probably at least 20 times too high.

The second question—what national action should be taken—is much more difficult to answer. There is no doubt that asbestos represents a major public health problem, one that extends beyond the large group of people who suffer from occupational exposure. Every possible way should be found to remove it from the human environment. But eliminating the substance from existing structures or from industrial applications may not be feasible for technical, economic, or political reasons. Meanwhile, there is controversy about the amount of asbestos exposure that is compatible with good health. Enforcing existing regulations, let alone more stringent ones, is difficult.

To date there has been no coherent, effective government program for dealing with the asbestos problem. Responsibility has fallen partly on the states and partly on several federal agencies. At a minimum, the federal government should be expected to take the initiative in developing a unified program to conduct research on asbestos diseases, measures to control exposures, and substitute materials. Technical advice and support should be offered to local control programs, and a policy should be developed for the future. Asbestos diseases become a medical problem only when it is too late to make them go away. Preventing these diseases is a political challenge, not a medical one.

Hazards of the Workplace

Home takes its place in the statistical records as a dangerous place mainly because we all spend so much time at home. There are just more opportunities for something to go wrong, and even relatively low levels of exposure to hazardous materials, like asbestos, can accumulate to present a relatively grave risk over the years.

Hazards of the workplace are somewhat different in character. Unlike homes, many work sites are supposedly regulated. But regulations can give a false sense of security. Enforcement may be weak or uninformed. Technological advance sometimes creates hazards more rapidly than they can be recognized and dealt with. The pressure to produce can lead people to take risky shortcuts.

Coal miners in the last century often took a canary into the shaft with them, because the bird, being more sensitive to poisonous gases, would give an early warning of a dangerous accumulation. Unfortunately, people must often serve as their own canaries—with all the tragic potential that such a situation implies.

Problems in the workplace sometimes arise because large quantities of dangerous substances must be handled: asbestos, solvents, and radioactivity are among the best-known examples. But health problems may also develop from the way work itself is organized. This aspect of workers' health is only now coming to be fully appreciated. Two examples covered in this chapter are the effect of shift changes on the biological clock and the influence of working with computer terminals—in themselves very safe devices—on vision, posture, and attitudes. Although the specifics of dealing with shift work or video display terminals don't apply to many work situations, the principles are broadly applicable. When work patterns are thoughtlessly designed, the consequences sometimes are quite serious.

Chemical exposures

Even tiny amounts of some chemicals can be extremely hazardous to health. The people most at risk of injury from these materials are, as a rule, the ones who handle them as a part of their work—people ranging from industrial workers to professional artists.

Toxic substances can enter the body by any of three routes—the mouth, the lungs, and the skin.

MOUTH Chemicals are often swallowed inadvertently when they contaminate hands, food, eating utensils, or cigarettes. Thus, a "safe zone" for eating should be designated and kept scrupulously clean; food should be kept out of the workspace. Pencils, paint brushes, and similar items should not be clenched between the teeth.

LUNGS Inhaling noxious dusts is a hazard for anyone who works with wood, stone, plastic, metal, or fibers. Direct damage to the lungs may be abrupt, and signaled by coughing, wheezing, or shortness of breath. It can also be a gradual process, leading to scarring and permanent damage, as is the case with exposure to silica or asbestos. Cigarette smoking is particularly dangerous for persons exposed to these last two substances; the risk of lung cancer due to asbestos exposure increases 10-fold for cigarette smokers. But all toxic chemicals that can be inhaled are considerably more dangerous to the smoker than to the nonsmoker.

Certain vapors are mildly intoxicating; combined with alcohol— say a beer or two at the end of the work day—they can produce severe symptoms, all out of proportion to the amount drunk. Some solvents act much like anesthetic gases, producing dizziness, fatigue, drowsiness, and even coma. Other solvents can seriously damage the bone marrow (benzene) or liver (carbon tetrachloride).

SKIN Although it is designed to defend us against poisons in our environment, the skin is actually the most common portal of entry for toxic substances. This is because various chemicals—including acids, strong alkalis, solvents, and bleaches—destroy the complex arrangement of fats and fibrous proteins in the skin that make it a barrier. Once a foreign substance penetrates the outer layer of skin, any of a variety of rashes can result. Potentially more serious is the possibility that skin-absorbed chemicals will be transported by the blood to internal organs. Over the years, a series of subtle chemical injuries could add up to serious complications, ranging from liver disease and cancer to reduced fertility, birth defects, and loss of bladder control.

When to suspect trouble

It is difficult to enumerate particular types of chemicals that are the dangerous ones while declaring others are safe. Instead of carrying a mental list of dangerous substances, workers and employers should pay attention to *situations* that signal a hazard.

Any change in standard routine can lead to unanticipated injury. For example, substituting one solvent for another in a washing process can create hazards that were not present before. Or a new catalyst in plastic manufacture may have health effects very different from the old one. Whenever a process is changed, both management and workers should ask, "What is this material? What are the risks?"

It can sometimes be quite difficult to answer those questions. Labels may be incomplete, because the precise contents of a package are a trade secret, because some ingredients are not listed, or because trade names obscure the true nature of a chemical. Fortunately, a "Material Safety Data Sheet" frequently is prepared by the manufacturer of a chemical. This information sheet may be less than perfect, but it contains a summary of what is known about the contents of the product. If the sheet is not distributed with the chemical product, it can be requested. In fact, for all potentially dangerous situations, the sheet should be requested because it indicates both the kinds of exposure to be avoided and what to look for as a sign of ill effects.

Many products are packaged with terse warnings: "Use only in a well-ventilated area" or "Avoid skin contact." Of course the warnings are frequently violated and often, after a single exposure, nothing happens. People are then inclined to think the warnings are meaningless. But the fact that a warning is present means that the product has been a hazard to someone at some time, and the label should serve as a red flag, a stimulus to go find out the whole story—especially if the substance is used repeatedly, in large amounts, or in a situation that allows it to be spread around.

Risks are often highest in relatively small operations, where safety precautions may seem too expensive. Risks are also high when the burden is placed on each individual worker to protect himself or herself—as by wearing respirators or protective clothing.

One of the most hazardous of all situations is when a person works alone, in a confined space, using a potentially toxic chemical. Nobody should enter such a setting without a "buddy" observer watching constantly, or a so-called "dead-man alarm" requiring repeated attention to keep it silent.

Hazardous art materials

One group of professionals who routinely work alone and who may be unaware of the many dangers in their workspace are artists. Most of the information about the dangers of particular art materials comes from research on their toxicity to industrial workers. Although artists usually work with lower concentrations, they may actually be exposed to greater amounts because their studios may have poor ventilation and lack safety precautions that are mandated for worker protection in industry. Moreover, many artists work at home, or live in the lofts they use as studios. This can mean round-the-clock exposure for them, as well as their mates and children.

The perils to an artist obviously depend on the particular medium he or she works in. Here is a quick survey of some of the major hazards posed by different media.

PAINTING At one time, many pigments were toxic. For example, there was arsenic in emerald green and cobalt violet, antimony and lead in Naples yellow, manganese in burnt and raw umber, and mercury in vermilion red. Lead is still present in certain pigments such as flake white, but for the most part many safe substitutes have been developed and are used by reputable manufacturers.

A major program to formulate standards and provide accurate product-labeling information, launched in 1983, should be increasingly evident in the years ahead. It was organized by manufacturers, concerned artists, and independent experts through the American Society of Testing and Materials. Participating companies must submit detailed information on product ingredients for evaluation by a board of toxicologists. This information is the basis for preparation of a certified label, which contains appropriate cautionary statements. The Art and Craft Materials Institute (715 Boylston St., Boston, MA 02116) will serve as the certifying organization for many smaller manufacturers.

CERAMICS Ceramic workers are at risk of lung damage from inhaling silica contained in dry clay dust and in certain colors and glazes. Glazes may also contain lead and asbestos, and colorants sometimes contain toxic metals such as antimony, chromium, manganese, or cadmium. A major danger is that of inhaling highly toxic fumes during the firing of pottery. Thus, adequate ventilation around the kiln is a health "must" for the potter.

SCULPTING/CONSTRUCTION Depending on what is used to make a sculpture, inhalation of stone dust, wood dust, or metal fumes may be a hazard. Welders may face electrical and heat dangers, eye damage, and exposure to a variety of noxious fumes.

Plastic workers take on a greater risk when they are working with materials used to make plastics (monomers, solvents) than when they are finishing presynthesized plastics.

PRINTMAKING The main problem here is solvent exposure, with benzene being the worst offender. Certain pigments and carbon black can be toxic. Etching requires the use of concentrated acids which can cause eye damage when splashed and lung damage when inhaled.

TEXTILES Spinners, weavers, and knitters are sometimes exposed to fiber dusts which can cause allergies or direct lung irritation. Dyers come in contact with many chemicals that can also serve as irritants. The dyes derived from benzidine predispose to bladder cancer.

Seeking safety

The best protection comes from using nontoxic materials in the first place. But when that is not possible, other steps should be followed to ensure worker safety:

- Provide for adequate ventilation when designing any workspace that will house noxious vapors or dusts. "Ventilation" does not mean fans. Fans just blow dusts and fumes around. Ventilation means using the equivalent of a filtered vacuum cleaner right at the source of the toxic materials.
- Be especially careful with storage and handling of flammable solvents.
- Carefully label toxic materials, store them in nonbreakable containers, and discard according to set precautions.
- Wash carefully with soap and water before taking a break.
- Do not eat or smoke when in contact with toxic materials.
- Vacuum or wet-mop dusts rather than sweep them up.
- Invest in specific protective equipment: air respirators for workers exposed to fumes, gloves for solvent-handlers, goggles for welders, and so forth.

It makes sense for workers to compare health notes, especially when a procedure is changed. "Coincidental" illnesses can be the first warning of trouble. Of course, there is always a possibility of overreacting, but the general tendency seems to be to wait too long before blowing the whistle. Workers should volunteer information about their work to examining doctors, who often forget to ask about occupational exposure.

Information can be obtained from Material Safety Data Sheets, the reference book *Clinical Toxicology of Commercial Products* (published by Williams and Wilkins, Baltimore, MD), local Poison Control Centers (sometimes), or the National Institute of Occupational Safety and Health (NIOSH) in Rockville, Maryland. A company, a union, or any three employees may submit a formal request to NIOSH's Health Hazard Evaluation Program for a study of a particular hazard. Federal regulations are enforced through the Occupational Safety and Health Administration or through state agencies devoted to occupational health.

Shift work

Approximately 15% of the female and 25% of the male work force in the United States must periodically adjust to work on the night shift. Such adjustments are not easy, for physiological as well as psychological reasons, and the result is fatigue, inefficiency, and, all too often, serious accidents.

At least three-quarters of the people who go through a major time shift experience serious disruptions of their sleep. They suffer insomnia, or they fall asleep when they should be awake. Thus, fatigue is a common result. Peptic ulcers or other gastrointestinal disturbances are well-known reactions to time-shifting. Digestive juices are secreted at the usual meal times; so after a time shift they continue to put in an appearance even when food is not present in the stomach. Without food to neutralize them, the digestive juices may act against the intestine itself. Many people rely on drugs, such as the caffeine in coffee or the amphetamines in pep pills, to get them through their new "day," but these drugs also have adverse effects of their own.

Work performance (or enjoyment of time off) is impaired by all of these factors—fatigue, digestive discomfort, drug effects. In addition, for most people the body is geared for peak performance during the day and is least efficient in the wee hours of the morning, say from 3 to 5 o'clock. If the work day is shifted to include these early morning hours, the unadjusted individual will be trying to perform well at his or her worst physiological time.

The major defect in performance at this hour affects "vigilance" or "alertness"—the ability to notice what is going on in one's surroundings. Attention drifts. "Silly" errors tend to occur, sometimes with grave consequences. The worker misses things he or she would normally respond to. Accident statistics reflect this fact. For example, truck drivers are most likely to have single-vehicle accidents (such as running into a bridge siding) at 5 o'clock in the morning. An isolated, but suggestive, example comes from Three Mile Island, where the famous accident occurred at 4 in the morning with a crew that had just started working the night shift.

As yet, there is not much good evidence regarding the effect on humans of prolonged, frequent time shifting. Animals exposed to weekly time shifts in long-term experiments die considerably earlier than others kept on a constant schedule. Recent studies suggest shift workers are more likely to have heart attacks than day workers. But until a major epidemiological study is done, we will not know the extent of the problem.

The cause

People find the adjustment to shift changes difficult because virtually every function in the body is timed according to a day–night cycle. This rhythm regulates not only the obvious things (such as activity, sleep, and eating) but also internal states (including body temperature, kidney function, and blood hormone levels). Although one might expect that these daily cycles would be governed solely by external cues—for example, by sunrise and sunset—they are, in fact, maintained by internal "clocks" that keep on working even when a person is removed from all external cues to time of day.

We come equipped with internal clocks to prepare us for events of the day. Thus, dawn doesn't take us by surprise; as a general rule, our bodies are ready to begin a new day before we awaken. Most people are set for peak performance in the early to middle part of the day, but at the extremes are "larks" (at their best near dawn) and "owls" (who come into their own after dark).

Most inner clocks (or pacemakers) are highly regular. If left to their own devices, they keep very good time. But the typical human pacemaker runs on about a 25-hour cycle; thus, it must be reset every day by time cues (external stimuli, such as light or mealtimes). As long as the time cues are not much out of phase with the pacemaker, the clock is easily reset and bodily rhythms are kept regular. But if the time cues are rapidly shifted by more than an hour or so, the pacemaker doesn't catch up immediately. Instead, it resets itself by about an hour each day until it is again synchronized with the external time cues. Jet travel is a well-known way to put body time out of joint with clock time. Less talked about, but a more common problem, is going to work on a night shift. For the night worker, important time cues may be altered by 8 hours—the equivalent of flying from Denver to Rome. Ordinarily, a whole week is needed to adjust to a change this big.

Compounding the difficulty of readjusting to such time changes is the fact that people do not have only one internal clock. There are at least two major pacemakers and other less important ones. Moreover, these internal clocks do not all respond to an external time change in the same way; one of them may reset by gradually advancing while the other responds by slowing down. Thus, during a period of readjustment, not only are we out of phase with the outside world, but some of our internal functions may be out of phase with others.

Minimizing the problem

Modern society depends on the willingness of certain people to work night shifts. In heavy industry and in hospitals, night workers are indispensable. In yet other situations, night operation is an economic advantage, if not a necessity. But any enterprise or institution should think seriously before starting round-the-clock operations, for there can be real drawbacks to both productivity and health.

In any case, it is probably best to assign workers according to their natural bent. Some people adapt rather easily to time shifts; others find it exceedingly difficult. The worst problems that have been observed with shift work occurred during World War II, when, because of the national emergency, large numbers of people had to work nights whether they liked it or not. Nowadays, although many people work at night, those who react most poorly probably seek other employment, and so the overall problem may not be as severe as it was during the war.

People who do not easily adjust to time shifts will suffer more and may present greater risk to the operation than those who quickly slip into the new routine. It is a common feature of labor contracts that workers are rotated through the night shift on a regular basis—often as frequently as once a week. This may not be a good idea; shifting so often may be more harmful than working at night for long periods. However, workers who stay on a night shift may go through a weekly time-shift anyway if they attempt to return to a "normal life" on Saturday and Sunday.

Schedules can be designed to minimize difficulty with time shifts, and workers can be taught how to adjust more comfortably (though any one solution is not ideal for everybody). Anyone who must go through a time shift can help to minimize his or her difficulty with a little planning. If the shift lasts less than a couple of days (for example, on a quick business trip), it is best to stick to one's old pattern—to pretend the shift hasn't occurred. Meetings should be scheduled for waking hours by the old time, and likewise meals and sleep—even if the result is bizarre by local time. If one has to stay longer, the best strategy is to switch to the new time as fast as possible: rise and eat meals according to the local time, get outside in the daylight hours, and so forth. The most important time cues influencing the internal pacemakers are mealtimes and light–dark cycles. Social cues may also play a role. Even so, the internal clock cannot be instantaneously reset to its new environment, and depending on the size of the discrepancy, the time-shifted individual should expect to spend a few days below par.

Video display terminals

Work will never be the same again for millions of people. Jobs that once called for filing, scribbling, telephoning, talking, typing, or flipping through books and ledgers now require workers to punch the keys of a computer terminal, read the words displayed on the screen and punch the keys some more. Video display terminals (VDTs) make many tasks easier; but do they make work itself easier, more pleasant, or healthier? There is some question.

Four types of health problems have been attributed to VDTs: alleged radiation hazard, visual disturbances, musculoskeletal difficulties, and job stress. This last category, though it sounds vague, may have the most significant long-term effects on both the emotional and the physical health of VDT users.

Radiation exposure

Alarm about the potential hazard from VDTs was triggered when two editors for the *New York Times* seemed to develop cataracts within a year after the newspaper shifted them to working with terminals. Subsequent cases of cataract in other settings were also ascribed to working with VDTs. In addition, women working with VDTs while they were pregnant reported miscarriages or abnormal offspring.

Both the cataracts and the reproductive problems have, understandably, been attributed to radiation leaking from the terminals. However, repeated measurements of radiation from VDTs have shown that leakage is well below present standards for occupational exposure. And certain types of radiation, such as x-rays or radio frequencies, have not even been detectable. In the meantime, new cases of cataract have not been reported at the rate one would expect if VDTs were causing them.

The question of reproductive difficulties is still unsettled. The Ministry of Labor in Canada has recommended that pregnant women be allowed to shift from operating VDTs to other kinds of work for the duration of pregnancy, but its task force has not cited any evidence, other than existing anecdotes, in support of their recommendation. In the United States, NIOSH has undertaken a large study of pregnant women who work with VDTs. It is well to remember that the overall rate of miscarriages (about 15% of all pregnancies) and birth defects (almost 2% of births) is sufficiently high that the clustering of reported problems is quite likely to be the result of a statistical accident, not VDT exposure.

In sum, on the basis of existing evidence, there appears to be *no radiation hazard* from VDTs.

Visual difficulties

People working with VDTs report discomfort or difficulty with their eyes more often than other workers with visually demanding jobs. More than half of VDT operators have eye complaints. Their eyes feel irritated (the eye appears red, is teary, or feels gritty) or fatigued (eyes are tired or ache, there may be headache, and the eyelids feel heavy), or they have difficulty with focus or accommodation (blurriness, difficulty seeing near or far objects). Fatigue is the most common complaint, and the one most likely to persist from the end of one day to the beginning of the next. Difficulty with focus usually ends within half an hour of resting the eyes.

In themselves, most VDT screens seem to meet basic requirements for visual work, although poor maintenance can allow defects to develop. Here are some current minimal criteria for the visual display:

- The image should not flicker.
- The entire display should be in sharp focus (no blurred edges).
- The contrast between light and dark areas should be at least 8 : 1.
- The characters should be formed in a 5 × 7 matrix of dots at the very least.
- All VDTs should have brightness and contrast controls that the operator can find and adjust.
- Dark characters on a lighter background may be somewhat easier to read than a negative image.

When VDTs create visual difficulties for operators, it is usually because they are located in improperly designed work areas. Too often, they are simply plunked down in an office that has been illuminated for work with "hard copy" (what we used to call "paper"). In this setting, light levels are usually too high for VDT work, so the operator must strain to see the relatively dim screen in a bright environment. Also, sunlight or poorly placed lighting produces glare on the screen, which makes the eye muscles work overtime to compensate for the distracting area of brightness.

Thoughtful design of lighting is crucial for the VDT operator to work comfortably and productively. If the operator must look mostly at the screen, room lighting should be quite low. On the other hand, if the operator is mostly reading from a paper and entering material into the computer, room illumination probably needs to be relatively bright. Someone whose eyes must travel back and forth between screen and paper may need low general illumination with a somewhat brighter light directed onto the paper.

Glare on the screen is often more of a problem for operators than inappropriate brightness of room lights. Simply blocking windows and dimming the lights is not a good solution; the resulting atmosphere can be too reminiscent of a mortuary or dungeon—not good for either morale or productivity. Filters placed over the screen can eliminate glare, but they also diminish both contrast and brightness of display. Hoods fitted over the terminal can be used to block sources of glare, but they make it hard for the operator to look back and forth from screen to documents. If a VDT cannot be located in a glare-free position, it may be necessary to redesign the lighting of a room.

Musculoskeletal difficulties

Because VDTs eliminate the need to move around (for files, a new piece of paper, an eraser), they also eliminate the opportunity to squirm, wiggle, and adjust that goes with such activities. Unfortunately, sitting stock still is bad for people. A long period of sitting puts a strain on the back and neck, slows circulation in the legs, and generally reduces muscle tone. To compensate for the exceedingly static nature of VDT work, frequent breaks are advisable, and they should include more movement than that required to transport a coffee cup from desk to lip.

Computer keyboards have an exceedingly fast action; it is impossible to "out-type" them. Repeated rapid striking of the fingers on a surface, if it goes on for hours, may lead to inflammation of structures in the hand and wrist. In some cases, a worker may experience carpal tunnel syndrome—pain, weakness, and tingling, usually involving the thumb and first two fingers.

Shoulder, neck, and back complaints are common in VDT operators. Sheer immobility, which weakens the postural muscles, probably contributes to these symptoms, but bad design of the work station is also a major factor.

VDTs should be equipped with a keyboard that can be detached from the screen. The keyboard needs to be relatively low, so that the arms and hands can be held at a comfortable angle. The screen should be high enough to be easily seen without excessive flexing of the neck (that is, the viewing angle should be less than 25 degrees). A screen and keyboard can be jury-rigged into the correct arrangement with the aid of a saw, a pile of old books, or other standbys. But in the long run, a better approach may be to purchase adjustable furniture for the work station.

An expensive chair is too often regarded as the mark of job status, rather than as an essential work tool. VDT operators, like other keyboard operators, should be equipped with chairs that are comfortably padded, fully adjustable, and designed to provide firm support to the lower back. The work station should be designed to fit the operator's job. Ideally, the operator should participate in planning it.

Job stress

Most VDT workers find that their jobs have enjoyable features, but over 75% of them also have physical or stress-related complaints attributable to the use of the terminal. The frequency of complaints about VDT use is higher than in any other work situation. VDTs themselves do not seem to be responsible. Rather, stress-related complaints are based on lack of planning.

Among the more common planning problems are the following:

- VDTs are often introduced to their users without adequate training. When employees are using the equipment inefficiently, they become frustrated.
- Too often, workload requirements tend to be set more by the capacity of the machine than that of its human operators. (This is not a new problem, as viewers of Charlie Chaplin's movie *Modern Times* may recall.) The fact that a computer can now process millions of bits of information in a minute does not mean that human capabilities have increased proportionately.
- The computer may be used to give a supervisor "too much" information about an operator's output. Constant monitoring and inflexible requirements for productivity can be exceedingly demoralizing. Everybody's ability to work varies in the course of the day and week.
- When a computer is introduced, many jobs are reduced in scope and become more monotonous. The VDT operator may be more isolated from colleagues. When the quality of a job is degraded in this fashion, both the worker and the employer suffer.

The VDT is not just another piece of office equipment; it changes the nature of the work people do. Most potential health problems caused by VDTs can probably be averted by planning that takes account of the operator's needs. Lighting and furniture at the worksite may need to be rearranged or redesigned to prevent eyestrain and postural stresses. Operators need to have frequent breaks, to be able to move about, to work at a variable pace, and to meet requirements set by human capacity, not a computer's. There are many ways to avoid becoming a "terminal case."

Radiation Exposures

Radiation is *the* metaphor for the dangers of modern life. And the prospect of nuclear annihilation makes that in some ways very appropriate. The relatively limited breakdown at Three Mile Island and the much more serious explosion at Chernobyl have also raised consciousness about radiation hazards. These are not, however, everyday occurrences and they are little subject to the control of individuals. Personal worry about radiation exposure in everyday life is sometimes realistic (as with the risk of household radon exposure in some areas of the country). Sometimes it is not. Here we take a look at several situations involving low-level exposure to radiation.

The first is use of microwaves, which are becoming a standard feature of the well-equipped kitchen. The second is medical use of x-rays, to which most of us will be exposed at one time or another in our lives. And the third is another form of medical exposure—the use of radioactive substances in health care and research, and the problems that have arisen from our country's failure to make decisions about disposing of the waste that results from this use of radiation.

Microwaves

Today microwaves cook our food, provide warnings against fire and burglars, and track ships, airplanes, and speeding cars. Teamed with relay towers or satellites, they send telephone conversations and TV and radio programs around the globe. Industry uses microwaves to dry and cure plywood, paints, inks, and synthetic rubber, to raise bread and doughnuts, control insects in stored grain, and to shuck oysters and clams. In medicine, microwaves provide deep-heat therapy for the relief of aching joints and sore muscles, and they have been used to reheat blood rapidly after certain types of surgery. Despite extensive use in all facets of life, however, research to date has been inconclusive about what—if any—health hazard is posed to humans exposed to small amounts of this radiation.

Animal experiments have suggested that exposure to *large* doses of microwave radiation may lead to cataracts, impairment of the central nervous system, and changes in the chromosomes, blood, and immune system—depending on duration of exposure, microwave strength, and wavelength. But it is difficult to draw conclusions about human exposure from experiments using animals because microwaves are absorbed differently by different types of tissue. Limited studies of humans have failed to settle the question. The debate continues over what effects large or small doses of microwave radiation can have on humans over long periods of time.

What are microwaves?

Microwave radiation is a form of nonionizing radiation and therefore should not be confused with atomic radiation. Atomic energy is so powerful that it can split molecules in the body into electrically charged particles (a process called ionization). If the molecules of DNA, which control the production of all substances the body produces, are ionized, changes will occur in the way the body functions, and serious disease can be the final result.

Microwaves are not as energetic as ionizing radiation. Microwave radiation increases the rate at which molecules vibrate but does not shake them so forcefully that they split apart. This vibration generates heat. In consumer products, such as microwave ovens, the ability of microwave radiation to generate heat is its most attractive property.

Microwaves have three characteristics that make them useful for cooking: they are reflected by metals; they pass through glass, paper, plastic, and similar material; and they are absorbed by foods. Microwaves are produced inside an oven by an electron tube called a magnetron. The beams bounce back and forth within the metal interior, which reflects them until they are absorbed by food. Microwaves agitate the water molecules in the food, and the resulting molecular friction produces the heat that cooks the food.

Microwave radiation can heat body tissue the same way it heats a steak. Exposure to levels of microwaves not ordinarily encountered in daily living can cause a painful burn. The lens of the eye is particularly sensitive to intense heat. Experiments with animals have shown that exposure to high levels of microwave radiation over a long period of time causes cataracts and can disrupt sperm production. But there is no proof that existing levels of microwave radiation encountered in the environment pose a health risk to people.

Behavioral changes?

Russian and Eastern European studies have reported behavioral effects of low-level microwave exposure on people working near a radiation source. These have included changes in electroencephalogram (EEG) patterns; perceptual changes, such as hallucinations; changes in the ability to hear and smell; headache, fatigue, general irritability, depression, hypochondria, antisocial tendencies, and a host of other undesirable symptoms. Western scientists have been critical of many of these studies because they fail to include specific information about the amount, power, and frequency of the radiation, and the physiological and psychological state of the human subjects.

Western studies have shown that some animals try to get away from microwaves. Other effects noted in experimental animals exposed to low levels of radiation include a decreased ability to perform certain tasks, chromosomal changes in cells, and an immune response as if the body were preparing to protect itself from a disease. The significance of these reactions for humans remains unclear.

It was discovered a few years ago that the Russians had been using microwaves to monitor activity at the U.S. embassy in Moscow between 1953 and 1976, and that personnel at the embassy had been exposed to low-level radiation for many years. Yet studies of those personnel performed by Johns Hopkins University showed no noticeable differences in death or disease rates between them and U.S. embassy employees in another country.

A study of 20,000 enlisted Naval personnel who worked at radar installations during the Korean War also showed no adverse effects as measured by mortality, hospitalization records while in the military or at the Veterans Administration later, or as reflected in VA disability compensation records.

Safety regulations and microwave products

Since October 1971, all microwave ovens in the U.S. have been covered by a safety standard that defines the limits of how much microwave radiation can leak from an oven throughout its lifetime. A new oven must not leak more than 1 milliwatt of microwave radiation per square centimeter at approximately 2 inches from the oven surface, and testing must prove that over the lifetime of the oven the leakage will not become higher than 5 milliwatts per square centimeter. The standard requires that ovens also have two independent interlock systems that stop the production of microwaves the movement the door latch is released. A monitoring system must be included that will stop the oven's operation in case one or both of the interlock systems fail.

The federal government has also set advisory standards for exposure to microwave radiation in the workplace. This guideline, set by the Occupational Safety and Health Administration, is higher (10 milliwatts per square centimeter) than the mandatory standards for microwave ovens.

There are no mandatory regulations in the U.S. limiting exposure of the general public to microwaves from such sources as radar installations and radio and television transmission stations.

Scientists agree that much more research is needed to determine the effects of microwave radiation on humans. While the verdict is not in, people who come in frequent contact with microwaves on their jobs should be aware of the possible effects of radiation and should inform their doctors of their occupational exposure.

Medical x-rays

Much more is known about the harmful effects of x-rays on human tissues. But x-rays can also be life-saving, either as a means of making a medical diagnosis or, at high doses, as therapy for cancer. There are, however, cases in which the value of an x-ray may seem less than obvious. In this era of anxiety about radiation, doctors are often asked whether a diagnostic x-ray is likely to do more harm than good.

The question is fundamental and important. We are all fortunate that it has been asked. As a result of concern about the potential harm of medical x-rays, there have been major improvements in radiation technology, sharply reducing the dosage delivered in many examinations, sometimes by as much as 10-fold. However, each individual x-ray must be considered as part of a risk-benefit calculation: Is the saving in health or life worth an increased radiation hazard, however slight? The hazard, with rare exceptions, does appear to be slight indeed.

The nature of the beast

X-rays belong to the class of radiation known as *electromagnetic*. They are no different in kind from ordinary light, radio waves, microwaves, or gamma waves. But the physical characteristics of x-rays and gamma radiation make them capable of penetrating tissue. If these forms of radiation are aimed at the body with just the right amount of energy, they proceed to knock electrons out of the atoms in tissue, much like a blast of wind carrying shingles off a roof.

X-rays are not the only form of radiation producing this type of injury. Free electrons may tear into tissue, like atomic bullets, as may alpha-particles, which are composed of two protons and two neutrons and might be compared to cannon-balls. These particulate forms of radiation usually don't have the penetrating power of x-rays; they travel very short distances before coming to rest, so they are more likely to be encountered as a result of inhaling or ingesting a radioactive material than from exposure to an outside source of radiation.

In any of these cases, the effect of a radioactive "hit" is to change the chemical relationships of the atom that is struck. One chemical compound more or less instantaneously becomes another.

This sudden change of chemical identity is potentially most damaging when it occurs in DNA. Because DNA is the coded master plan of a cell, the slightest change in its chemical integrity may result in a drastic misreading of the genetic code. Other molecules, when messed up, can usually be disregarded or dispensed with. But scrambled DNA persists, to serve countless times as a false blueprint for the cell's machinery. A system for repairing minor damage to DNA exists, but it is not fail-safe. Above a certain dose of radiation, these mechanisms are overwhelmed and may simply fail to recognize a new error in the code.

Altered DNA may produce one of three unlucky consequences. (1) If the DNA is contained in a sperm or ovum, the damage may have no immediate effect. But now this DNA carries a mutation with the potential to pass on a genetic change. This is quite improbable, but it may be terribly serious when it does happen. (2) If damage occurs to DNA in a fetus, its development during gestation may proceed abnormally. (3) Finally, irradiated adults are susceptible to another disorder of cell development: cancer.

Protection

The practice of shielding the gonads (ovaries or testicles) during an x-ray serves to protect our progeny from the first type of damage. Obviously, some x-rays simply can't be taken with such a shield in place. The need for the x-ray must then be balanced against the (statistically *very* low) risk of causing genetic damage.

Preventing exposure of a developing fetus is somewhat harder. Approximately 1% of all pregnant women have abdominal x-rays taken during their first trimester. Sometimes the exposure is accidental (because neither the woman nor her physician knew she was pregnant); sometimes it is intentional, after physician and patient have weighed risks and benefits. In either case, the actual dose of radiation delivered to the fetus proves to be very slight in the great majority of cases, and if there is an increase in miscarriages, malformations, or other abnormalities it has not been possible to detect (perhaps because so many other, more common hazards, such as alcohol and cigarettes, viral infection, or hereditary defects account for a much larger proportion of fetal damage).

The risk of cancer, the main potential hazard for adults, will persist as long as x-rays are used, but this risk can be minimized. Certain tissues are known to be more sensitive than average to the effects of radiation—breast tissue being one of them, bone marrow another. A recent attempt to assess the effect of diagnostic radiation on these two sensitive tissues concluded that as many as 1% of all cases of leukemia and less than 1% of breast cancers could result from exposure to diagnostic x-rays. (The actual number could well be much lower; it almost certainly is not higher.) Most of the leukemias are estimated to occur in people aged 69 or older; the majority of the breast cancers in women over the age of 75. Obviously, it's important to minimize the dosage delivered to bone marrow or breast tissue. Reducing total-body exposure is a matter of choosing x-rays judiciously, using equipment that has been designed to yield the most information for the least exposure to radiation, and using whatever shielding is consistent with getting a useful picture.

Certain aspects of human biology work in our favor, when it comes to x-ray exposure. The body handles any given amount of radiation better when it is delivered slowly over a period of time rather than all at once. If our lifetime total of x-rays were all taken at a single moment, we would be much more likely to suffer damage than we are in the real world.

Younger people are less vulnerable than older people to radiation damage. Since children also have fewer x-rays than adults, on the whole, medical x-rays play a vanishingly small role in the list of hazards affecting them. With age, sensitivity to radiation damage increases, and so does exposure to x-rays. But since there is usually quite a long period of time (many years to decades) between the moment of initial damage to DNA and the point at which a cancer appears, x-rays taken near the end of life, as most of them are, are not likely to have any adverse effect on survival.

On the other hand, females are somewhat more sensitive than men to radiation, and they must receive higher doses for some examinations (as with a chest x-ray, which requires a higher dose of radiation to compensate for the presence of breast tissue and get a clear image of the lungs). In this case, biology does not work in our favor. And because it does not, mammography, which is advocated as a screening test for breast cancer, has been subjected to severe scrutiny. Although mammography is intended to protect women from cancer of the breast, it has a theoretical potential to induce the very sort of cancer it is being used to detect. However, current technology results in exceedingly low levels of radiation exposure, particularly with the method known as *film-screen* mammography. And mammography is generally reserved for older women, who are unlikely to be affected by a process of carcinogenesis requiring upwards of 20–30 years. There is currently no evidence to suggest that the incidence of breast cancer among women who have undergone mammography is any higher than in those who have not. Most authorities concur that the minute risk of developing a fatal cancer from mammography is vastly less than the benefit of early detection in women who are already at high risk of the disease.

Perspective

Medical x-rays should also be placed in the context of our total experience with radiation. We are all exposed to a fair amount of natural "background" radiation of all three types: electromagnetic, high-energy electrons, and alpha-particles. The amount averages out to about 100 mr a year. (The abbreviation *mr* stands for *milliroentgen*, meaning 1/1000 of a roentgen, which is a standard way of measuring x-ray energy. The unit is named after the man who discovered x-rays in 1895.) People who live at high altitude are exposed to a somewhat higher background, because less of the radiation from outer space ("cosmic" radiation) is deflected by the atmosphere. Those who live near natural sources of radiation in the earth, such as uranium deposits, are also exposed to a somewhat higher background. As we noted earlier in this chapter, seepage of radon gas from soil and rock into homes has also been recently recognized as a significant source of radiation exposure in some regions of the world, including sections of the United States.

Radiation produced by human activities annually adds 7 mr or so to the background. The major fraction of such radiation comes from fallout caused by above-ground nuclear weapons tests conducted before 1962. Other, minute sources include television sets, airport inspection systems, radio-luminous watch faces, and odds and ends of occupational exposures (for example, electron microscopes).

What do medical x-rays contribute, by comparison with the background? A single chest x-ray delivers 0.04 mr to a man's testicles; every year general environmental radiation exposes them to about 2,500 times that amount. A woman's ovaries receive about 0.2 mr during a chest x-ray, likewise a small fraction of the amount from background sources. X-rays of the skull and the extremities, which are that much further from the gonads and permit effective shielding, expose the gonads to very little radiation. But x-rays of the abdomen and lower back, which are thicker and closer to the genital area, produce much higher exposures, 12 mr in men— the equivalent of about 300 chest x-rays—and 125 mr in women —the equivalent of about 600 chest x-rays. These are comparatively high values—worth weighing whenever the need for such an x-ray is assessed. On the other hand, many people make transcontinental air flights without ever considering that the gonadal dose of radiation will be the equivalent of 60 chest x-rays in a man, 12 in a woman.

Guidelines

People concerned about the safe use of medical x-rays in themselves should keep the following suggestions in mind.

▪ If you do not understand why x-rays are being ordered, do not hesitate to ask why.

- You can ask for quantitative answers. The radiologist or technician supervising your x-ray examination should be able to give you a comparison—for instance, to the amount of radiation received from a chest x-ray.
- Women of childbearing age should not have any x-ray of the abdomen taken during the first 14 days of the menstrual cycle, unless there is an urgent reason for the examination. The object is to avoid any exposure to the embryo of an unrecognized early pregnancy.
- Any nonessential x-ray of the abdomen should be avoided during pregnancy.
- Young adults should avoid any repetitive exposure of the testicles or ovaries to x-rays, unless there is a clear medical reason for breaking this rule.
- One good way to minimize exposure to x-rays is to keep a good record of the date and location of any x-ray examinations. At a later time, these x-rays may provide information that reduces the need for others to be taken.
- No medically important x-ray should be refused on the grounds that the radiation dose is "too high." The theoretical risk of dying from even relatively high-dose x-rays is much smaller than that of riding in a car for a few hundred miles.

Low-level radioactive waste

Despite 6 years of political maneuvering, the United States still does not have a permanent system for disposing of low-level radioactive waste (LLRW). This situation has serious implications for health care, but the implications are not the ones you might imagine.

Low-level radioactive waste has become a major byproduct of medical care, though often the use of radioactive material occurs at some distance from the person being cared for. Most commonly, the radioactivity is required for laboratory measurements made behind the scenes, and thus never comes in contact with a patient. If these radioactive substances are carelessly handled or disposed of, they have the potential to injure people. But if they were not available, many kinds of diagnosis or therapy would be forfeited.

Sometimes medical treatment requires exposing the patient directly to a radioactive material. Iodine-131 is the most familiar example. When a thyroid gland is overactive, the patient can be given a drink of this *isotope,* a radioactive version of the ordinary material. Because iodine is avidly taken up by thyroid tissue, and by virtually no other tissue, the iodine-131 is rapidly concentrated in the gland. Radiation released by iodine-131 travels a very short distance—1–2 millimeters—and thus affects only the active thyroid tissue that has absorbed it, and not innocent tissue in the immediate neighborhood. There are one or two other situations in which radioactive substances can be used in this way. But by far the major application of isotopes is in diagnosis and research.

The value of radioactive material in diagnosis is twofold: on the one hand, isotopes are handled by the body exactly as though they were a substance that is normally present; on the other hand, because they are radioactive, they can be easily detected. For example, minute doses of a radioactive *tracer* can be given to a patient; then where it goes can be followed by a machine known as a *scanner,* which produces an image revealing the size, activity, or function of a body tissue. Certain cancers can be sought in this way; they appear either as an overactive "hot spot" or as an empty space in otherwise normal tissue. Malfunction of an organ, such as a lung or liver, can also be evaluated with scanners. Currently, though, the most common diagnostic use of radioactive materials is in test tubes. When a substance is sought in blood or urine, it is likely to be present in very small amounts. Accurate and sensitive measurement is then possible only with methods employing its radioactive twin.

The need for radioactive tracers may be even greater in medical research. To take one example, when a new drug is being developed, the way it is processed by the body must be studied. This is virtually impossible without using radioactively labeled forms of the drug. Thus, if we are to have new drugs, we are dependent on the use of radioactivity. At a more basic level, virtually all the chemical processes of the body, normal and abnormal, can only be unmasked through the use of tracers, many of which have to be radioactive.

The beauty of working with tracers is that detection methods are extremely sensitive. Thus, the quantities of radioactive material required for any one procedure are minute. Also, virtually all of the commonly used isotopes emit their radiation over very short distances. Little or no shielding is needed to protect workers from the emissions. As long as the material isn't swallowed, inhaled, or injected, no radiation exposure occurs.

Moreover, unlike radioactive materials in power plants or weapons, medically useful tracers have a very short life. Typically, half of the material has decayed to a nonradioactive form in hours to days. Iodine-131 has a *half-life* of 8 days; thus, after 10 half-lives, or 80 days, the amount of radioactivity is less than one-thousandth of the original level—and is virtually undetectable. (By comparison, plutonium-239, which appears in nuclear fuel and is used for weapons production, has a half-life of 24,000 years, and neptunium, a byproduct of plutonium production, has a half-life of up to 2 million years.) The point here is that the radioactive materials used in medicine and research will, in a relatively short time, decontaminate themselves.

The need for disposal sites

Some materials can simply be stored in a hospital or laboratory until they have decayed to background levels of radiation, and then they can be disposed of as nonradioactive materials. But this approach is almost always expensive and in many instances impractical. For hospitals and research laboratories, the problem isn't so much with levels of radiation, which tend to be exceedingly low, as with the bulk of the materials that need to be stored. Protective gloves and gowns, glassware, fluids in which the radioactive material has been carried, organic material, bedding from animal cages—all of these materials have to be disposed of safely, even though the level of contamination is minimal. To cope with this problem, producers of LLRW have been learning how to reduce the volume of material they generate. One hospital in the Boston area has cut its output to about 10% of what it was just a few years ago. Using materials more judiciously and compressing the waste in a trash compacter have helped to make this difference.

On the other hand, isotope manufacturers, on which hospitals and researchers depend, have to deal with larger quantities of radioactive material. On-site storage can become not only impractical but illegal for them, because there are limits to the amount of each type of isotope they are permitted to have on the premises. If the levels of an isotope in stored waste approach the legal limit, production must cease until the waste material has been disposed of. In such a situation shortages could occur.

Medical and research facilities produce about one-fourth of the total volume of LLRW generated in the United States. Some materials could be incinerated, because the amount of radioactivity released to the air would be well below the levels generated by natural processes. However, the least expensive way to dispose of these materials is to bury them near the surface of the ground. Disposal sites must be selected for soil type and drainage properties that minimize the risk of leakage from the area.

Spread through soil is slow, because the soil itself tends to bind and hold radioactive compounds. In the meantime, of course, their radioactivity continues to decay. Nevertheless, from time to time worrisome leakage outside disposal sites has occurred. In response, engineering techniques have been developed that are more effective at confining the materials. Contaminated wastes are often not merely buried but first embedded in something like asphalt or concrete to immobilize them. Trenches can be constructed with linings that further prevent leakage. As levels of waste are added, they are covered with soil. Then the trenches are capped with more soil and covered with clay or plastic. Finally, a permanent marker is placed to indicate the location, volume, and amount of radioactivity of contents. The question is not really *whether* we are able to build safe disposal sites, but rather how much we are prepared to spend for a margin of safety.

Currently, in the United States the LLRW originating annually from medical and related uses would require two 10-foot-deep trenches, each about the size of a football field. To meet this country's needs until the end of the century would require 5 disposal sites, each of about 100–200 acres. The sites must be closed off and monitored for leakage, vandalism, and accidental intrusion. After 20–30 years it is expected that such a site will have reached capacity. The trenches will then be filled and capped. At this point, no radiation would be detectable at the surface. Control of access would have to continue for about 100 years, and monitoring for another 200. In the unlikely event that someone were to move onto one of these sites after a century and derive all water and food from it, his or her total level of exposure would be little more than 3–6 times the typical exposure of a U.S. resident to background radiation, and it would be well below any level known to cause harm.

The current situation

The United States currently has only three sites for storage of LLRW. Two of those were closed temporarily in 1979 but then reopened. The states where the sites are located—Washington, Nevada, and South Carolina—have objected to being the nation's sole repositories for LLRW, and in the past have also complained about carelessness in the packaging of material transported to their burial sites.

The temporary closure created a crisis for research and medical institutions, as well as for the industries that also produce LLRW. Congress responded by passing a law that required the states to take care of their own LLRW problems. The states were encouraged to form regional associations, or "compacts," which would negotiate disposal sites and pay for construction and maintenance. A political stumbling block of this legislation is that once it is in a compact, a state cannot veto the location of a disposal site; it has only one vote among the states in that group.

The law had a 6-year deadline and expired in January of 1986. At that point, no new site had been established, and in some regions, including the Northeast, which is a major producer of LLRW, very little progress had been made. Congress then permitted a 6-year extension of the period for developing a waste-disposal plan but this time built in a series of checkpoints. If any state had not made a specified amount of progress by one of these checkpoints, its access to the existing disposal sites would become more expensive and could eventually be cut off. This provision may create the incentive needed for the states to solve a problem that is more political than technical.

The problem will not, however, remain purely political. Unless it is solved in the fairly near future, the effects will be felt in all aspects of medical care. At least 4 years are required to prepare an adequate disposal site. If negotiations continue at their current sluggish rate, we may well find that our national commitment to better health care at a reasonable cost is sabotaged on both counts. Medically important radioactive materials may not be produced because of the storage problem. And those that are produced may become prohibitively expensive.

4 | On the Surface: Skin, Hair, Nails, Teeth, and Eyes

The tendency to equate the superficial with the trivial just doesn't hold for the human body. Our most superficial tissue, the skin, for example, is more than just a wrapping; it's really an intricately designed space suit, compliments of Mother Nature, that protects us from our environment. It serves as a barrier against germs and toxic materials, it prevents excessive loss of body water to dry surroundings, and it helps to keep our body temperature within a very narrow range despite fluctuations in the weather. Skin even has nutritional value: it synthesizes vitamin D and stores extra albumin, a critical component of the blood.

Eyes originate from the same primitive embryonic tissue—the ectoderm—as does skin. Of all the sensory organs, none tells us more about the world around us. The special surface that makes vision possible is the retina, a complex network of nerve tissues at the back of the eye that records images from the outer world and transmits them to the brain.

Teeth, hair, and nails also began as embryonic ectoderm. Anyone interested in sustenance of a firmer texture than applesauce can appreciate the special function of the teeth. On occasion, profound weight loss in an older person can be traced to poorly fitting dentures that cannot handle the foods customarily eaten over the years. Hair and nails were also present in our predecessors for a good biological reason. But whatever warmth-retaining function hair may have once provided has been rendered quite unimportant to human survival by the availability of thick clothing, warm furnaces, and home insulation. Likewise, fingernails and toenails, vestiges of the powerful claws used by other species to hunt and protect themselves, have only rudimentary use, at best, for most of us.

But biological function is not the whole story. Because of an aesthetic sense that has evolved along with intelligence, all of these surface structures have taken on an additional role in most of our lives. Their shape, color, texture, and cleanliness determine to a large extent how presentable we are to others. Indeed, this cosmetic importance can acquire cosmic importance in the mind of a person looking for a job, a lover, or a satisfying reflection in a mirror. For these reasons, this chapter, "On the Surface," deals with both the health and the appearance of tissues that are the interface between a person and the world.

Skin Care

Beauty may be only skin deep, but that's deep enough to support a multimillion-dollar industry in over-the-counter skin-care products. The old standbys—soaps, suntan lotions, and deodorants—are now sharing shelf space with more exotic preparations, such as antibiotic ointments and steroid skin creams, in the never-ending battle against dryness, itching, inflammation, odor, sun exposure, and just plain dirt. When over-the-counter approaches fail, as in severe cases of acne and psoriasis, several new therapies requiring a doctor's prescription can often provide dramatic relief.

Over-the-counter products

It is easy to become bewildered by the variety of nonprescription skin-care products and their even larger variety of claims. Usually these claims, as well as the item's price, are rather poorly correlated with effectiveness. Sometimes experimentation with a number of brands is the only way to find the preparation that meets one's individual needs.

Soaps and dry-skin products

Soaps help to dissolve (really to emulsify) greasy or oily substances in water. Thus, they are useful for removing oils and foreign particles from the skin. Their detergent and alkaline properties, however, can cause irritation. One common sign of soap damage is chapping—rough, red, dry, and cracked skin. Until July 1979, no study had compared different commercial soaps for their safety and irritant potential. Soaps had been called "mild" on the basis of their manufacturers' beliefs, wishes, or commercial interests. But then a report published in the *Journal of the American Academy of Dermatology* showed that the irritant properties of many products bore no relation to the label's description of them as neutral, superfatted, or "for dry skin," nor to other characteristics such as transparency and cost. According to this study, which measured the irritant effect of 18 well-known toilet soaps, Dove was by far the mildest, whereas Zest, Camay, and Lava were the most harsh.

Soaps, solvents, and disinfectants cause chapping by damaging the skin's ability to serve as a barrier to the loss of water. In fact, repeated exposure to these agents can accelerate the skin's water loss to 75 times the normal rate. Other factors that may lead to deficient moisture in the skin are certain skin diseases (psoriasis, eczema, ichthyosis); excessive sun exposure; dry air (especially from winter heating systems); and dry, cold wind, which literally pulls water from the skin. Wearing gloves or mittens, using humidifiers, and avoiding excessive washing all help to prevent dry skin.

To repair dry skin, the moisture level must first be raised and then maintained. And the outer layer of skin must be restored to its normal texture. The most effective way to correct dryness is to soak the affected area in water for 5–10 minutes, then apply a greasy ointment such as petrolatum (Vaseline) or lanolin, or somewhat lighter preparations (for example, hydrophilic petrolatum, Eucerin). Less oily but still effective are oil and water emulsions (for example, Keri, Lubrex, Lubriderm, or Nutraderm grease or lotions; Nivea cream). After they are applied, the water evaporates, leaving a thin film of oil on the skin.

Urea and lactic acid, it is claimed, have a softening and moisturizing effect, and they may increase the skin's capacity to bind water. Aquacare HP, Carmol Ten, and Nutraplus contain 10% urea; Carmol has 20% urea. Lacticare lotion and Purpose Dry Skin Cream contain lactic acid. U-lactin lotion has both.

Bath oils are added to tub water on the theory that the skin absorbs a portion of the oil along with a surfactant also in the fluid. The oil makes the skin feel smooth and may prevent water from evaporating. Bath oils come in two types: those dispersed in the water (Alpha-Keri, Domol, Lubath, Jeri-bath) and those that lie on the surface to coat the body as one steps out (Surfol). Even though these products are designed to promote skin comfort, some people feel more itchy after they have taken a bath with one of them.

A person may need to experiment to find the preparation that works best; products with fancy names, high prices, and exotic ingredients are no more effective than many others. Furthermore, moisturizers on the face may lead to an acne-like condition. Also, lanolin or any of the many other ingredients in these preparations may cause allergic reactions.

Sunscreens

Sunscreens contain chemical substances which absorb ultraviolet light (UVL) and thereby decrease or eliminate some of the adverse effects of sunlight exposure. Conscientious application of sunscreens beginning in childhood would not only prevent acute sunburn but would also reduce the carcinogenic potential of chronic UVL exposure by as much as 75%.

All sunscreens display a numerical sun-protection factor (SPF) on their labels. The SPF value is the ratio of the time required to produce faint sunburn (redness) through a sunscreen product to the time required to produce the same degree of redness without the sunscreen. Thus, for a person who normally develops redness after ½ hour in the sun, the use of an SPF 15 sunscreen would make it possible to stay outside for 7½ hours (½ hour × 15) and obtain the same minimal response.

Although sunscreens protect very well against sunburn, which is produced by mid-range ultraviolet light (UVB), they do not absorb longer wave ultraviolet light (UVA). UVA produces adverse effects also, such as degenerative changes in the skin's connective tissue. So while a person may stay on the beach all day without sunburning while using the SPF 15 sunscreen, the process of "photoaging" is still taking place.

Sunscreens contain multiple ingredients and are marketed in many different forms (high- and low-alcohol lotions, creams, lip protectors, and so on). For individuals allergic to some sunscreen components, such as paraaminobenzoic acid (PABA) or its esters, non-PABA products are now available. Everyone should be able to find an effective sun-protective agent in a form pleasing to use.

Antiperspirants and deodorants

Many people are troubled by sweat because it stains their clothing or they find the odor unpleasant. Both heat and emotions can stimulate sweating from armpit glands, and the two together cause the

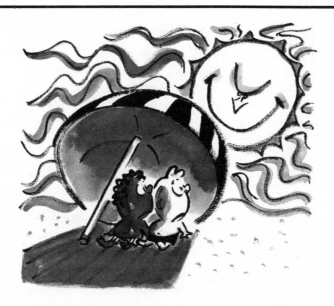

Even darkly pigmented skin can get sunburned. Although black skin doesn't suffer as much sun damage as lighter skin, it is not immune. Black babies, in particular, need protection for hands, feet, and the backs of their legs. Sunscreens with a high sun-protection factor (SPF 15–19) are recommended.

most intense perspiration. Aluminum compounds are reasonably effective at inhibiting sweating, and they are the main ingredient in all over-the-counter antiperspirants. Even so, the armpit sweat glands are relatively resistant to antiperspirants; agents that reduce sweating by 100% on most areas of the body achieve only a 50% reduction in the armpits.

Although no published study has actually compared the various brands of commercial antiperspirants, most work reasonably well for most people. But when armpit sweating is particularly troublesome, more drastic measures may be taken. A saturated solution of aluminum chloride in alcohol, kept in place overnight under an airtight wrap, will almost eliminate sweating for a few days. The preparation, known as Drysol, requires a prescription. Occasionally, mild tranquilizers help. For some people with uncontrollable sweating, the best course may be surgical removal of the armpit skin that contains sweat glands—a relatively simple procedure.

Armpit odor is not caused by sweat itself so much as by bacteria that grow in the warm, moist environment the armpit provides. Successful deodorants, then, must prevent the bacteria from growing. The aluminum compounds in antiperspirants are moderately effective against bacteria and thus reduce odor by diminishing both the output of sweat and the growth of bacteria. Some people who cannot tolerate the usual antiperspirants or deodorants may be helped by antibacterial soaps such as chlorhexidine (Hibiclens), solutions such as povidone-iodine (Betadine, Efudine), or by topical antibiotics such as Neosporin cream (which requires a prescription) or ointment (which does not). Drugs to inhibit the nerves that stimulate sweat glands, whether applied to the skin or taken by mouth, are usually ineffective.

Products for skin infections

BACTERIAL Skin infections such as impetigo and folliculitis, which are superficial and caused by bacteria, may be treated with topical ointments—either antibiotics (such as bacitracin) or antiseptics (such as the iodine-polymers Betadine or Efudine). Neomycin-containing ointments are also effective, but they often cause a contact allergy. Before using one of these ointments, it is helpful first to soak the area and then gently remove crusts and debris. If the infection is angry-appearing or widespread, medical attention should be sought, because antibiotics by mouth or injection will most likely be necessary.

FUNGAL These infections are most common in warm parts of the body where the skin is kept moist with sweat, such as between the toes (athlete's foot) or in the groin (jock itch). But fungal infections may also affect the scalp, trunk, hands, and nails. Drying thoroughly after bathing, using a talcum powder, and wearing sandals and absorbent clothing help to prevent and cure fungal infections. Treatment with nonprescription agents is often quite effective. Most commonly recommended are miconazole (Micatin) or tolnaftate (Tinactin and other brands). Powders and ointments containing undecylenic acid (such as Desenex) have long been used and are also effective.

VIRAL Few over-the-counter items are very effective in treating the most common viral infections of skin—recurrent oral and genital herpes simplex, herpes zoster (shingles), and warts. Most preparations recommended for recurrent herpes may decrease discomfort, but they have no effect on healing time and do not delay recurrence. Acyclovir (Zovirax) ointment is effective in shortening the course of first-episode genital herpes. Oral acyclovir can be a useful suppressant for persons plagued by frequent, recurrent oral or genital herpes infections. The callus covering a wart can be reduced and sometimes the wart itself eliminated slowly by remedies containing skin-softening agents, such as Compound W and various corn-plasters.

Steroid skin creams

Drugs related to the adrenal family of hormones (steroids like cortisone and prednisone) can produce dramatic relief in a wide variety of human ailments, including skin problems, because of their powerful anti-inflammatory effects. But because they act in so many different parts of the body, steroid preparations were long available only by prescription. Once it was established that these drugs are much less likely to produce systemic (body-wide) effects when applied to the skin as topical treatment, the Food and Drug Administration allowed mild versions of steroid skin medications to be marketed over-the-counter. Several products based on one particular steroid, hydrocortisone, are now available without the cost and inconvenience of a prescription. Although these over-the-counter creams and ointments should prove useful for many minor skin irritations, several words of caution are in order.

Steroids act by curtailing the body's inflammatory response, thus reducing itching and irritation. This produces initial improvement in almost any skin problem. If the cause of the problem is an underlying bacterial or fungal infection, however, the improvement may be short-lived, and interference with the body's appropriate response could be harmful in the long run. Indeed, using steroids on herpes simplex infections may dramatically worsen the condition. Such creams should never be used for infections around the eyes unless approved by a physician, because steroid treatment of herpes infections of the eye can lead to blindness.

The dose approved by the FDA for over-the-counter sale—up to 0.5% strength—may be effective for only very mild irritations, and the 0.25% strength of some preparations may be no more effective than a placebo. Topical steroids of any type seldom provide relief from severe cases of poison ivy, oak, or sumac; oral steroids must be used for significant improvement.

Acne—a treatable disease

The basic problem with acne starts in small structures known as *pilosebaceous follicles,* which are found in large numbers on the face, back, and chest. Each follicle consists of a tiny but active sebaceous gland (which secretes a waxy substance known as sebum) in association with a hair remnant and a narrow channel leading to the skin surface (*see illustration*). Acne occurs when these channels either leak or become plugged with sebum, causing the follicles to expand into visible lumps known as comedones. If a comedo stays closed at the skin surface, it becomes what is called a whitehead; if it opens, exposed pigment causes the comedo to become a blackhead, a discoloration that is caused by oxidation, not dirt. If excessive pressure within comedones produces leakage into the surrounding skin, disfiguring cysts and abscesses can form.

The real question, of course, is why all of this happens. Final answers are not in—though the following factors are known to be important:

HORMONE STIMULATION   Acne is almost unheard of before the arrival of puberty, when increased levels of male hormones (androgens) stimulate secretion by sebaceous glands. Females produce less of these hormones, but they do produce some in their adrenal glands, which explains why girls also get acne—though usually less severely than boys.

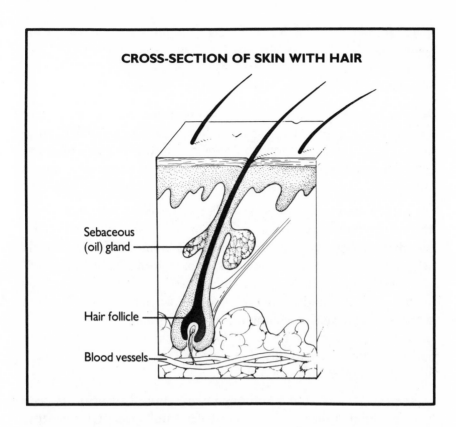

CROSS-SECTION OF SKIN WITH HAIR

Sebaceous (oil) gland

Hair follicle

Blood vessels

BACTERIA   While their exact role is not understood, there is evidence that certain normal skin bacteria contribute to inflammation by causing the breakdown of skin fats into irritating chemicals. The effectiveness of antibiotics in treatment tends to confirm the importance of bacteria in causing acne.

OTHER FACTORS   Although hormone stimulation and bacterial action are thought to be major causes of acne, other factors may contribute to the process—including excessive humidity, various cosmetics, exposure to oils or greases which may plug up skin ducts, and medications such as steroids, iodides, and the anticonvulsant drug Dilantin. Birth control pills can work in either direction: they cause acne in some women and relieve it in others. Occasionally, a woman will develop acne only after she stops the pill.

It has been well established that chocolate, cola drinks, and other foods do not cause acne. However, if any particular dietary item seems to contribute to acne in a given individual, common sense suggests avoiding it—if just for peace of mind. Emotions *can* aggravate acne.

Treatment

Although the exact causes of acne are unknown, making prevention impossible, excellent treatment methods are now available. Adequate control of acne should be expected in the majority of cases. The following methods of therapy are listed in the usual order of use, as the severity of acne increases:

GENERAL MEASURES   Special dietary measures are usually not helpful or necessary. Facial creams and moisturizers should be avoided, as they may block off skin ducts. Some contain chemicals which induce whiteheads and blackheads to form. Tight-fitting articles of clothing—such as headbands and turtleneck sweaters— may also block glands. Although washing when the skin feels oily is advisable, compulsive scrubbing with soap and water can make acne worse. Contrary to myth, hair length does not affect acne unless it contributes to oily skin. Exposure to sunlight can be very helpful in milder forms of acne.

BENZOYL PEROXIDE   Although many topical agents have been tried in the treatment of acne, most dermatologists prefer benzoyl peroxide—which apparently acts both by reducing bacterial activity and by promoting the healing of comedones. Initial treatment usually consists of once-a-day application of a 5% gel preparation—but other preparations are available as needed. In many cases, benzoyl peroxide will be the only treatment necessary. In a small number of persons, it will cause a contact sensitivity reaction and will have to be discontinued.

ANTIBIOTICS   Most authorities feel that antibiotics should never be given as the sole treatment for acne. However, when the above measures fail to control acne—and especially when acne becomes inflammatory, with the development of pustules, abscesses, and scarring—antibiotic therapy can make a critical difference. The most commonly used drug today is low-dose tetracycline, which has been adequately studied for long-term effectiveness and safety. Tetracycline should not be used by pregnant women.

ACCUTANE   Sometimes the pocket of sebum and associated materials (bacteria, hair, keratin) ruptures and spreads into surrounding skin. This can result in inflammatory masses (ranging from small pimples to large abscesses) that are collectively referred to as cystic acne. This form of acne is usually the most severe and is often resistant to antibiotic therapy. The introduction of isotretinoin (Accutane), which is quite effective in the treatment of cystic acne, has been of tremendous value to many patients.

Accutane is a synthetic form of vitamin A chemically known as 13-cis retinoic acid. This particular member of the vitamin A family has been approved because (unlike many other forms of vitamin A) it is quite safe when used orally. Taking large amounts of ordinary vitamin A, on the other hand, can be very dangerous.

Accutane use may cause the skin to become quite dry and the lips chapped. A side effect of more concern is the drug's tendency to elevate blood fats (triglycerides and cholesterol). People taking Accutane should be monitored for a significant rise in blood fats. And finally, *Accutane can cause extremely serious birth defects and should never be taken by women who are pregnant or who are contemplating pregnancy.* A pregnancy test should be given before the drug is started, along with careful counseling about this side effect of the drug, the woman's reproductive plans, and her method of contraception.

In most cases, severe acne will come under complete control after one 5-month course, and in many instances the disorder will not recur. Most dermatologists are rightly hailing this new drug as an important addition to the acne arsenal—and for treatment of some other, less common skin conditions. It will undoubtedly be misused in mild cases. But for the person with disfiguring acne, studies clearly indicate that the drug can make a dramatic difference with relative safety.

ESTROGENS   In women with severe acne not responsive to the above measures, estrogens (given as birth control pills) may be useful in counteracting the effects of male hormones. Estrogens are not used for men because of unacceptable side effects.

SURGICAL MEASURES   Various procedures to drain and remove acne skin lesions can be helpful in carefully selected cases. Most dermatologists rely on nonsurgical treatment except when pustules or abscesses become very large. Dermabrasion techniques are used only for severe scars left by old acne, and should never be directed to active, inflammatory areas. These are sometimes treated with steroid injections directly into the infected skin.

New light on psoriasis

At least 5 million Americans are affected by psoriasis. Each year, they lose some 56 million hours of work and spend over a billion dollars in treatment. Fortunately, treatment is improving.

At its most typical, psoriasis appears as patches of skin with a thickened, scaly surface. Under the scale, the skin is reddened and inflamed. Such a patch of abnormal skin is referred to as a *plaque*. Psoriasis often affects just a few areas of the skin—particularly the elbows, knees, or base of the spine. When confined to the scalp, it may be confused with another condition known as *seborrheic dermatitis*. Sometimes psoriasis may extend to the fingernails, which develop tiny pits on their surfaces, or it may affect the palms and soles. The tip of the penis, the vulva, or the area around the anus may be involved. In many people, psoriasis never gets worse than the periodic recurrence of isolated patches, but others suffer from bouts that involve large areas of their skin. In addition to the skin disease, psoriasis is sometimes accompanied by an arthritis that most typically affects the joints of the fingers.

The basic skin abnormality in psoriasis is not fully understood, nor is it known why minor injury (a scratch or abrasion) or even a bacterial infection can serve to trigger an attack at a new skin site. However, it *is* known that the rate of skin formation—as measured by production of new cells—is greatly accelerated in plaques of psoriasis. What causes this acceleration is a matter of intense research. An immunological abnormality or a basic flaw in the control mechanisms of skin cell replication may be responsible.

Psoriasis isn't contagious. Rather, it appears to be a built-in abnormality of a person's skin. Psoriasis runs in families, but exactly how it is inherited has not been worked out. A parent with a presumed gene for psoriasis has a 50–50 chance of passing it on to each child, according to the prevailing theory, but there is also only about a 50–50 chance that the gene will become active in any individual. So each offspring has roughly a 25% chance of developing the disease if one parent has it. Psoriasis occasionally puts in an appearance during infancy; more commonly it develops in adolescence or young adulthood, but many cases begin even later in life.

Treatment

Psoriasis is not the kind of disease that has one best treatment. The coming and going of major outbreaks is extremely unpredictable, even when no treatment is given. Periods of remission, in which the plaques simply go away, often occur without any particular intervention.

When psoriasis is persistent, severe, or otherwise troubling, treatment is indicated. In each case, the patient and doctor need to work as a team to find the best approach. What works for one person does not always work well for another. In mild cases that run a fairly steady course, patients can often take over routine management of their own disease. More severe cases, with ups and downs, need close professional supervision.

For very mild psoriasis, with small areas of abnormal skin, prescription-strength steroid cream (cortisone and its relatives) may be adequate therapy. Over-the-counter steroid preparations are unlikely to work because they are not strong enough. Often, however, the plaques become resistant to steroids after a while, and other treatment is needed.

The simplest therapy for psoriasis is sunlight, because the ultraviolet component causes psoriatic skin to slow down its overly rapid rate of proliferation. Sunlight seems to work best if the skin is covered by an oily material, such as petrolatum (Vaseline), which helps the rays penetrate beneath the surface. Uninvolved skin should redden slightly, but a painful sunburn should be avoided because burn injury can actually stimulate skin growth.

For reasons that are not known, "tar" (a complex of thousands of chemicals derived from petroleum) helps to heal psoriasis. Because tar is an unstandardized substance, various preparations may not be equivalent, and a dermatologist may need to experiment a little to find the most effective one. Tar preparations are often used in the bath, as topical applications, or in shampoos for psoriasis of the scalp. An alternative to tar is a chemical, anthralin, which can be very effective when applied to involved skin for several hours at a time. This treatment is somewhat difficult to manage, because the anthralin must not be allowed onto normal skin, which it irritates, and it also stains clothing. A variety of recent improvements have made anthralin easier to use. In certain severe cases, oral medications that destroy proliferating cells (such as methotrexate or or hydroxyurea) are used, but side effects are important limitations.

When psoriasis is extensive, artificial ultraviolet (UV) radiation, rather than natural sunlight, is often used. Light for phototherapy is produced by lamps inside a booth where the patient is positioned for a specified time. Two types of UV are used in phototherapy:

UVB and UVA. UVB is the type of light that causes typical sunburn. When used with lubricants (such as mineral oil), it is an effective treatment for psoriasis. Tar preparations are also used with UVB phototherapy in some centers: this is the Goeckerman regimen, named after the physician who developed it. In recent years, many victims of severe psoriasis have benefited by a new type of therapy, nicknamed PUVA, because it uses UVA light. Two hours before treatment, the patient takes a medication (psoralen) that penetrates the skin and is then activated by exposure to UVA. PUVA can be very effective, even in cases that fail to respond to other treatments. It is important to recognize, though, that accelerated aging of skin and increased susceptibility to skin cancer are problems with the UV light therapies. In an effort to reduce the risk of such problems, even newer approaches that combine one form of UV therapy with another or with various oral medications are under investigation.

Prevention

A person with psoriasis should avoid trauma to the skin and keep it moist and lubricated. In winter, a humidifier may be especially helpful. Certain drugs given for other conditions (such as oral steroids, lithium, and beta-blocking drugs) can aggravate psoriasis. Excessive alcohol intake probably worsens psoriasis as well.

Dietary theories of psoriasis have always been popular, but there is no evidence that diet plays an important role. Health food stores have promoted lecithin or vitamins for psoriasis, but these agents have not lived up to the promises made for them. Although stress is sometimes considered to be a factor in provoking episodes, its precise role remains uncertain.

Beauty versus Health: The Safety of Cosmetics

The manufacture and use of cosmetics must be among the oldest of human activities—and among the most likely to persist. But how safe are beauty products?

For the most part, cosmetics—a category which includes soaps, shampoos, lotions, make-up, perfumes, deodorants, and antiperspirants—are safe in the sense that they don't put users in any serious danger. But they can cause quite a few adverse reactions. How many, and their exact causes, are difficult to determine, primarily because the industry is not regulated in the same way that the drug industry is.

The difference between a cosmetic and a drug is not nearly as clear as the Food and Drug Administration might have us believe. According to the FDA's formal definitions, a drug is a "product intended to affect the structure or any function of the human body," whereas a cosmetic is intended to be "rubbed, poured, sprinkled, sprayed on, introduced into, or otherwise applied to the human body or any part thereof for cleansing, beautifying, promoting attractiveness, or altering appearance." It's not hard to see that there can be considerable overlap, despite this legal distinction. A manufacturer can put anything into a cosmetic, including a hormone, as long as no claims are made that it affects the structure or function of the body. The manufacturer doesn't have to prove that the stuff is effective or safe, or even say that it's in there at all.

Consequently, all cosmetics have many hidden components, a fact that complicates the problem of discussing reactions to them. For instance, sunscreens are present in many kinds of make-up to absorb ultraviolet light and prevent it from breaking down the product. Antibiotics are often used to retard growth of bacteria. Vitamins C and E are also used as preservatives. When a cosmetic label says "natural, no preservatives," chances are the product contains one or the other of these vitamins, which work very well for the purpose.

No federal regulatory agency requires that cosmetics and their ingredients be registered and tested either before or after they go on the market, and the FDA doesn't have a formal mechanism for collecting complaints. Only in the event that a cosmetic creates a problem after distribution will it come under scrutiny for possible removal from sale. Consequently, the number and type of adverse reactions to beauty products is thought to be seriously under-reported. In one study, 11 dermatologists with an interest in contact dermatitis (inflammation of the skin caused by substances touching it) saw at least 145 cases of cosmetic-related rashes a year, nearly one-third as many as the *total* number of complaints about cosmetics reported to the FDA annually from all sources. Hair products and facial make-up were by far the most common offenders, and the agents in them that were most likely to cause a reaction were fragrances, preservatives, and lanolin.

Even though the federal government does not require it, the cosmetic industry itself uses a series of pre-marketing tests to weed out products that may be irritating, sensitizing, or downright poisonous. Smaller companies tend to contract this kind of testing to outside laboratories, whereas the larger cosmetic firms maintain in-house research and development facilities. Use of animals in this type of testing has been heavily criticized by proponents of animals' rights and has helped generate opposition to *any* laboratory use of animals.

When a cosmetic that is already on the market comes under suspicion, the firm is often cooperative in supplying not only the product but its individual ingredients for a physician to use in skin testing. To protect proprietary secrets, these ingredients are usually not identified to the physician unless a reaction is noted during the testing process.

Rashes

The rashes described by the 11 dermatologists mentioned above were caused by irritation, sensitization, and photosensitization.

Irritation reactions are typified by rashes or redness of the skin occurring within minutes to hours after the product is first applied. This type of response is usually due to a direct chemical action damaging the surface of the skin.

Sensitization, or allergy, occurs when the body develops an immune reaction to the product. The resulting inflammation reflects this reaction rather than any direct injury from the chemicals themselves. Typically, the initial application is not followed by any problem. It is only on one of the subsequent exposures that a rash or redness develops. Sunscreens are known to produce sensitization reactions—and it may be difficult to tell whether the person is sunburned or reacting to the sunscreen. People will often come into the doctor's office with a story of developing a rash on the skin exposed to the sun. Their initial response is to apply more sunscreen, on the assumption that they have been burned. The result is even more intense inflammation.

Some substances cause a skin problem only when the skin and the chemical are simultaneously exposed to sunlight or other sources of ultraviolet light. This process is referred to as *photosensitization*. Here's a common example: Sometimes sunbathers apply lemon or lime juice to hair to lighten it. Ascorbic acid in the juice is probably responsible for this effect. But the juice also contains psoralens, which are photosensitizing substances. If the juice drips down onto the skin, the area it touches will develop an exaggerated sunburn. Substances in beauty products that commonly interact with sunlight include musk ambrette, bergapten (used in fragrances), angelica root, cumin oil, orange oil bitter, rue oil, sandalwood, cedarwood, lavender, and verbena oil.

In addition to causing these three kinds of rashes, make-up can also induce pimples to form. Some components of make-up alter the way skin grows and may encourage clogging of facial pores. Lanolin and D&C red dyes (used in blushes) are common offenders.

Other adverse effects

The effect of most cosmetics is superficial, but there are exceptions. Some cosmetic creams contain the hormone *estrogen,* which can penetrate the skin to produce feminizing effects. There are reports that a 10-month-old girl and a 5-year-old boy who were exposed to hair cream with estrogen developed enlarged breasts. Breast development has also been observed in older men, and vaginal bleeding in post-menopausal women, as a result of using estrogen-containing cosmetics.

Because cosmetics are not registered with any government

agency, no one really knows how many cosmetics containing estrogen are sold in the United States. Moreover, no governmental mechanism requires manufacturers to specify on the product label the type and concentration of estrogen contained in their preparations. But efforts are under way to achieve better labeling of these products. In the meantime, the FDA has issued a statement to the effect that the levels of hormones used in cosmetics sold over the counter are inadequate to make skin "younger looking," as is sometimes claimed—but obviously the amounts can be enough to produce significant side effects.

Some *carcinogens* can be detected at very low levels in a variety of cosmetic preparations, but they probably do not constitute a cancer risk. Nitrosamines, which are potent carcinogens, have been found in very low concentrations, probably introduced as an impurity during the preparation process. Evidently they are absorbed through the skin, as nitrosamines have been detected in the urine of people who have applied cosmetics containing these chemicals. However, the concentrations are much, much lower than those required to cause liver cancer in mice. And no connection of cosmetic use to liver cancer or any other type of cancer has been observed in people.

Another carcinogen, 1,4-dioxane, finds its way into cosmetics from the raw materials. Dioxane is a known carcinogen, but because it is so volatile, it probably evaporates before it ever penetrates the skin of a cosmetic user.

Some hair dyes have another kind of potential carcinogen in them—so-called coal-tar dyes. There is clear evidence that these dyes are absorbed into the body, but levels that build up in the blood stream are so low that concern hardly seems warranted. And, again, there has been no evidence from epidemiologic studies to suggest a link between hair dyes and cancer.

Absolutely no association between the use of cosmetics and skin cancer has been found.

People at special risk

Fair-skinned, blue-eyed people are more vulnerable than average to reactions to skin products and so should be more aware of the possibility that a cosmetic could be responsible for causing a rash.

People with acne should be very careful about applying facial products. And people with known allergies, especially skin allergies, should be sure to check out the labels of any products they plan to apply to their skin.

Given the sheer amount of cosmetic products sold in this country, there are remarkably few reactions. Those that we do see appear to be a small price to pay in the pursuit of beauty and eternal youth. How effective cosmetics may be in achieving those goals is another question, however.

Hair Care

The covering (or the lack of one) on their pate is of concern to many people. According to the Roman historian Suetonius, even Julius Caesar combed his hair across a bald spot on the top of his head. Other people are disturbed by excess hair growing in the "wrong" places. And still others worry not so much about their scalps as about *being* scalped—wooed by the advertisements into paying more for hair-care products than is necessary for either beauty or health.

Normal hair growth

Each hair we see above the skin is a strand of dead protein tissue. The hair follicle, which resides just below the skin surface (*see illustration, p. 197*), is the essential growth structure of a hair. As dividing cells at the bottom of a hair follicle are pushed upward, they eventually die and become the visible product we know as hair. If a hair follicle is destroyed, no new hair will grow. The total number of hair follicles in an adult has been estimated at about 5 million, of which about 100,000 are in the scalp. The number decreases with age.

In humans, each follicle grows hair in cycles, and the duration of the cycle is different in each part of the body. In the scalp, for instance, each hair grows steadily and continuously for 3–5 years. Growth then stops, and 3 months later the hair is shed. After another 3 months of a resting phase, a new hair starts to grow from the same follicle. On the eyebrows, however, the growing phase is only about 10 weeks and thus the hairs can never grow very long. Scalp hair grows about one-third of a millimeter each day (one centimeter per month, one inch in 2–3 months). Since there are about 100,000 scalp hairs, this growth produces about 100 feet of practically solid protein the thickness of one hair each day (7 miles per year). People who tend to grow long hair have long growth periods (6–8 years), but their hair does not grow any faster than that of others.

Normally, about 90% of scalp hairs are in a growing phase and 10% are resting. The resting hairs stay in place for several months, but when a new hair is formed and begins its own growth cycle, the old one is pushed up and out. We normally lose 50–100 scalp hairs per day as old hairs are shed to make room for their successors.

Many events can change the hair cycle. A temporary increase in the rate of shedding may occur 3–4 months after childbirth, or following a high fever, major illness, major surgical procedure, blood loss, or severe emotional stress. Accelerated hair loss is also seen in association with rapid-weight-loss diets involving severe restriction of calories (less than 800 per day) or protein. In these situations, hair will literally come out by the handful, but it always regrows some months later. Various drugs can also cause hair shedding.

At times, hair thinning can be due to *inadequate replacement* of hair shed at a normal rate. This can occur as a result of thyroid disease, cancer chemotherapy, or iron deficiency, and is also seen in some cases of diabetes.

Baldness

The common type of hair thinning that occurs in men is a normal process, not a disease, and so it's difficult to think of treatments in the conventional sense. There is no deficiency of vitamins or excess of hormones to be corrected, no infection to clear up. In women, on the other hand, thinning hair more often reflects a hormonal imbalance and can sometimes be influenced by medication.

Balding is fundamentally related to the growth cycles of hair follicles. Some follicles appear able and willing to continue these cycles indefinitely. But a certain group of them are inclined to shut down after a while. In men, these follicles are located predominantly on the temples and at the crown of the head. In women, they are distributed more diffusely across the top of the scalp (*see illustration*). As time goes on, each period of active growth gets shorter

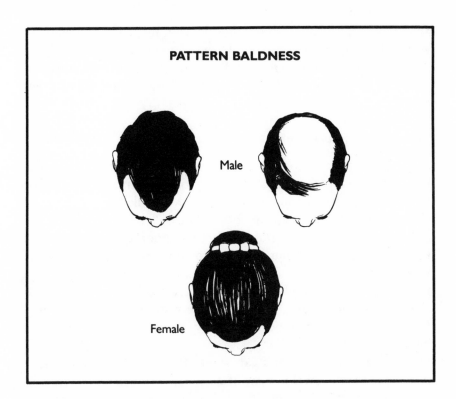

PATTERN BALDNESS

Male

Female

and shorter, the diameter of the hair diminishes, and pigment is lost. Ultimately, a fine, short, colorless, nearly invisible hair remains. This process must overtake nearly half the follicles in any given area of the scalp before thinning becomes noticeable.

Normal balding occurs when two conditions are met. First, the person must be carrying genes for baldness. Thus, the tendency runs in families and also varies from one race to another. Caucasians are most susceptible, Asians least so. The exact way in which baldness is inherited has not been worked out. Contrary to an old belief, the tendency to baldness does not run exclusively on the mother's side of the family; it can be passed along by either the mother or the father.

The second condition is the presence of male hormones, or androgens, such as testosterone. Men who lack these hormones, for whatever reason, tend to keep their hair. But going bald is not a sign that a man has extra amounts of male hormone, and keeping hair is not a sign of deficiency.

The scalp of most women gets somewhat more sparse with age,

although usually not as conspicuously as in men. Those women in whom thinning becomes noticeable sometimes have slightly higher than average levels of male-type hormone (which is normally produced by a woman's adrenal glands and sometimes also by her ovaries).

The myth of prevention

At present, there is no very satisfactory way to prevent baldness. Folk remedies and the sort of product promoted through the mail or in the back pages of some magazines are worthless.

Procedures to maintain a "healthy scalp" have no effect. For example, baldness does not result from poor circulation to the scalp, so there is no point in trying to stimulate blood flow. Likewise, baldness does not result from excessive oiliness or from dryness of the scalp, and efforts to treat these conditions won't retard thinning. Vigorous brushing may cause resting hairs to fall out—but they would soon come out anyway, and brushing doesn't cause balding.

Nothing you eat or don't eat, short of malnutrition, will make a difference to the development of common baldness. The vitamins and other products promoted for "healthy" hair are not effective. Indeed, the Food and Drug Administration is now developing a campaign to force such products off the market, but it will be a while before the agency can go through the required legal process.

In the meantime, though, it is safe to assume that commercial offers to sell you anti-balding remedies are slightly less trustworthy than offers to sell you shares in the Brooklyn Bridge.

Medical approaches

When medical attention is sought for hair thinning, the first thing to do is to make sure that the problem isn't something besides the common or "pattern" baldness that we've discussed.

At a hair clinic in an academic center, a lot of tests may be done—but at present most of these have more value as research tools than in direct application. The basic tests performed by a dermatologist or other physician are likely to include measurements of male and female hormones (more useful in women than men), thyroid hormone (which markedly influences texture and abundance of hair), and iron stores (because thinning hair is occasionally associated with a deficiency). A careful review of medications is worthwhile. Anti-clotting agents, such as heparin and warfarin, cause some hair loss in about half the people who receive them, and amphetamines, L-dopa, oral gold, and propranolol (Inderal) have sometimes been linked to this side effect. Other potential causes of hair loss include poisoning from thallium (a component of pesticides), boric acid (from some mouthwashes or from occupational exposure), mercury compounds, or excessive doses of vitamin A.

Much more often, though, no cause can be identified, and the diagnosis offered is "common baldness." Until a few years ago, nothing whatever could be done to slow, stop, or reverse this process. Now there are a few rays of hope for the incipiently bald. New drugs that alter the body's response to male hormones were the first medical advance. Various agents have the ability to block the effect of male hormones, and thus to "protect" hair follicles. Unfortunately, none of the available ones can simply be rubbed on the scalp with the assurance that their action will be limited to the skin. They all are absorbed into the whole body and thus can have feminizing effects. For obvious reasons, these agents are more useful for women than men, and in any case the benefit is pretty minimal. One of their greatest limitations is that they do not stimulate regrowth of fully developed hair; they simply prevent a further shift to the nearly invisible kind, and they only work as long as they are taken regularly. Thus, they slow the progress of balding, but they cannot reverse it.

Minoxidil is a new drug that has recently been approved as an anti-balding agent. Its effect on hair growth was first suspected because patients taking the drug to treat high blood pressure began to notice that their bodies were becoming hairier. It was then discovered that minoxidil would stimulate hair growth when rubbed on the skin. Since absorption into the system is minimal when it is applied this way, side effects (such as low blood pressure) do not appear to be an important problem for healthy adults. The striking fact about minoxidil has been its ability to *reverse* the balding process and not just to arrest it.

As soon as that is said, however, a number of qualifications are needed. Minoxidil is not a wonder drug. It works best for people who need it least—those who have been balding for less than 10 years and whose bald area is less than 4 inches in diameter—and it doesn't consistently work for all of those. It is only effective as long as it is applied regularly, usually twice a day. The kind of hair growth produced is far from lush in most cases. Currently, the treatment can be expected to cost $20–25 a week for an indefinite period—as long as the individual wants to keep his or her crop of regrown hair.

Other routes

The majority of bald people will not benefit from any drug old or new. Their quest for a remedy can be very expensive. Some hair pieces—wigs—look very good. The better they are, though, the more they cost. A related approach is to attach additional hairs to those still present in an area of thinning—but this procedure is time-consuming, expensive, and limited by the fact that the anchoring hair will grow, so the whole routine needs to be repeated at relatively frequent intervals, and at an ultimate cost running to thousands of dollars.

Hair transplantation, another costly procedure, does work, and if skillfully done it can look quite natural. It succeeds because hair follicles that are moved to the top of the head don't become sensitive to male hormone. So if a small plug of skin, about 4 millimeters in diameter, is removed from the back of the head and placed in the bald area, its follicles will continue to produce full-sized hairs. This procedure, which costs about $15 per transplanted plug does, however, run into money.

A very dangerous procedure, which has now been largely stopped, involved attaching bits of acrylic hair directly to the scalp with sutures. Infection and scarring were frequent complications of this procedure.

On the whole, our ability to "treat" baldness is still pretty limited. For the present it may be more worthwhile to work on attitudes, as there is nothing unhealthy or shameful about hair loss. Indeed, the tenth-century monk Hugbald of St. Amand reportedly was moved to write a poem praising the dignity of baldness.

Hair removal

Hair growing excessively, or in the wrong places, can be more aggravating than baldness. Usually the only significance is cosmetic, and the cause is genetic—a "family tendency." But very occasionally, an unusual growth of hair signals a hormonal or other medical problem which should be attended to by a physician skilled in endocrinology.

Excessive fine hair can be bleached to make it less obvious. The most common preparation is 6% hydrogen peroxide (commonly known as "20-volume peroxide"). Adding about 10 drops of ammonia to an ounce of peroxide immediately before it is used will make the bleaching action more intense.

There are several ways to remove hair. Plucking is painful but effective. Since each pluck starts another growing cycle in the hair root, this is not a permanent method. Wax depilation is essentially widespread plucking. Warm wax is placed on the skin, allowed to dry, and then peeled off with the hairs attached. Shaving is quick, easy, and effective, and it does not cause hair to grow back more abundantly or rapidly. However, it does leave the cut shaft of hair in place. Rubbing with a pumice stone or some other mild abrasive also removes fine hair.

Depilatories cause hair to disintegrate even though they leave the roots and thus permit regrowth. By disintegrating chemical bonds in the hair shaft, a depilatory turns it into a gelatinous mass, which is then wiped away. Because these agents dissolve protein, they also affect the skin and can irritate it if left on too long. Two types of depilatory are available. The sulfide types (such as Magic Shaving Powder and Royal Crown Shaving Powder) are more effective, but their odor is pungent and they are more irritating. The thioglycolate types (such as Better Off, Nair, Neet, and Sleek) must be left on longer, but they are more easily perfumed and are not so irritating.

Electrolysis is the only *permanent* method of hair removal. With this procedure, the hair bulb is destroyed by an electric current so that hair cannot regrow. However, electrolysis may be complicated by temporary irritation from the procedure or, later, by pitlike scarring. Also, incomplete destruction may allow hair to grow back. As with everything, the quality of the results depends on the skill of the operator; both cost and skill vary but not necessarily together.

Shampoos and rinses

The many commercial varieties of shampoo on display usually advertise themselves as being for dry, normal, or oily hair, but clinical trials reveal that these fine distinctions are meaningless. Also, there is little or no connection between the cost of a shampoo and its usefulness as a cleansing agent.

People with scaling disorders of the scalp, such as dandruff or seborrheic dermatitis, often find medicated shampoos useful. In these conditions, the skin is replacing itself too rapidly, so excess amounts are shed from the scalp. Medications that control (not cure) these conditions usually work by slowing down cell division to a near normal rate. The most effective shampoos are those containing 2½% selenium sulfide (available only by prescription). Then, in descending order of effectiveness, are those containing zinc pyrithione (for example, Danex, Head and Shoulders, Zincon); salicylic acid and sulfur (Ionil, Sebulex, Vanseb); tar shampoos (Ionil, Sebutone, Pentrax, Zetar); and finally, nonmedicated shampoos, particularly those containing surfactants (detergents), if used at least every other day.

Physical and chemical injury to hair occurs all the time in our culture. Hairs are exposed to sunlight, to the physical trauma of brushing and curling, to heat and tension, and to a variety of chemical insults. These can result in brittle and unmanageable hair, with a rough, irregular surface. Protein-containing rinses temporarily fill in the defects on the surface of the hair shaft, making it smoother and thicker. For some people, these products are of benefit in caring for their hair, but they do not cause hair to grow.

Nail Care

Most of us don't give fingernails or toenails much thought unless we're trying to change their color, keep them from splitting, or use them for a task that would be better done with a pocket knife, pair of tweezers, or small screwdriver. Actually, few products improve the health and texture of the nails. But nails have quite an interesting life of their own.

The normal nail

The nail itself, technically called the nail plate, is about half a millimeter thick. It is made up of a tough protein, keratin, which is also the main component of hair and the outer layer of skin. The nail plate itself does not contain living cells, but is produced by a special

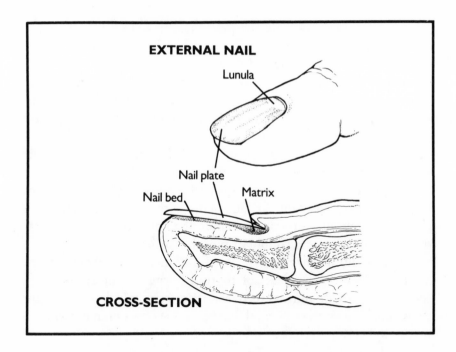

EXTERNAL NAIL

Lunula

Nail plate

Nail bed

Matrix

CROSS-SECTION

group of cells, called the *nail matrix*. This matrix lies under the whitish half-moon (or *lunula*) that is at the base of each nail and is most easily seen on the thumb (*see illustration*). The matrix cells continually produce the keratin that makes up the nail plate.

Nail growth is unique because it is directed toward the tip of a finger or toe instead of perpendicularly, the way hair grows. This is due to the fold of skin that surrounds its base. The nail lies in this sheath of skin the way a letter lies in an envelope, and the direction of its growth is thus constrained.

Skin under a nail has a "fingerprint" of ridges and grooves, but unlike the skin on the pad of the finger, which has various loops and whorls, the nail skin is arranged in straight parallel lines. The cells of this skin are attached to the nail and seem to be responsible for guiding the nail along its course.

A nail grows constantly, unlike a hair, which tends to grow for a couple of years and then rests for a while. On average, a fingernail grows one-tenth of a millimeter each day, which adds up to one-eighth of an inch a month or 1 inch in 8 months. Nobody knows why, but the longer a finger, the faster its nail will grow. Thus, the middle fingernail grows fastest, whereas nails on the thumb and pinkie are slower. Toenails grow only one-third to one-half as fast as fingernails.

A lot of energy is required to grow nails, relative to the small amount of tissue actually involved. And this high level of metabolic activity is rather sensitive to outside influences. Nails grow more slowly as one gets older, and they can slow down very abruptly during an illness. This effect is so dramatic that it can show up as a depressed groove (called a "Beau's line") across the nail plates. If you see such a groove running crossways on all 10 of a person's fingernails, chances are that he has had a fairly serious illness with fever or perhaps has gone through major surgery. If you see that the grooves are about half way out along the nail, you can guess that the event took place a couple of months earlier.

Some conditions make nails grow faster than usual. Among them are pregnancy or an excess of thyroid hormone. Injury to a nail speeds its growth during recovery. Psoriasis, which makes skin grow much faster than normal, has the same effect on nails when it involves them.

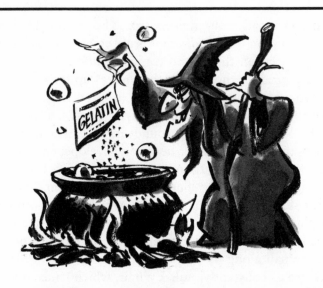

Eating gelatin will not strengthen your fingernails. In fact, nothing you eat helps (unless you've been suffering from malnutrition). The most common cause of brittle, breakable nails is water exposure.

One of the oldest, and wrongest, superstitions around is that you can make nails grow faster or stronger by eating gelatin (or various other products). No particular food or nutrient you can consume will force your nails to grow differently from their usual way. Of course, if you have been badly malnourished, your nails will have suffered right along with the rest of your body. Resuming a normal diet will correct that, but adding supplements to an otherwise healthy diet will not make any difference at all.

The funny-looking nail

Certain disease states change the appearance of the nail, and the sharp-eyed clinician will use these clues. Cirrhosis of the liver tends to produce an abnormally opaque, white nail (instead of the normal pink conferred by blood in the skin below a translucent nail). Sometimes, chronic kidney disease leads to a nail that is pink near the tip but white across the base. Chronic accumulation of lymph fluid may be associated with a yellowish color, though tobacco staining is a much more common cause of yellow nails. Poisoning with excess copper or silver can make the nails blue. Iron deficiency leads to a spoon-shaped (somewhat concave) nail, instead of the normally curved surface. Psoriasis sometimes causes little round pits to appear in the nail. An overactive thyroid may cause the nails to separate from the underlying skin. Prolonged oxygen deficiency (due to lung or congenital heart disease, as a rule) make the fingertips get thick and soft; the nail gets a "clubbed" shape and feels a little squishy when the skin at its base is pressed.

Most of these abnormalities are relatively unusual, however. The really common reason for a groove across the nail, for example, is injury, say from overly vigorous use of an orange stick during a manicure. Such pressure on the nail matrix may cause it to interrupt its activity temporarily. The result: a slight deformity of the nail. Many other oddities of appearance are just that. Grooves, ridges, bumps, spots, and what have you, are usually just variants of the normal nail.

Common complaints

Many people complain about the brittleness of their nails. Sometimes a chronic illness, such as anemia or poor circulation, makes nails brittle, but mainly it is direct injury to the plate or bed that does the damage. Probably the chief cause of brittle nails is frequent, prolonged exposure to water. Although nail protein looks tough and is physically hard, it is extremely permeable to water or solvents. Water can move through a fingernail 100 times faster than it can penetrate the outer layer of skin. Because nails are so porous, they can be injured in a variety of ways by fluid. Plain water does its damage by causing the nails to swell during immersion. They then dry out and shrink after the hands have been taken out of water. This accordion-like cycle of shrinking and swelling disrupts the structure of the nail and makes it easier to break. Thus, bartenders, surgeons, cooks, swimmers, homemakers, and others whose hands are moist a good deal of the time are very likely to complain of nails that split or break near the end.

An irritating or allergenic substance applied to the nails can rapidly penetrate them and set up a reaction in the underlying skin. As a result, the nail becomes misshapen, brittle, or soft. Once in a while, a nail-care product that contains an ingredient such as formaldehyde gets on the market. The result is a minor epidemic of contact dermatitis affecting the nails, which lasts until the product is withdrawn.

Fungus infections of the nail are fairly common, and are tedious to treat. Filaments of the fungus grow right in the nail plate, which provides it with both support and access to nutrition. As fast as the nail plate grows out, the fungus penetrates the newly formed area. Antifungal drugs, such as griseofulvin or ketoconazole, can be given to stop the fungus from growing, but they have to be continued until the nail has completely grown out—4 to 6 months for a fingernail, a year to a year and half for a toenail—in order to be sure that the infection will not start up again. Neither drug is cheap, and both have to be taken by mouth, because topical therapy is ineffective. Side effects, though rare, can occur. So the decision to treat a fungal infection of a nail, as opposed to just living with it, involves balancing the discomfort and unpleasant appearance of an otherwise harmless disease against the drawbacks of therapy.

Ingrown toenails develop when the nail gets caught in its own groove—usually as a result of being cut back too far, but sometimes because the nail itself acquires too much curvature (generally a problem of older people). Simple surgical treatments can be used to fix ingrown toenails. In general, the earlier they are treated, the simpler the procedure.

When psoriasis affects the nail, it cannot be treated with the usual topical methods that work on skin. For some reason, nails with psoriasis are very resistant to sunlight, tars, ultraviolet light, and other direct therapies. Thus, if the problem is severe, a systemic treatment has to be considered.

Nails are easier to protect than to treat. Avoiding direct injury to the finger tips, keeping water exposure to a minimum, and using cosmetic products sparingly, if at all, are the best ways to keep nails looking natural and healthy.

Tooth Care

Once upon a time, most people lasted longer than their teeth. Problems with decay and destruction often made it seem a matter of luck or good genes to escape dentures later in life. Although many people still bring dental plates to their dinner plates, an enormous amount of progress has been made in the field of prevention and treatment of tooth and gum disease. Young people can generally look forward to fewer cavities, thanks to fluoridation, and stronger teeth, thanks to improved nutrition. Newer methods to achieve healthy tooth alignment are now available. More aggressive attention to combating periodontal disease is keeping teeth tight within their sockets in later life. And the field of tooth implantation is maturing rapidly, so that even when primary tooth-preserving strategies have failed, a permanent replacement with artificial teeth can be considered.

Sealing out tooth decay

For several decades, fluoridation has played a major preventive role in the battle against tooth decay. Another powerful technique for making teeth impervious to decay has recently become available. The process, called dental sealing, places a durable material on the biting surfaces of teeth so that all the pits and fissures can be closed off and bacteria that cause decay excluded.

Two areas of a tooth are especially vulnerable to cavities. The smooth surface of the side facing an adjacent tooth is one of these; food and bacteria lodged between two teeth create the environment that leads to acid formation and decay. Cavities in this location are very effectively prevented by fluoride. The other prime location for decay is the biting surfaces of the back teeth. In most people these teeth acquire tiny defects in the enamel surface even as they form. The pits and fissures are the perfect place for trouble to begin once a tooth has emerged through the gums. Unfortunately, fluoride is not very good at preventing cavities in this location.

Devising a technique that would really seal these pits and fissures has not been as simple as the basic idea, however. First you need a nontoxic material that does not let anything through. Then you have to find a way to get it to bind to the tooth enamel (which resists adherence of most substances). Finally, you have to be able to apply the material rapidly and easily, so as to make sealing a practical method. These difficulties have been overcome, however, and sealing of teeth is now a straightforward and painless procedure that can be used on a wide scale.

The dentist or a trained assistant thoroughly cleans the tooth and then applies a very dilute solution of phosphoric acid to the surface. This step makes the enamel microscopically rough so that the sealant will bind to it. Next the tooth is completely dried. As the last step, the sealant, a type of plastic, is simply painted onto the prepared surface of the tooth with a fine brush. It dries in minutes, and that is all there is to it. This artificial surface is highly durable, and even though the upper layer wears away in time, the plastic that has slipped into the pits and fissures remains to lock out decay-producing material.

For whom?

Sealing should be standard practice with all growing children, and should be considered by some adults. There is ample evidence from a variety of studies that this method is highly effective in preventing decay. One of the best of these was conducted in Colombia, where one group of children had their teeth sealed and another did not. After only 2 years, the treated group showed a 65% reduction in caries, compared with the untreated group.

The ideal time to seal a tooth is when it first erupts from the gums, before decay has time to start in the pits and fissures. A sensible practice would be for a child to have a dental appointment for sealing shortly after each of the 16 permanent back teeth comes in.

Although sealing produces the greatest protection right after the tooth emerges, it can still be worth doing throughout the teenage years. Indeed, many college students develop new cavities because they acquire a typical college eating pattern (frequent snacking on foods that predispose to caries). A parting gift to the student going away to college might well be a visit to the dentist for sealing. The number of new cavities usually diminishes in adult life, but adults who find themselves suffering from cavity formation—perhaps because of changed eating patterns—can benefit from sealing, too.

Maintenance

Well-conducted trials, such as the Colombia study, have demonstrated that sealing will eliminate the large majority of cavities that would otherwise form on the biting surfaces. And a single treatment usually lasts for a lifetime. However, about 15% of the time the seal comes off, or less commonly it gets loose without falling off. This situation is easy to recognize and can be fixed at the next visit. Thus, it is important to continue with regular dental examinations twice a year to make sure, among other things, that the teeth have remained properly sealed and to reseal the failures.

Beyond braces: the new orthodontics

The teenage mouth full of glittering metal is a familiar image. Many of us may not realize that the image is obsolete, and that in the last few years orthodontics has moved past its own adolescence as a science.

The most common orthodontic procedure is still correcting crowded or crooked teeth in an otherwise normal jaw. But now more severe deformities of the facial features can be corrected. Orthodontists, working with surgical specialists, have new techniques which can align jaws that have failed to grow symmetrically, relocate misplaced eye sockets, and correct cheekbones or chins that are too far back or protrude. These procedures can often be performed in infants and children, before emotional damage is done. In the past, some children of normal intelligence had to live in institutions simply because their appearance and handicapped functions made them unacceptable to others. Although they still cannot be made into "beautiful" people, it is often possible for such youngsters to go to school with an ordinary appearance, one that does not distract attention from what they do or say.

Surgeons can now cut bone and reposition it because they know how to maintain a blood supply to the jaw. Teeth and sockets are thus kept alive while they are being moved around, and continue to grow once surgery is finished. New information about these growth patterns has made it possible to tailor a procedure to take advantage of favorable growth tendencies, or to interrupt undesirable ones. Scarring, which limits growth, is now much better understood than in the past, and therefore many of the disappointments that were once encountered are avoided. For example, surgery for cleft palate used to limit growth of the upper jaw, thus leaving the individual with a receding appearance along the upper lip. This result can now be avoided (and it can be surgically corrected if it has already occurred).

As a general rule, most people undergoing orthodontic treatment can expect better results with less discomfort than in the past. Those who were told 5 or 10 years ago that an abnormality could not be corrected may well find out that it now can be. And individuals whose previous treatment has left them with a functionally or aesthetically poor result may find that the newer methods can improve it.

Crooked teeth

Abnormally located teeth affect not only appearance but health. Most people's teeth fall short of the textbook ideal, to be sure, and mild crowding (the most common abnormality) is not likely to cause loss of teeth. Tightly crowded or tipped teeth, on the other hand, may be impossible to keep clean. In time, caries (tooth decay) or periodontal (gum) disease leads to loss of these teeth. Or, if the stresses caused by chewing work at an angle instead of straight along the tooth, bone in the socket may be damaged.

The braces used today are lighter, smaller, easier to clean around, less irritating to wear, and less likely to produce damage of their own. The main reason is that they can now be anchored—actually glued—right to the tooth. Two major developments have made these advances possible: adhesives that bond the brace directly to the tooth, and plastics that can be used instead of metal to form parts of appliances. In some instances, brackets can be placed on the inside surfaces of the teeth so that the appliance does not show during normal conversation. And because it is no longer necessary, as a rule, to put a metal band around all teeth being moved, there is less need to extract teeth in order to make room for the braces.

Periodontal disease

Periodontal disease is a process that damages tissue surrounding a tooth and eventually erodes the bone that forms its socket (*see illustration*). It is the major cause of lost teeth after the age of 35.

Dental caries (tooth decay), when treated with modern techniques, can progress pretty far and yet a working tooth can be saved. However, if supporting tissues are destroyed by periodontal disease, even a good tooth may be lost. As periodontal disease begins, the gum turns from its natural pink to red, and then a little space forms between the gum and the tooth. At this stage, the gum disease (technically termed *gingivitis*) is not necessarily painful. Gingivitis may linger on for many years without progressing, but as a rule it goes on to *periodontitis* (meaning "inflammation around the tooth"). At this stage, the gum peels away from the surface of the root and crown of the tooth to leave deep pockets where bacteria accumulate and destroy the socket of bone that supports the tooth. This infection may also penetrate the space between the tooth and its socket. Once infection invades the root, it destroys the fibers (or ligaments) that anchor tooth to bone. After the tooth has been loosened and its supports eroded, it cannot be kept in place.

If the open end of a pocket becomes sealed off, an abscess, or

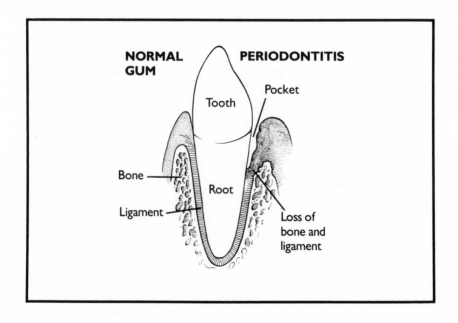

enclosed infection, develops. Such gum abscesses are entirely distinct from the root abscesses of dental caries, and they are not preceded by pain or sensitivity to hot and cold as root abscesses are. But once gum abscesses form, they are painful indeed.

Standard approaches

Like caries, periodontal disease is caused by bacteria (although of a different type), so all accepted forms of prevention are aimed at preventing the accumulation of bacteria adhering to teeth and of the gelatinous material that covers them. Removing these *plaques* is what brushing and flossing are all about. Both are mechanical efforts to remove bacteria from the gum margin. Even with a fairly good program of home care, though, some plaques form and with time become calcified. This material (called either *tartar* or *calculus*) should be removed by a dental hygienist at regular intervals. It was once thought that mechanical irritation from the tartar was the principal cause of gingivitis, but the bacteria themselves are now thought to be the main problem; housed in and upon the tartar they have made, they attack the gum tissue.

Established periodontitis, with its pockets of infection and areas of weakened bone, defies home treatment. There are two standard approaches to the problem:

SURGERY   With surgery, a periodontist or dentist cuts open the pocket to expose the area of infection. Now able to see directly, he or she then thoroughly cleans out the diseased material and removes all evidence of infection. The gum is then put back in place, usually with the gum line somewhat closer to the root than it was, so that the pocket is now shallower. When results are good, this procedure allows a patient to keep the disease under control with the usual home-care methods (brushing and flossing). Without proper and continuous maintenance care after the surgery, it is likely that the pockets will return to their presurgical depths within 2 years.

But sometimes problems persist. Very deep pockets cannot always be eliminated, and they may develop again. Thus, the area may need to be cleaned by the dentist at fairly frequent intervals. Surgery may again be required, even though the procedure was expertly done in the first place.

DEEP SCALING   An alternative to surgery is a procedure known as *deep scaling*. At frequent intervals—perhaps as often as every 2–

3 months—the patient must have pockets curetted (scraped) by a dentist or a hygienist working with a dentist. It is important for the dentist or periodontist to make sure that the deepest areas have been properly cleaned each time. If the base of the pockets can be reached, and if the procedure is done frequently enough, surgery can be avoided, but even the most experienced periodontists may have difficulty cleaning out deep pockets.

Of these two approaches, surgery is more likely to provide a long-term solution for deep pockets. But patients may refuse surgery because it frightens them. Or if periodontal disease is located near the front teeth, surgery—which is likely to expose the roots of the teeth—may be avoided for the sake of appearance. Deep scaling, done skillfully and frequently enough, is then an acceptable alternative to surgery.

Getting at bacteria

Because bacteria are the cause of periodontal disease, a good deal of attention is being focused on ways to kill the offending organisms.

Scrupulous oral hygiene should be the cornerstone of prevention. Unfortunately, many people find it difficult or impossible to keep up adequate motivation for proper home care. Periodic cleaning by a dental hygienist is thus very important. Although a period of 6 months between cleanings is the standard recommendation, the frequency of visits should be a matter of individual need. But it is also apparent that we must look for other approaches to prevention.

Mouthwashes containing *antimicrobials* (substances that kill bacteria) have shown reasonable promise in the treatment of gingivitis. In principle, this approach is a good one, but there are practical problems. For example, chlorhexidine, one effective antimicrobial agent, stains teeth if it is used for long periods of time. As yet, the Food and Drug Administration has not approved any antimicrobial mouthwash for use in this country, but studies conducted abroad have been encouraging. Material impregnated with a drug and then stuffed into the pockets of infection can deliver antimicrobials directly to the site of bacteria without coating visible surfaces of the teeth. Research on this approach is in progress.

In general, it is more practical to give antibiotics as pills. But if they must be given for long periods, as is likely in cases of periodontitis, questions of dosage, side effects, and possible resistance of bacteria become important. So far, the most promising antibiotic is tetracycline, which has already been shown to be safe for the long-term treatment of acne. But many questions must be resolved before it can be accepted as a standard therapy for periodontitis.

The so-called Keye's technique attempts to monitor microscopically the types of bacteria in the pockets and adjust the treatment regimen according to the findings. Such treatment includes the conventional scaling and curetting of the root surfaces, irrigation of the pockets with antimicrobial solutions, and the home application to the gums of a mixture of sodium bicarbonate, sodium chloride, magnesium sulfate, and hydrogen peroxide. Whether this treatment program for moderate periodontal disease gives better results than conventional treatment and home-care procedures is not clear. In more advanced cases with deep pockets, it is doubtful that this approach can substitute for surgery.

Long-term animal studies have demonstrated that the non-steroidal anti-inflammatory drugs (Motrin, Indocin) are capable of slowing down the destruction of bone around periodontally diseased teeth. A clinical trial is currently in progress to determine the efficacy of such drugs in humans with advanced periodontal disease.

At present, it seems unlikely that a vaccine can be developed for periodontal disease because a variety of different bacteria cause it. Caries, on the other hand, is caused by just one species, and so there is hope of developing a vaccine for that disease.

Dental implants

The phrase "false teeth" has long evoked the image of a disembodied smile resting overnight in a glass of water. In the last few years, however, major developments in technique have made it possible to attach artificial teeth permanently to the jawbone—often with considerable improvement in convenience, comfort, and stability. But the field is still new and even better methods can be expected.

The principle of dental implantation is fairly simple. A conventional crown or bridge of artificial teeth is held in place by a support that is fixed to the jaw. Once it is in position, such a bridge usually cannot be removed by the person wearing it, and it comes to be treated much as though it were a set of natural teeth. Implants take one of several basic forms. Supporting screws or cylinders may be placed in the jaw, or a blade-like support may be inserted. Another approach is to mold a frame to the shape of the underlying bone and use that as the support for teeth.

Actually making these devices work, and work reliably, has been much more difficult than it might sound. Until the last few years, the techniques in use were quite unpredictable, and for most people the risk of failure was not acceptable. What caused the failures was a tendency for fibrous tissue instead of bone to grow in around the implanted support. When this tissue grew in too thickly, the implant was likely to be unstable and subject to infection.

Basically, what happened was analogous to acquiring advanced periodontal disease, and the bridge then had to be removed. As it turned out, there was no single secret for encouraging bone to grow. Several measures, which had all been tried but not all together, had to be applied simultaneously. When they were, reliability of implants increased to greater than 90% during follow-up periods lasting as long as 10 years.

First, for maximum stability and longevity an implant cannot be installed all at once, because the forces created by chewing delay healing. So the implant has to be inserted in two stages. The supports are placed, and then several months are allowed for healing before the bridge is secured to them. Second, a high-speed drill cannot be used to cut bone to insert the supports. The heat of drilling burns the bone, which then will not heal adequately. Third, the whole procedure must be sterile; if bacteria invade, chances of healing are seriously reduced. Fourth, the choice of material is very important. It must be fully compatible with living tissue, so that there is a greater likelihood of bone growing around the implant and becoming firmly attached.

The current scene

Although dental implants have been a form of treatment available to people in the United States for the past 35 years, it is only recently that this therapy has become widely used. Much of the current success can be traced to 20 years of work conducted by a Swedish researcher, Per-Ingvar Bränemark. Bränemark was largely responsible for recognizing the importance of protecting the bone from heat, infection, or premature force. He also designed a two-stage implant of pure titanium that proved to be very successful. It is claimed that his device, when implanted with proper technique, will become chemically bonded to the jawbone. This may indeed be the case, but unequivocal clinical evidence is lacking.

Bränemark's report of his achievements triggered rapid growth in implant dentistry. But the Bränemark device is not the only implant design accepted by people in the field, and it is not regarded as the appropriate choice in all situations. Currently, a variety of effective dental implants are available for use in settings where the Bränemark implant is not ideal.

In a clinical situation, the first problem is to decide which implant to use. There are two major manufacturers, although many others are entering the market. One company is producing and marketing the Bränemark implant itself. This company has placed certain restrictions on purchasers. Theoretically, it limits sale to members of specified dental specialties. It requires purchasers to take a 3-day course. And the package it sells—implants, drills, and other equipment—is very expensive.

The Bränemark company can, however, make a very important point: this package comes with solid support from a couple of decades of research—including a follow-up period of 10 years on this device when used in patients without remaining natural teeth. The academic dental community feels very strongly that such evidence is valuable; it's a standard that health research should always aim for. On the other hand, if we wait around for 10 years' worth of follow-up on every modification of the original device, progress is going to be exceedingly slow. At some point, insisting that these original research results be duplicated every time seems only dogmatic.

Another implant, developed by Dr. Gerald Niznick, a prosthodontist from California, is the Core-Vent implant; it is a device incorporating principles very similar to those on which the Bränemark is based but is by no means identical in design (*see illustration*). The Core-Vent implant does not have the same kind of research to back it up, but it's clear from clinical experience that the Core-Vent can be a very useful device, with advantages over the Bränemark in some situations. For example, the Bränemark is hard to insert if any natural teeth remain in the jaw, whereas the Core-Vent can be used in this situation. There is, however, no way to know at present whether the Core-Vent will indeed prove just as

THREE COMMON DENTAL IMPLANTS

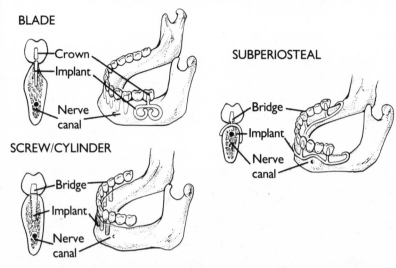

BLADE

Crown
Implant
Nerve canal

SCREW/CYLINDER

Bridge
Implant
Nerve canal

SUBPERIOSTEAL

Bridge
Implant
Nerve canal

In each of these diagrams, the implant is shown as it would appear in a lower jaw and also as it would appear in cross-section.

Top left: The blade implant is often used when natural teeth remain in the jaw, as illustrated here. This kind of implant is also favored when previous loss of bone has reduced the amount of support available.

Lower left: When screw or cylinder implants are used, 6 supports are typically placed in the front portion of the jaw, as shown here. The size of the supports requires a fairly normal thickness of jawbone. (Common examples of this implant are Bränemark and Core-Vent.) In the illustrated example, a full bridge of teeth is anchored to the supporting screws.

Right: When so much of the jawbone has been lost that the remaining surface is very close to the nerve canal, implants cannot be inserted into the bone. In that event, a frame can be molded to the surface of the bone and then implanted under the covering membrane, or periosteum; hence the name "subperiosteal."

durable as the Bränemark. Meanwhile, many other devices, which promise to solve a variety of dental problems, are under development, and the same questions must be asked about them.

Some basic principles

- In general, placing implants is least complicated when a jaw has no natural teeth, although there are certainly situations in which implants can be made compatible with remaining teeth or even used to replace a single tooth.
- Although the patient should have completed growth before an implant is attempted, age is generally not an important consideration. Teeth lost in an accident, as well as those lost to decay or periodontal disease, can be replaced. Anyone who is able to go through the procedures required to place a fixed bridge can tolerate the implant procedure. Lowered resistance to infection (as in people treated with steroids) raises the risk of complications.
- The cost of an implant may range from little more than $1,000 to as much as $15,000 for one jaw. Many factors enter into this wide disparity in price. In general, the cost of an implant is about equivalent to the cost of placing a fixed bridge to solve the same problem. Indeed, the major component of cost is usually the bridge or crown, and not the implantation procedure.
- There is no question that the Bränemark device has demonstrated the best results, where it can be used and when it can be afforded. But other implants may best solve certain problems, or may be more easily afforded. When chair-side decisions are made, having alternative devices may be a real advantage.
- Placing an implant is not something that happens as a single event. It requires repeated visits; so whenever quality care is available close to home, that's the best place to seek it.

Eye Care

Good eyesight is taken for granted by most who have it, and when vision fails, depression may not be far behind. Three common conditions can lead to visual deterioration, especially later in life—glaucoma, cataracts, and macular degeneration. But by far the most common eye problems in this country involve so-called refractive

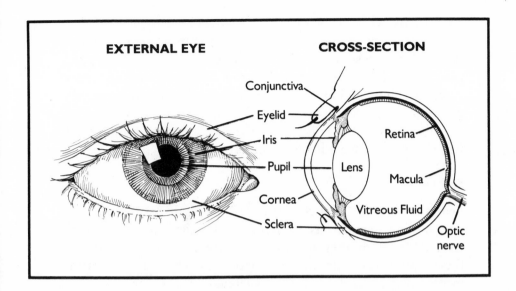

EXTERNAL EYE   CROSS-SECTION

Conjunctiva

Eyelid

Iris

Pupil   Lens

Cornea

Sclera

Retina

Macula

Vitreous Fluid

Optic nerve

errors—meaning that the front parts of the eye (cornea and lens; *see illustration*) do not bend light rays correctly so as to focus them on the retina, the "film" at the back of the eye. If rays focus in front of the retina, the person tends to bring objects in closer and is said to be nearsighted; if rays focus behind the retina, the person will hold objects farther away and is labeled farsighted. Fortunately, both of these common problems are easily corrected with additional bending power placed in front of the cornea—in the form of either glasses or contact lenses.

Contact lenses

Strictly speaking, contact lenses are prosthetic devices that come in intimate contact with the eye for long periods of time. They should be used with care. Three main types of contact lenses are now in use: hard, soft, and gas-permeable lenses.

Hard lenses

The first successful contact lenses, developed about 40 years ago, were made of plastic and were quite large. Techniques for fitting them were cumbersome and successes were few. Then, in the late 1940s, contact lenses that covered only the cornea (the transparent membrane at the very front of the eye) were introduced. These early hard lenses were all made of PMMA (polymethylmethacrylate), and the greater success with them resulted from modifications in design. Hard lenses continue to be widely used because they offer good vision (especially when the patient has astigmatism), ease of care, durability, and low cost. For most contact-lens wearers, however, hard lenses have been replaced with lenses made of new materials that have not only increased the success rate of fitting contact lenses but also have allowed more people to wear them.

Soft lenses

Lenses made from plastics such as HEMA (hydroxyethylmethacrylate) or similar materials are more flexible than the older PMMA lenses. As a result, they are more comfortable than hard lenses, and they require very little time for adaptation. They can be worn for many hours without producing swelling of the cornea.

Soft lenses have some valuable advantages, but they also have limitations. Vision is frequently not as sharp as with conventional glasses or hard lenses. Because bacteria and fungi can grow on the surface of soft lenses, they must be disinfected with a heating unit or antiseptic and rinsing solutions, which add to potential complications and expense. Many ophthalmologists believe that, even with proper cleaning, soft lenses carry a slightly higher risk of causing eye infection. They are also associated with a higher rate of allergic reactions to the solutions or to protein build-up on the surface of the lens. These problems have been significantly reduced by the use of enzyme cleaners and by the introduction of solutions which either do not require preservatives or which use preservatives that have a much lower incidence of allergic reactions.

Once begun, an infection may lead to corneal ulceration, a condition in which the outermost surface of the eye becomes eroded and swollen. Corneal ulcers can be painful and difficult to treat; they may result in permanent scarring with resultant loss of vision. A red, painful eye signals the need for immediate evaluation in any circumstance, but particularly in a patient wearing any type of contact lens.

Soft lenses do not work well for *corneal astigmatism,* a condition in which the cornea has a somewhat irregular shape, rather than a perfectly smooth curve. This common problem can be corrected by conventional eyeglasses or by rigid contact lenses because they automatically compensate for slight distortions in the shape of the cornea. Soft contact lenses, however, conform to the slight distortions of the cornea and thus do not provide correction.

Toric soft lenses have been developed in an attempt to rectify this problem, but they have met with only limited success to date. They work best for some cases of low-to-moderate degrees of astigmatism. Fitting fees and replacement costs for these lenses tend to be significantly higher than for conventional soft lenses.

Soft lenses are, in general, damaged in more ways than hard lenses, so they require fairly frequent replacement, which entails inconvenience and expense.

Gas-permeable lenses

A new generation of lenses is being made from plastics such as cellulose acetate butyrate (CAB), pure silicone, or a polymer made by mixing silicone with PMMA in various combinations. These lenses resemble hard lenses in their high optical quality, durability, and ease of care, but they permit more oxygen and carbon dioxide to pass through them. This is important because the cornea must "breathe" directly from the air. In addition, CAB lenses are more flexible than hard lenses and thus allow for better pumping of tears across the eye's surface. They also transmit heat more readily—a property that may have some advantages during long-term wear. These lenses tend to be more comfortable than conventional hard lenses but not as comfortable as soft lenses. Silicone lenses resemble soft lenses in their optical properties, but they are more easily cared for and more durable.

Continuous-wear lenses

The introduction of high-water-content soft lenses and gas-permeable lenses has made it possible for people to wear their lenses

24 hours a day. While the initial interest in the use of continuous-wear lenses centered around the needs of patients who had undergone cataract surgery (*see below*), the increasing safety and success of lenses that are implanted directly into the eye of cataract-surgery patients has diminished this need considerably.

A tremendous advertising campaign is under way to encourage the use of continuous-wear lenses in "normal" patients who simply wear their lenses for the correction of their nearsightedness or farsightedness. In most instances, this mode of wear is primarily for convenience.

Patients with certain types of corneal disease (dry eyes, chronic infections of the eyelid or eyeball) or who do not have easy access to medical care should not be fitted with continuous-wear lenses. Every patient considering continuous-wear lenses should be evaluated by an ophthalmologist for the presence of any medical reasons not to wear them.

Special problems

Because failures still occur with *all* types of contact lenses, a fitting should be preceded by an evaluation and counseling about the type of lens that is best in a given situation. This evaluation should include an examination of the entire eye to discover any abnormality that might make wearing lenses hazardous.

Fortunately, relatively few serious problems are associated with contact lenses. Irritation from the "overwearing syndrome" that occurs with hard lenses is temporary and heals completely—albeit with considerable discomfort. It can be prevented by wearing gas-permeable or soft lenses. Warping of the cornea (the development of an irregular curve on the surface of the eye) rarely occurs in a patient who is properly fitted and followed. Blood vessels are not normally present in the cornea (where they could interfere with clarity of vision), but they may grow in if the cornea is deprived of oxygen for a long time. Contact lenses can have this effect, but it is extremely rare with proper fitting and follow-up.

Some abnormalities are actually *better* suited to contact lenses than to conventional glasses. Keratoconus, for example, is an unusual hereditary disease in which the cornea gradually thins, protrudes, and acquires fine scars; eventually the diseased cornea may have to be replaced by a transplanted one. Glasses do not correct the visual defect, whereas contact lenses usually work well (unless

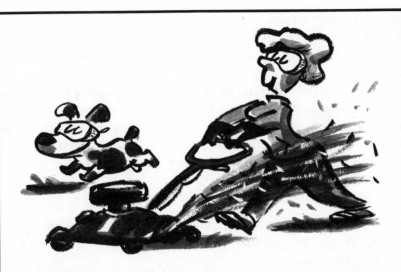

High-speed rotary tools (lawn mowers, sanders, power saws) can easily strike off a particle of wood, metal, or stone and send it deep into the eyeball. A hammer striking a chisel or wedge can do the same thing. Plastic eyewear, preferably formed with side pieces, is inexpensive and readily available. Do yourself a favor: wear a pair.

the condition is severe), thus postponing or even eliminating the need for a transplant.

An injury to the cornea can also produce irregular scarring, for which spectacles are of no value, but with contact lenses it may be possible to correct vision. For the patient who has had cataract surgery, contact lenses can provide vision very close to normal, whereas the thick lenses of cataract glasses result in annoying magnification, distortions, and limitation of peripheral vision. But because vision with contact lenses is so different from that with cataract glasses, switching back and forth creates problems. Also, uncorrected vision after cataract removal is so poor that patients have great difficulty preparing, inserting, and removing contact lenses. The most popular solution these days is an artificial lens implant. When, for whatever reasons, an implant is not desired, continuous-wear contact lenses can be an enormous boon.

Bifocal contact lenses have been available for many years as hard lenses but have met with very limited success and acceptance. Soft bifocal contact lenses, which were recently introduced, have not yet become any more popular. Fitting fees and replacement costs are significantly higher than those with conventional single-vision lenses.

Many older patients who require a separate reading prescription have benefited from an approach known as *monovision*. The dominant eye is corrected for distance and the nondominant eye is corrected for near vision with conventional single-vision contact lenses. This approach works for most but not for all patients.

The future

New materials offer exciting prospects for the future, including inexpensive lenses that can be worn for a month or so and then simply thrown away.

And here is a more speculative possibility: instant contact lenses. Imagine a liquid polymer available in a range of different viscosities. Conceivably, if we knew the curvature of a patient's cornea and the power of the lens required (easy information to obtain), we could select the appropriate polymer, put a drop of the material onto the eye, and watch it flow and harden into the shape of the desired lens.

Glaucoma

Glaucoma can be simply described as an increase in pressure within the eyeball sufficient to damage the optic nerve that carries nerve impulses from the eye to the brain. Glaucoma is one of the leading causes of blindness in the United States, afflicting an estimated 2 million Americans, and 25% of them are not aware of it. The most common form of glaucoma (over 90% of cases) causes damage to the eye without any warning symptoms until visual loss occurs. This is tragic because the damage is permanent and could have been prevented by early diagnosis and treatment. The true hazard of glaucoma is not knowing that one has the disease until it is too late.

Types of glaucoma

A complete classification for glaucoma includes over 30 different types. Glaucoma can occur in infancy or childhood, but more commonly it is a disease of middle and older age groups. While everyone agrees that increased eye pressure is the underlying problem in glaucoma, there are many reasons why such increases may occur. Glaucoma can result from injury, cataracts, or inflammation within the eye. In predisposed eyes, even medical treatment with steroids or certain drugs that dilate the pupil can cause glaucoma. The vast majority of adult cases, however, are of the so-called chronic open angle variety, which occurs in 1–2% of the population over the age of 40.

Acute glaucoma is due to obstructed fluid drainage from the outer chamber of the eye. It is relatively uncommon, but at its onset it can represent a true emergency since permanent visual loss may occur within hours. Fortunately, this type of glaucoma almost always produces symptoms pointing to serious trouble: blurring of vision, colored rings or halos around lights, plus severe eye pain and redness. (These symptoms should not be dismissed as *conjunctivitis*—"pink eye"—in which such discomfort and visual changes do not occur.) An ophthalmologist should be consulted at once. Although medical treatment may initially be effective for acute glaucoma (and is actually the treatment of choice for chronic glaucoma), surgery is generally recommended as a permanent cure for the acute, painful variety.

Unfortunately, the much more common type of glaucoma—chronic or open-angle—has no dramatic warning symptoms, and it is this type that will be the focus of the rest of this discussion.

Screening and diagnosis

Because vision lost from glaucoma cannot be regained, it is imperative that the diagnosis be made early, before such loss has developed. Although several different methods of examination are used, the following are the most important:

TONOMETRY   Most eye physicians recommend that people over 40 be screened for increased eye pressure periodically (approximately every 2 years). Those with a family history of glaucoma, or with a known history of previous eye injury or disease, should begin their regular check-ups earlier and be re-examined somewhat more frequently. The instrument most commonly used by physicians other than medical eye specialists is the *Schiotz tonometer,* which is placed directly on the front surface of the eye after anesthetic drops have been instilled. Ophthalmologists typically use a method known as *applanation tonometry,* in which a pressure probe is applied to the front surface of the eye, also in a painless manner after anesthetic drops. This technique is more accurate than Schiotz measurement, but is not widely available for screening purposes. Another device increasingly used for glaucoma detection by technicians and nonmedical eye specialists is the *air-puff tonometer*, which measures the eye pressure with a small painless burst of air against the eyeball.

EXAMINATION OF VISION AND THE EYE   When glaucoma is suspected, an ophthalmologist will examine many aspects of eye function and structure. Not only is the central vision measured by a reading chart, but the peripheral portion of the visual field is inspected for evidence of hidden areas of damage. If glaucoma is found, peripheral vision will be monitored periodically to ensure that baseline vision is preserved during treatment.

Each of the patient's eyes is then thoroughly examined in a painless manner. *Gonioscopy* involves the use of special lenses and lights to examine the internal drainage system of the eye. This examination will tell whether the pressure increase in the eye is due to angle closure (in which case surgical treatment might be necessary) or whether the drainage system is open. Appropriate treatment is based on what is revealed by gonioscopy.

The complete examination will also include an examination of the back of the eye after dilating the pupils. In particular, the eye physician will be looking for possible damage to the optic nerve and will often be able to correlate the area of visual loss with the appearance of the optic nerve and surrounding tissues. The blood vessels of the eye and the retina will also be examined to be sure that no additional disease is responsible for potential visual loss.

It is important not to label someone as having glaucoma on the basis of a single pressure reading. This is particularly true when the Schiotz or air-puff tonometer is used. Since a diagnosis of glaucoma almost automatically leads to treatment, it is important to confirm it by additional tests administered by an ophthalmologist.

Treatment

The vast majority of people with chronic glaucoma can be successfully treated with daily medications. There are several classes of drugs that are designed either to increase fluid drainage from the eye or to decrease the amount of fluid produced by the eye.

DRUGS THAT CONSTRICT THE PUPIL (MIOTICS) Until recently, the most widely used drugs for the treatment of chronic
glaucoma have been those that improve the drainage system in the
eye. Pilocarpine, the most frequently used miotic in the United
States, usually causes no significant side effects, although it may be
associated with visual blurring, especially in young people and in
older people with cataracts, because it makes the pupil small. In
addition, the small pupil lets in less light to the back of the eye,
which may cause "darker vision" in poorly lit surroundings.
Pilocarpine drops are used 3–4 times daily, usually a matter of only
slight inconvenience to the patient on a day-to-day basis.

DRUGS THAT DILATE THE PUPIL Epinephrine, another eye
drop often used to treat glaucoma, reduces the fluid produced in the
eye. This drug, too, may affect the pupil size—characteristically
dilating or widening the pupil, making vision slightly blurred and
perhaps unduly bright. It has the advantage of longer action, often
requiring use only once or twice daily. Although epinephrine is
usually well tolerated, some patients develop allergic or irritative
reactions to this medication; because the drops may be absorbed
into the circulation, heart palpitations or nervousness are sometimes experienced.

BETA-BLOCKERS In addition to its other properties (see Chapter 7), this group of drugs inhibits the secretion of the eye's aqueous
fluid and thereby reduces pressure in the eye. The drugs are administered in drop form. The majority of patients who have used
them have found the treatment comfortable, effective, and without
significant visual side effects. However, beta-blockers can be absorbed into the circulation, and care must be used in treating patients with heart disease. The first beta-blocker drops approved for
glaucoma, Timoptic, became available in 1979. Recently, several
other preparations have been introduced. Betagan can be used on a
once-a-day basis, as contrasted with the more frequent instillations
usually required for Timoptic. Betoptic causes fewer cardiac and
pulmonary side effects than Timoptic, but it may be less potent as
an anti-glaucoma drug.

As with the other eye drops, some patients will show a great
improvement in pressure and others will have very little response.
Curiously, a beta-blocker may work for just a few weeks and then
lose its effectiveness.

CARBONIC ANHYDRASE INHIBITORS   Carbonic anhydrase inhibitors such as acetazolamide (Diamox), taken by mouth, act to decrease eye-fluid production. Because of long-term side effects such as kidney stones, weakness, lethargy, and gastrointestinal disturbances, these medications are usually reserved for those in whom drops do not adequately control the intraocular pressure.

LASER SURGERY   In patients with chronic open-angle glaucoma that cannot be controlled on any medication program, laser surgery to the internal drainage system of the eye may improve its drainage capacity. Approximately 70% of patients with chronic open-angle glaucoma will have a significant lowering of the intraocular pressure after such laser treatment, often to the extent that medications may be reduced or eliminated. After several years, though, the pressure appears to build back up in a minority of the patients who have been helped. The laser treatment is applied in one or two sessions through a contact lens. As opposed to conventional surgery, there is no risk of internal infection, hemorrhage, or the development of cataract. Most ophthalmologists utilize the laser treatment only when well-tolerated medications are ineffective in controlling the pressure.

INVASIVE SURGERY   More traditional surgical techniques are reserved for glaucoma patients whose eye pressure cannot be controlled with medications, taken singly or in combination, or by laser treatment. A variety of techniques, referred to collectively as *filtration surgery,* are available to establish new drainage routes whereby fluid can leave the eye. *Cryosurgery,* a form of freezing tissues, has been used to decrease fluid formation. Glaucoma surgery is effective in decompressing the eye in well over 90% of patients.

Cataracts

A cataract is an opacity or clouding of the normally transparent lens, which is located within the eyeball, just behind the pupil and iris (*see illustration, page 231*). Such clouding often prevents the proper focusing of light onto the retina. This opacity results in the principal symptom of a cataract—blurring of vision that is often influenced by light and glare. Because there may be other reasons for visual blurring, one should have an examination by an eye physician to ensure that glaucoma, inflammation, retinal detachment, or some other disease is not present within the eye. Any one of these conditions might require more prompt attention and treatment than a cataract.

Although cataracts may be present at birth or occur in childhood (as a result of a variety of metabolic problems, injuries, or other eye diseases), the overwhelming number occur in later life. Even though certain medications, radiation, endocrine imbalances, and diabetes can cause cataract formation, most cataracts seem to occur on their own, without any evident contributing causes. *Senile cataract* is a term given to lens opacification that occurs as part of the aging process, and it should not be taken to imply any loss of mental faculties.

Treatment

Surgery remains the only definitive treatment for cataracts. Although various drops and ointments have been promoted to arrest or dissolve cataracts, none are effective. In a few instances, patients may see slightly better after their pupil has been dilated with drops; this allows them to "look around" their central cataract. But the cataract remains unchanged. In recent years, a possible role for aspirin in stabilizing early cataracts has been proposed, but further studies are needed.

The major indication for cataract surgery is vision so poor that it significantly interferes with a person's enjoyment of life. Fortunately, with the current safety and effectiveness of cataract surgery, one need not wait many months or even years until a cataract is "ripe"—a term used for a cataract so dense that nothing can be seen through it. Obviously, the desire and need for surgery will vary from person to person, depending upon his or her visual requirements. Early cataracts that cause little or no visual blurring usually are not removed and require no attention beyond a periodic examination by an eye physician. People such as draftsmen, truck drivers, and watchmakers might well require cataract surgery long before a person who is not bothered by slight visual blurring.

Although there are many different techniques for cataract removal, all require an incision into the eye, all require a period of several weeks for complete healing, and all have potential risk, such as infection, bleeding, and anesthetic complications. Fortunately, these complications are rare, and cataract surgery is successful in

95–98% of cases. There are two basic types of cataract surgery. *Intracapsular extraction* is a procedure that removes the entire lens. Often a freezing probe is used to extract the cataract through an incision into the eye near the margin of the iris. The *extracapsular extraction* method involves the removal of the central portion of the lens via a suction device. The "back" of the lens capsule, ordinarily clear, is left within the eye. In past years, the intracapsular operation was more frequently used. However, because of improved technology in the extracapsular technique, many ophthalmologists have recently shifted to this type of procedure. Occasionally, the back part of the capsule that is left behind becomes cloudy with the passage of time and needs to be opened either by a small second operation or by laser therapy. *Phacoemulsification,* a special type of extracapsular cataract operation, requires a smaller incision. The cataract is sucked out through a special needle whose tip vibrates at high frequency, fragmenting the cataract as it is removed.

Each of the different techniques for cataract extraction has particular advantages for special circumstances. The most common form of cataract surgery today provides the patient with a rapid convalescence and low risk because of new instrumentation and suture material. The decision as to which operation is best in a given patient will certainly depend upon individual considerations. The age of the patient, the type of cataract, and the presence of coexisting eye disease will often dictate the best type of operation. Where options exist, the ophthalmologist is obliged to discuss them and to point out the relative hazards as well as possible advantages of each technique. Any cataract operation, as routinely performed today, has an extremely high success rate—almost always producing an improvement of vision when no other eye disease is present.

Vision after cataract removal

Since the eye's own lens has been removed or destroyed in cataract surgery, some other method of focusing light upon the retina must be used. Glasses, contact lenses, and intraocular lenses are the three methods of providing this focusing power to the eye.

For many years, spectacle lenses were the only available way to bring the world into focus after cataract surgery. But these lenses, because of their thickness and extra power, cause objects to appear to be significantly larger and closer than the normal eye's vision.

After a cataract operation in one eye only, this difference in image size, approximately 30%, prevents the patient from using both eyes simultaneously. Thus, he may wear a spectacle correction for either the operated eye or his unoperated eye but he cannot fix an object with both eyes simultaneously, as the brain cannot bring the two disparate images together into a single three-dimensional picture.

If a contact lens is placed on the surface of the cornea of the operated eye, the image disparity between the two eyes will be reduced from the 30% level to approximately 8%, a difference that the brain can merge into a single, three-dimensional image. Also, the contact lens allows the perception of the environment as normal-sized.

Contact lenses have been so improved over the past few years that almost all patients can, with proper instruction, use them. In fact, the eye that has had cataract surgery often tolerates the contact lens better than the eye that is fitted to a contact lens for purely cosmetic reasons. Quite recently, contact lenses have been developed that may be worn not only for days but for weeks or months without removal (*see above*).

Another new and increasingly accepted method of correcting vision after a cataract operation is the *intraocular lens* (IOL). The IOL is a small, plastic lens that is placed within the eye to restore the focusing power previously provided by the patient's lens before the cataract formed. This, in theory, is the perfect solution, as there is no need for either a contact lens or glasses after cataract surgery. Indeed, many elderly patients are extremely pleased with the often dramatic improvement of vision afforded by these artificial implants. Although one might wish that such results would occur in every patient, the fact is that there are well-recognized complications caused by placing the artificial material within the eye. On a national average, the frequency of these complications is greater with IOL implantation than are the risks and failures of cataract surgery alone. Although there are many "models" of intraocular lenses, none is ideal and free of complications. Generally, IOLs are not used in eyes with other diseases or in individuals who have only one eye. In summary, when these lenses work well, as they usually do, they are fantastically effective—but when they work poorly, they may be catastrophic to the vision and even to the eye itself. Obviously the decision for an intraocular lens should not be made lightly, either by the patient or the ophthalmologist.

Glasses, contact lenses, or the intraocular lens? Again, it is necessary that the patient and his eye physician discuss thoroughly the relative advantages and disadvantages of these different methods of optical correction. All are usually successful.

Macular degeneration

One of the most familiar facts of life is that in good light, to see something most clearly, you have to look right at it. For example, you cannot read out of the corner of your eye, no matter how hard you try. The reason for this is that the eye is designed to perceive most visual detail right in the direction of gaze and to give only a general impression of the surrounding area.

Light coming into the eye is focused by the lens onto the retina, which is a thin sheet of light-sensitive cells lying against the back portion of the eyeball, somewhat like a piece of film inside a camera. But there the resemblance to a camera ends. Each of the cells in the retina acts as an independent detector, which continually tells the brain about the brightness and color of the tiny patch of light that is falling upon it at any given moment. The light detectors are most densely packed in an area that is about the size of this "O" and is located on a direct line behind the center of the lens. Called the *macula lutea* (Latin for "yellow spot"), this portion of the retina receives and analyzes light only from the very center of the visual field. The remainder of the retina has relatively few light detectors for any given area and thus cannot provide such detailed information.

A second, and extremely unhappy, fact of life is that in some people the macula is inclined to break down after 50 or 60 years of service. The reason for this is poorly understood. In almost three-quarters of cases, all that can really be said is that the macula gets thinner and its cells degenerate. Little can be done to prevent, stop, or reverse the process. However, in about 1 out of 10 cases of macular degeneration, the damage is initiated by abnormal leakage of blood from the vessels that lie beneath the retina. Subsequently, new and abnormal blood vessels form in the same area, and these new blood vessels lead to further deterioration of vision.

In 1982 a national study group of ophthalmologists showed that this type of macular degeneration can be arrested or slowed with a laser. Eye surgeons now use pinpoint beams of high-energy light to

---

▪ The sunglasses syndrome ▪

Summertime numbness and unpleasant sensations beneath the eyes, over the cheeks, inside the nose, and eventually around the upper front teeth may signal the "sunglasses syndrome." Its cause is almost certainly compression of a sensory nerve that emerges from the bone a little below each eye and about half an inch away from the nose. The rims of sunglasses, which tend to have larger lenses than ordinary glasses, may rest right on this pair of nerves, producing a special version of the pinched-nerve syndrome. This one could befuddle sunbelt doctors and dentists if they are not aware of the connection between sunglasses and numb gums.

---

cauterize the leaking vessels, thus sealing them off and deterring new vessels from forming.

The treatment only works in a minority of cases, and then only if it is applied soon after the first symptoms appear. Most people with macular degeneration, 80–90%, will not benefit from laser treatment. Those who can be helped must be identified very early, before the damage is done.

Even if laser treatment is not possible, however, there are ways to improve one's daily life. Large-type books and newspapers, bright light, and certain kinds of magnifiers or other lenses can help. No vitamins, drugs, or special diets have been shown to be effective, and there is currently no known reason to use these approaches in treating macular degeneration.

You can test yourself for possible indications of macular degeneration by asking whether fine detail in the center of vision, such as words on a page, have begun to appear blurred while the remainder of your visual field seems unchanged. You can look to see whether straight lines, for example on a piece of graph paper, appear distorted where you are looking, but not near the edges. However, these are not definitive symptoms. An ophthalmologist should be the one to make the diagnosis. Regular visits to an eye physician are a good idea after the age of 40 or so—earlier if your family tends to develop eye problems.

5 | Sex and Its Complications

Social changes and scientific advances pose both problems and possibilities in matters sexual. Birth control is a case in point: While new techniques mean more "control" over the reproductive process, these same techniques have caused concern about side effects, birth defects, and product liability. Advances in fertility treatment in recent years have raised ethical and legal questions undreamed of a generation ago. And some observers have charged that the explosion of new diseases associated with sexual activity involve as many social as medical issues.

The following discussions do not attempt to address these troublesome questions directly. Rather we simply hope to present an up-to-date factual framework for the consideration of the many personal choices that can now be made by both men and women.

Birth Control

A perfectly safe and effective method of birth control that would be acceptable to everyone has yet to be devised. But the wide range of less-than-perfect methods available can nevertheless meet the medical and social needs of most people. The following survey presents their relative advantages and disadvantages, including safety, reliability, cost, convenience, and side effects.

Least invasive, least reliable

Three of the safest and least expensive ways in which people have traditionally attempted to avoid pregnancy while still having intercourse are (1) withdrawing the penis before ejaculation (coitus interruptus), (2) flushing semen from the vagina after intercourse (post-coital douche), and (3) breast feeding (lactation). Each of these methods will reduce somewhat the chances that pregnancy will occur, but they are all extremely unreliable in the long term. Couples using these methods of birth control run a very high risk of becoming parents.

Rhythm

An equally safe and inexpensive approach is simply to avoid intercourse during the time of a woman's cycle when it might lead to pregnancy. This rhythm method of contraception is used by many couples because it is the only one approved by the Roman Catholic Church, but it is much easier said than done.

A woman is infertile at all times during her cycle except around the time of ovulation, when the egg is released from the ovary. Intercourse does not have to occur precisely on the day of ovulation to lead to a pregnancy, however. Sperm can live for 3 days or more once they are safely inside the woman's cervix, uterus, or fallopian tubes. So intercourse during the 3 days or so preceding ovulation puts a woman at risk of becoming pregnant.

Pinpointing the time of ovulation is the key to success with the rhythm method. Recording basal (morning) body temperature may help establish that ovulation has occurred, because body temperature normally rises about 0.5–0.7 degrees F within 24–36 hours after ovulation (*see p. 270 for a fuller description of the BBT*). However, determining the precise time of ovulation is difficult, even in women with regular cycles, and becomes almost impossible in women with irregular ones. And women who are usually regular will occasionally ovulate early—ovulation is not unheard of even during menstruation. Consequently, the practice of refraining from intercourse starting at 3 days prior to the time the woman is expected to ovulate may, in some cycles, put her at risk of pregnancy.

Because of these uncertainties, users of the rhythm method often err on both sides: not having sex during most of the first half of the menstrual cycle, just to play it safe, and inadvertently engaging in sex during times when the woman might become pregnant. The outcome is a high rate of unplanned pregnancies among couples who rely solely on the rhythm method.

CERVICAL MUCUS MONITORING   In an attempt to establish the time of impending ovulation, some women supplement the BBT with a daily inspection of mucus taken from the area around the cervix. Cervical mucus undergoes a number of changes over the course of the menstrual cycle, but the change that takes place just prior to ovulation is, in some women, the most dramatic. As ovulation approaches, the cervical mucus becomes first clear and slippery, and then (a day or so later) very elastic; if a bit of it is held between the thumb and forefinger, and if the thumb and forefinger are then separated, the mucus will stretch into a string. This is a sign that ovulation is about to occur.

Unfortunately, daily inspection of cervical mucus is not a practical approach to birth control for most women. It requires instruction in how to evaluate changes in cervical mucus, as well as a high degree of conscientiousness in monitoring the changes and then abstaining from sex when there is any doubt. This is not likely to become a popular or very effective means of birth control, despite its advantages over rhythm alone.

Other methods of pinpointing "safe" periods for intercourse are often promoted, but their long-term track records are, at best, mediocre.

Improving the odds

Contraceptives that work by killing sperm or presenting a barrier to their entry into the uterus are more effective than the traditional methods described above, though less effective than the pill, the intrauterine device, and sterilization (*see table*). Barrier/spermicide methods are in general also quite safe, not very expensive, and usually free of side effects. They do have disadvantages, however.

Condoms

Condoms can be psychologically distracting, they can dull sensation, and, rarely, they can break or leak. But condoms offer a good measure of protection from sexually transmitted diseases, and are simple to use and inexpensive to buy. Using a condom is also one of the few steps the *male* partner can take to prevent an unwanted pregnancy.

Spermicidal agents

A wide variety of vaginal creams, jellies, foams, and suppositories kill sperm directly or present a physical barrier to their passage.

▪ How sure is your method? ▪

Method	Lowest observed annual rate of pregnancy (%)	Annual pregnancy rate among typical users (%)
Sterilization (vasectomy or tubal ligation)	0.4	0.4
Pill		
Combination estrogen/progestin	0.5	2
Progestin only (mini-pill)	1	2.5
IUD	1.5	5
Condom (no spermicide)	2	10
Sponge	9–11	10–20
Diaphragm (with spermicide)	2	19
Spermicide (alone)	3–5	20
Rhythm	2–20	24
Withdrawal	16	23
Douching	—	40
Chance (no method)	—	90

Source: Planned Parenthood.

Despite the claims of their manufacturers, these spermicides are not a reliable method of birth control when used alone. But used in conjunction with a condom or diaphragm, they can be quite effective. The tablets and suppositories require several minutes for adequate distribution throughout the vagina before protection is afforded. Some women will experience local tissue irritation from these agents, but in general side effects are not a problem.

Diaphragm

Used in combination with a spermicidal preparation (jelly or cream applied to both sides of the diaphragm), this device offers good protection from pregnancy. Its disadvantages are that it requires careful fitting by a physician, it must be inserted before intercourse, and the cream or jelly entails a certain degree of messiness.

Contraceptive sponge

In the spring of 1983, yet another kind of contraceptive came on the market—the sponge. Sold under the trade name Today, it is currently available throughout the United States; it is relatively safe and uncomplicated to use.

The device is exactly what its name suggests: a sponge (one size fits all), which is made of polyurethane. The plastic framework of the sponge is permeated with nonoxynol-9, a spermicide. Once the sponge is thoroughly moistened and becomes sudsy with the activated chemical, it is ready for use. Over the next 24 hours, the spermicide continues to be released, providing protection for that period. There is no need to put any further medication in the vagina, even if the woman has intercourse more than once. The sponge should be left in place for at least 6 hours *after* the last intercourse, but not, according to recommendations, for longer than 24 hours. However, if intercourse occurs at 24 hours, the sponge should be left in place for 6 more hours.

The advantages of this product are that it can be bought over-the-counter, without a physician's prescription; it is easy to use; and it is less messy than other vaginal preparations. Moreover, complications appear to be quite minor. Local irritation of the vagina is the most common complaint from users. Less frequently reported problems are fragmentation of the sponge and difficulty removing it. Use of the sponge according to directions has not been associated with any greater risk of toxic shock syndrome than use of standard tampons.

Although the sponge is clearly better than nothing, and in many ways more convenient than other forms of contraception, it is not as reliable as some of the other methods. Pregnancy rates have been reported to be as high as 20% in women who rely on the sponge. As with most vaginal methods, the more compulsively one uses the product, the more effective it is.

Higher tech

IUD

When IUDs (intrauterine devices) were first popularized as a form of female contraception in the 1960s, some advocates were almost euphoric in suggesting that IUDs were the "ideal" form of contraception—safe and effective. Now, several decades later, the record indicates that IUDs are neither perfectly safe nor completely effective in preventing pregnancy. However, reports concerning the dangers of IUDs may also create misleading impressions.

IUDs rank second only to the pill in practical effectiveness, but they are not foolproof. About 5% of women using them will become pregnant. However, that degree of effectiveness, combined with the fact that no further action is required once the IUD is inserted, has made the IUD the contraceptive choice for between 15–20 million women worldwide.

Since January 1986, the only IUD available in the United States has been the Progestasert—an IUD which contains a synthetic female hormone (progestin) that is slowly released for added contraceptive effect. However, unlike medicinal IUDs containing copper, which had to be replaced only every 3 years, the Progestasert IUD must be replaced yearly to maintain its contraceptive potency. Therefore, before removal of the copper IUD from the marketplace, it was favored over the Progestasert IUD by a 20:1 margin.

Copper-bearing devices—and Lippes Loops—were withdrawn by manufacturers from the U.S. marketplace because of liability concerns and difficulty obtaining insurance. Some experts predict an increased pregnancy rate in this country as women use other, less reliable methods of contraception; some American women are traveling to Canada and other countries to obtain the IUD of their choice.

The past record of IUD safety can be put in perspective by pointing out that the overall risk of dying from pregnancy or delivery is about 20 times greater than that of dying from complications associated with IUD use. However, this "perspective" should not divert attention from the real dangers of IUD use, including:

BLEEDING AND CRAMPING While not life-threatening, these complications lead to the removal of the IUD in about 1 out of 5 women during the first year of use. The addition of either copper or progestin (for added contraceptive effect) permitted smaller IUDs to be designed, making insertion easier and causing less bleeding and cramping.

INFECTIONS On average, women using the IUD have a 3–5 times increased chance of pelvic inflammatory disease (PID), compared with nonusers. These infections of the reproductive tract are usually easily treated, but they may lead to subsequent infertility, chronic discomfort, and, very rarely, death. Because of the risk of infertility—and because infections are more likely to occur in younger women who have not had children—many experts advise other forms of contraception for women under age 25 and those who wish to have children at a future date.

PERFORATION The exact incidence of perforation (puncture of the uterus by the IUD) is unknown but is thought to be quite rare— approximately 1 per 2,000 users. The reason that the incidence is unknown is that perforation may cause no symptoms and go undiscovered until the next check-up. Abdominal surgery to remove the IUD may be required.

The pill

The introduction of "the pill" in the late 1950s revolutionized birth control in this country and throughout most of the world. However, by the 1970s the pill had fallen into relative disfavor as serious side effects among pill users began to appear. Now, in the 1980s, the medical reputation of the pill is being rehabilitated by newer evidence suggesting that, in modern versions, it is not only safer but may actually offer protection against some serious health problems.

The contraceptive pills prescribed in the United States today contain combinations of the female hormone estrogen and the synthetic hormone progestin (a close relative of progesterone, the other major female hormone). This combination of hormones prevents pregnancy by upsetting the normal sequence of events that lead to ovulation (release of the egg from the ovary).

In women who are not taking birth control pills, the ovary produces precise amounts of estrogen at precise times during the first half of the cycle. The pituitary gland is stimulated by these bursts of estrogen to produce other hormones that, in turn, trigger ovulation. Following ovulation, the ovary produces progesterone, which prepares the uterus for the implantation of a fertilized egg. When the sequence of events leading up to ovulation is upset by the added hormones contained in birth control pills, the pituitary gland does not respond properly and ovulation does not occur.

Because the female reproductive system is so complex and so tightly regulated, the addition of very little extra hormone can unbalance the system and suppress ovulation. Consequently, the amounts of estrogen and progestin used in most birth control pills available today are much less than those in the original pill released in 1959. This reduction of hormones is expected to reduce the risk of possible side effects, which can include the following:

STROKES   There is a slight, but definite, increased risk of blood-clot formation in women who use the pill. Put in perspective, the overall risk of death from blood clots in pill users has been about 1.5 per 100,000 under age 35 and 4 per 100,000 over age 35, versus 0.2 and 0.5 respectively in those who do not use the pill. This small excess risk must be weighed against the overall death rate from pregnancy and delivery (excluding illegal abortions), which is about 22 per 100,000, and against the fact that the pill, properly used, is the most effective reversible method currently available for preventing pregnancy.

HEART ATTACKS   Data from British studies suggest that women over 40 using the pill are at higher risk for heart attacks, especially if traditional risk factors, such as smoking and high blood pressure, are also present. However, other studies suggest that smoking is the major culprit and that the increased risk of a heart attack attributed to the pill occurs almost exclusively among smokers using the pill.

TUMORS   Animal and human studies have indicated that certain female hormones may cause changes in breast and uterine tissue. However, the evidence to date indicates that the combination birth control pill currently used does *not* cause cancer of either organ. Since growth of certain tumors of the breast is stimulated by hormones, the use of birth control pills is not advised for women with a past history of breast cancer.

Tumors (adenomas) of the liver have been reported in women who have taken oral contraceptives for many years. These tumors are rarely malignant, but they can be dangerous because of their tendency to bleed into the abdominal cavity. In some instances the bleeding has been fatal. The incidence of liver tumors is exceedingly rare, but any woman taking the pill should be alert to the fact that onset of severe pain in the upper right abdomen demands prompt medical attention.

OTHER EFFECTS   Many other side effects may be caused by the pill—including high blood pressure, obesity, depression, headache, nausea, breast engorgement, and acne (although in some women the pill can have just the opposite effect and improve acne). Often these side effects can be eliminated by changing to a different pill. But women with the following problems should not use any form of oral contraceptive:

- A strong family history of stroke
- Evidence of vascular disease of the brain
- Heart, liver, or kidney disease
- Thrombophlebitis
- Breast or uterine cancer

Women should not start using the pill until a thorough medical history has been taken and a physical examination performed.

THE BENEFITS   New information from ongoing studies of pill risks indicate that the pill may actually *protect* women against some conditions. Although details vary, there is consistent evidence that pill use reduces the risk of ovarian and uterine cancers by about half; the Centers for Disease Control recently estimated that pill use prevents almost 4,000 cases of these cancers in the U.S. each year. Taking the pill may also protect against benign breast tumors.

Pill users appear to develop infection of the reproductive tract (pelvic inflammatory disease, or PID) at one-third to one-half the rate of nonusers. And since PID can lead to considerable and chronic discomfort as well as infertility, this benefit is of major

---

▪ Missing a pill ▪

Can a woman get pregnant if she misses only a single contraceptive pill? Doctors have tended to doubt this claim when made by patients who are taking the combined low-dose formulation that is now commonly used. But a recent study indicates that missing a pill, especially during the first 7 days after a new pack is begun, could indeed be all it takes to permit ovulation. The authors suggest that a woman who misses a pill during the first week of a new cycle use an additional means of contraception during that cycle. Simply taking two pills the next day, as is usually recommended, may not provide adequate protection. A missed pill later in the cycle probably is not so significant but also requires using another method of contraception to maximize protection.

importance. Also, for reasons not clear, pill users have about one-quarter the risk of toxic shock syndrome.

Some observers believe that pill use may protect against rheumatoid arthritis—perhaps one of the reasons why the frequency of this disease has decreased among American women since the mid-1960s.

In addition, the pill reduces the pain and bleeding of menstruation for some women. Indeed, the pill is often prescribed for this purpose rather than for contraception as such.

Other types of birth control pills

Birth control pills other than the estrogen-progesterone combination have been developed in recent years. Their mode of action is different from that of the conventional pill, in that they interfere with pregnancy at a later stage than ovulation. The personal dilemmas and societal controversies raised by the problem of preventing or terminating an unwanted pregnancy are likely to be intensified by these new pills.

MINI-PILL   This pill is composed of small amounts of progestin alone. The exact way in which it prevents pregnancy is not known —instead of suppressing ovulation, it may prevent implantation of the fertilized egg or it may work in some other way. In any case, it is not as reliable as the combination pill, but it is an alternative for women who cannot tolerate estrogen. The only disadvantages are a slightly higher pregnancy rate and, in most women, irregular bleeding and spotting.

MORNING-AFTER PILL   This birth control pill contains diethylstilbesterol (DES) and is taken for 5 days *after* unprotected intercourse, before a woman knows whether or not she has conceived. DES is thought to prevent pregnancy by interfering with implantation of the fertilized egg in the uterus. Most women develop nausea from these pills. Moreover, DES can cause abnormalities in a fetus whose conception the drug fails to prevent. When this happens, some women may wish to consider a therapeutic abortion.

MISSED-PERIOD PILL   These pills are taken within a few days after the first missed period signaling that a woman is possibly pregnant. If a woman *is* pregnant, the pills cause an abortion by blocking the action of the hormone progesterone, which normally prepares the lining of the uterus (endometrium) to accept the fertilized egg and then nourish it throughout the pregnancy. If the progesterone level falls during pregnancy, or if the hormone is blocked from acting on the endometrium, menstruation will be triggered and the embryo will be sloughed along with the uterine lining. The active ingredient in missed-period pills brings about just this sequence of events by occupying the endometrium's receptor sites for progesterone, and thereby causing a miscarriage.

The medication which has received the most attention thus far is RU 486, a synthetic anti-progesterone. This drug, when taken very early in pregnancy, is both safe and effective in most women. As medications of this type become available, they will make possible the "home abortions" that pro-choice proponents advocate and anti-abortionists oppose. RU 486 is not yet approved for sale in the United States.

Sterilization procedures

Tubal ligation in females (procedures that interrupt the continuity of the fallopian tubes which transport the eggs to the uterus; *see illustration, p. 268*) and *vasectomy* in males (procedures that block the vas deferens which transports sperm from the testis; *see illustration, p. 267*) are described as methods of "permanent contraception." Both procedures offer the great advantage of almost 100% effectiveness with no further concern about contraception. It is now possible to "reverse" as many as 70% of vasectomies and 30% of tubal ligations by micro-surgical techniques. But persons undergoing these procedures should regard them as permanent and should not expect them to be reversible.

Both procedures are relatively safe, although bleeding and infection sometimes occur. In general, a vasectomy is a simpler and less costly procedure than tubal ligation. Some males experience psychological impotence after a vasectomy until they understand that the procedure does not involve any impairment of male hormone levels or physical sexual performance.

The concern that vasectomy might predispose to atherosclerosis—and a consequent increased risk for heart disease—arose a few years ago, based on studies performed on monkeys. Good data from long-term studies on human subjects have recently become available, and they strongly suggest that men differ from monkeys, at least as far as vasectomy risks are concerned. Among men enrolled in the University of Washington Exercise Testing Registry, those who had undergone vasectomy (on average, 15 years prior to the study) showed no higher risk for coronary disease than non-vasectomized subjects.

In another report, investigators who examined 10,590 vasectomized men could find no increased risk of heart disease in comparison with matched controls. Over 2,000 of the subjects were studied more than 10 years after vasectomy. Vasectomized men were also found to have no increased risk for a variety of diseases believed to be caused by immunological disturbances. (These diseases were looked for because antibodies to sperm appear after vasectomy, and there has been speculation that such antibodies could somehow trigger an attack on the body's own tissues.) The only apparent problem that could be attributed to vasectomy was local inflammation of sperm ducts (epididymitis), but this complication was infrequent and usually of brief duration.

Sexually Transmitted Diseases

Even as recently as the 1960s, the subject of sexually transmitted diseases (STDs) was considered straightforward. Venereal disease (so named for Venus, the goddess of love) encompassed 5 well-known diseases, the two most important being syphilis and gonorrhea. The identification and treatment of these diseases may have been difficult for social reasons, but they were reasonably well understood medically.

The 1970s, however, produced a revolution in "venereology." Currently, over 20 different germs associated with sexually transmitted diseases have been identified. And concern is now directed toward the role of STDs in causing birth defects, infertility, long-term disability, and death.

Gonorrhea and NGU

Unlike syphilis, gonorrhea still cannot be detected with a blood test, despite years of intensive research. Therefore, accurate diagnosis of gonorrhea requires obtaining material (via a cotton-tipped swab) from appropriate locations and then looking under the microscope or, particularly in women where microscopic examination is often unreliable, growing the bacteria from specimens under laboratory conditions.

Because of these more cumbersome diagnostic techniques, past practice often boiled down to treating suspicious symptoms (painful urination and milky discharge—a condition called *urethritis*) with penicillin. However, three developments have called this approach into question:

- the emergence of strains of gonorrhea resistant to penicillin;
- the realization that both men and women can harbor gonorrhea without obvious symptoms; and
- the rapid spread of another sexually transmitted disease, *nongonococcal urethritis* (NGU)—inflammation of the urethra that cannot be traced to the bacterium that causes gonorrhea. Up to half of all cases of NGU are caused by the chlamydia organism (*see below*), which does not respond to penicillin but can be treated with other antibiotics.

The safest course for sexually active men and women to follow is to be screened periodically for gonorrhea, whether or not they show symptoms of STD. If the culture for gonorrhea is negative in a person who has symptoms, treatment for chlamydia or one of the other organisms that can cause NGU should be undertaken. Most cases of NGU respond to tetracycline or erythromycin.

Chlamydia infections

Chlamydia is currently the major cause of sexually transmitted disease in the United States. Estimates are that over 10 million cases of STD are caused by this organism—sometimes in conjunction with other diseases, such as gonorrhea, syphilis, or herpes.

Men

Men with chlamydia are most likely to develop inflammation of the urethra (urethritis). Mostly, they feel burning on urination, and a mild discharge may be apparent. Traditionally, this complaint has suggested gonorrhea—which is, to be sure, a reasonable diagnosis. However, gonorrhea causes but a fraction of all cases of urethritis; chlamydia causes more.

Up to a third of all men with chronic chlamydia infections of the urethra have no symptoms. Untreated, they continue to transmit the disease. About half the cases of infection of the epididymis, the tube that leads out of the testicle, also result from chlamydial infection—that's about 250,000 a year. Rectal infection with chlamydia can also occur as a result of anal intercourse.

Women

Women develop nagging infections with chlamydia—most commonly in the cervix. About half of all cases of cervicitis (usually the form known as *mucopurulent cervicitis*) are caused by this bug. About 3–5% of *all* young, healthy women have chlamydia in the cervix, as do 5–10% of pregnant women, and 25% of women visiting STD clinics. The infection is especially likely to occur in women who are young, economically disadvantaged, very active sexually, and on birth control pills.

Symptoms of chlamydial infection may include vaginal discharge, intermittent vaginal bleeding, abdominal discomfort, or pain on urination. But there may be no symptoms, and this is the major danger.

A chlamydia infection may travel upward into the uterus, where it can remain symptomless ("silent") for some time. Then, during labor or shortly after a woman has given birth, the infection may flare up and cause complications. About 60–70% of infected mothers pass the organism along to their baby during the birth process. A fairly minor infection of the baby's eye (conjunctivitis) is the most common result, but pneumonia serious enough to require hospitalization is also possible. Chlamydial pneumonia affects around 30,000 newborns in this country every year.

When chlamydia ascends further, to the fallopian tubes and ovaries, it produces a chronic infection known as *pelvic inflammatory disease* (PID). Current estimates indicate that chlamydia accounts for 250,000–500,000 cases of PID each year in the United States. PID, especially if it is prolonged or repeated, can lead to scarring of the tubes and infertility.

About 10% of women become infertile after 1 bout of PID, 30% after 2 episodes, and 50% or more after 3. When PID is caused by chlamydia, the rates of damage are thought to be even higher. Accurate numbers are hard to come by, because chlamydial infection is so often silent. That very fact is what makes the infection so much more destructive than other types of PID (such as gonorrhea). Diagnosis and treatment are often delayed until after scarring of the fallopian tubes has occurred.

Sometimes, tubal scarring from PID can lead to an ectopic pregnancy—meaning that the embryo has implanted outside the uterus. If implantation occurs in a tube, the embryo—and often the tube—will have to be surgically removed. Tubal pregnancies that are not promptly diagnosed and terminated go on to rupture the tube and produce potentially life-threatening hemorrhage.

The symptoms of chlamydial infection seem disproportionately mild, compared with the danger it represents for a woman's reproductive health. Some women have high fevers, severe abdominal pain, and vomiting, but others may have only vague discomfort—or none at all. The major unanswered question at present is whether screening asymptomatic women at the time of a Pap smear, and treating those with chlamydia, would reduce the rate of subsequent infertility. Research addressing this problem is under way.

Diagnosis and treatment

One important clue to the presence of chlamydial infection is a negative result when specimens are cultured for bacteria by standard techniques. Because chlamydia organisms refuse to grow outside human cells, they can only be detected by special methods. Finding another STD germ on culture doesn't prove that chlamydia is absent, however. Chlamydia too often goes unnoticed because something else seems to explain the symptoms.

Chlamydial infection of the reproductive organs can be effectively treated, but relapse is common for several reasons. Among antibiotics, tetracycline and erythromycin are the mainstays of therapy; sulfa drugs can also be used. These drugs are taken orally for 1–3 weeks, depending on the condition being treated. Failing to take a full course of drug can lead to relapse. Sometimes, though, antibiotics fail even when taken properly—probably because they do not reach a few chlamydia organisms that are resting inside cells. Also, natural defenses against these bugs are not terribly vigorous and thus don't help the antibiotics do their job.

Another important reason for treatment failures is the high likelihood that a patient's sexual partner or partners will continue to carry chlamydia. Everybody who is interacting sexually has to be treated to eradicate the organism, and for a variety of practical or emotional reasons, this can be difficult to achieve.

Obviously, chlamydia should be considered whenever other genital infections are found. But cultures for chlamydia are expensive and aren't always positive even when the organism is present. Since treatment is inexpensive and generally safe, the best course may be to treat all people who are at high statistical risk—those who have gonorrhea or PID, women who have mucopurulent cervicitis, and the sexual contacts of people who have symptoms suggesting chlamydial infection.

Herpes simplex infections

The herpes simplex virus is increasingly implicated as a common cause of STD. The herpes family includes many viruses. The two that often go by the casual name of "herpes" are herpes zoster, which causes chickenpox in kids and shingles in adults, and herpes simplex, which causes clusters of small red lumps that soon turn into painful blisters. The simplex viruses are further divided into two types: usually, type 1 (HSV-1) is associated with blisters around the lips (where they are known as cold or fever sores), while type 2 (HSV-2) is found in blisters on the genitalia and sometimes the buttocks and thighs.

Up to 10 million Americans harbor the HSV-2 virus, and it is easily spread by sexual contact. Indeed, HSV-2 is now a contender for the most common sexually transmitted disease in this country. Unlike gonorrhea, which can usually be eradicated by simple antibiotic treatment, there is no effective cure for herpes. However, the introduction of acyclovir therapy has reduced the suffering of many victims of genital herpes.

Available since February 1985 (under the trade name Zovirax), oral acyclovir, like its predecessors, speeds the healing of the initial attack of genital herpes. In addition, the capsules have a special role in protecting against recurrences of herpes. For people who suffer frequent and severe herpes attacks, continued daily use of acyclovir capsules may markedly reduce the number of episodes. Episodes that do occur are more likely to be mild.

Acyclovir works by preventing the herpes virus from spreading to uninfected cells. It does not eradicate the virus. Once the drug is discontinued, attacks start up again, and the first such episode is often notably severe. As with almost all drugs, infrequent side effects may occur. Such problems have included occasional headaches, stomach upsets, dizziness, muscle aches, fever, rash, and sleep disturbances.

The possibility that acyclovir will be used widely and indiscriminately raises the worry that resistant strains of the virus will soon emerge. Just as some bacteria have become resistant to penicillin, viruses such as herpes can elude the effects of antiviral drugs. The greater their exposure to these drugs, the more rapidly viruses acquire this talent. In fact, some degree of resistance to acyclovir has already been noted, and only time will tell just how important the problem will become.

Many investigators have speculated that acyclovir capsules could be used to protect against transmission of the herpes virus during sexual intercourse. As yet, there is no evidence to show that by taking acyclovir the person with herpes can become less infectious to a sexual partner than would otherwise be the case. And no data support the notion that someone who has not been infected could use acyclovir the "morning after" or "evening before" to protect against acquiring the disease.

At present, oral acyclovir is approved only for the treatment of severe, first attacks of herpes and for suppressing flares that are both frequent and disruptive. Milder forms of herpes should not be treated with the drug.

Pregnant women and nursing mothers should not take acyclovir because the effect on the fetus or infant is not known. It *is* known, however, that herpes infection acquired during passage through the birth canal can cause severe, permanent neurological damage—and even death—in the newborn. Therefore, a cesarean section is strongly recommended if active herpes is present in the birth canal at the time of delivery.

It has long been recognized that cervical cancer is more common among women who have intercourse with many partners or begin sexual activity at a very early age. Many researchers now think that HSV-2 is one of the infectious links between sexual intercourse and cervical cancer. Women infected with HSV-2 are 8 times more likely to develop cervical cancer than women not infected. Therefore, periodic Pap smears are particularly important for this group.

Acquired immunodeficiency syndrome (AIDS)

- In 1978 AIDS was unknown.
- By the beginning of 1987, 30,000 cases had been reported in the United States, with over 17,000 fatalities.
- Approximately 300,000 persons are expected to develop AIDS by 1991, if its growth rate remains unchecked.

The principal route of spread of AIDS is through sexual intercourse, although it can be transmitted by blood or blood products. Infected men can transmit it to women through either vaginal or anal intercourse. It is now established that women can also transmit it to men through sexual intercourse; how frequently this happens is unknown and is a matter of intense debate.

For every person in the United States who has AIDS, there are 40–50 who are carrying the virus but do not know it. In this situation, preventing spread of the illness will obviously be very difficult, particularly as two main routes of transmission are sexual intercourse and drug use via shared intravenous needles.

Implications for the sexually active

Ultimately, a vaccine will be the surest way to prevent infection with the AIDS virus. Research efforts are under way, and there is reason to hope that a vaccine can be produced. But it isn't a sure thing, and development may very well take a long time. Pending development of a vaccine, prevention of the virus' spread is the only way that the scope of this tragedy can be limited.

The first recommendation that is usually made is to reduce one's number of sexual contacts. In itself, as a strategy of self-protection, this approach has somewhat limited value in the group at highest risk. Although multiple sexual contacts were a typical feature of the homosexually active men who originally developed the disease, this behavior pattern is no longer a consistent feature of patients with AIDS. When the virus was still rare, obviously the people who had most opportunities for exposure were most likely to encounter it. But as the virus has become more prevalent, exposure is likely to occur after progressively fewer contacts with potential carriers. Thus, in recent surveys, the number of sexual contacts reported by homosexually active men with antibodies to the AIDS virus does not appear to be significantly greater than the number reported by men without evidence of exposure to the virus.

- The AIDS virus is transmitted by blood, semen, and (probably) vaginal fluid. Physical contact does not transmit the virus without exposure to one of these fluids. Thus, casual, occupational, or household contact is safe.
- There is no known reason to fear spread by insects, by objects that an infected person has touched, or by coughs and sneezes.
- Transmission through IV drug use can be prevented by not sharing needles or by sterilizing needles and syringes with Clorox solution or boiling water.
- Intercourse, anal or vaginal, is the sexual practice most likely to transmit the virus.
- Sexual activities that do not involve exposing a mucous membrane (rectum, vagina, mouth) to body fluids are presumed to be safe.
- Completely monogamous relationships between uninfected people are safe.
- "Knowing your partner" is not as easy as it sounds. Establishing whether a partner has been, or is likely to have been, exposed to AIDS is very difficult. Screening tests are fallible.
- Use of condoms is strongly encouraged. Laboratory evidence indicates that an intact condom prevents the virus from passing. How much safety condoms provide during actual use is not known. However, it seems very probable that they work well when properly employed. Condoms should not be used with oil-based lubricants, which dissolve the latex. If the condom is not snugly fitted to the penis, it may be more likely to break.
- A single behavior may be regarded as "low, but not zero, risk." If such behavior is frequently repeated, the cumulative risk of transmitting the virus increases.
- Much remains to be learned about AIDS prevention.

Whether the same evolving pattern of risk is repeating itself with heterosexually active people is not clear. Currently many prostitutes in large metropolitan areas are infected with the AIDS virus. The principal reason may be simply that prostitutes are exposed to many sexual partners. If so, then as the virus becomes more prevalent, the proportion of affected women with fewer sexual partners will begin to increase. On the other hand, if prostitutes are affected by other factors, such as drug use with shared needles, that trend may not be observed.

What this implies is that diminishing the number of one's sexual contacts in itself is likely to be a partially effective strategy of self-protection in populations where the AIDS virus is rare (currently still the case among heterosexually active individuals). As carriers of the virus become more common, however, reducing the number of one's new sexual contacts to any number greater than zero no longer provides much protection.

It is true that celibacy or strictly monogamous relationships are strategies that will effectively prevent transmission of AIDS. But it is at best naive to rely on advocating these forms of sexual conduct as the principal public health measure against AIDS. Nothing in the history of sexually transmitted diseases suggests that upholding certain social or moral ideals is sufficient to prevent these diseases from spreading.

PRACTICAL GUIDELINES   The AIDS virus is transmitted in body fluids that are likely to be exchanged during sexual contact. People who are sexually active (that is, having sexual relations outside a securely monogamous relationship of several years' standing), and those with a single partner who may be sexually active, should take measures to protect themselves from transfer of body fluids. In essence, this means avoiding oral exposure to semen and using a condom during intercourse, as there is reasonably persuasive evidence that condoms provide a barrier to the transfer of viruses. Whether anal intercourse is more likely than vaginal to damage the condom membrane and reduce the level of protection is not known. Spermicidal creams are sometimes germicidal; whether they destroy the AIDS virus when used during intercourse is not known, but in conjunction with a condom they may add a measure of protection. Use of petrolatum-based lubricants (such as Vaseline) with condoms is not recommended, as the oil dissolves the latex of the condom.

Infertility

The expectation of parenting is usually implicit in the decision to marry. When the time arrives to conceive a first (or second) child, failure usually comes as a rude shock. Cycle after cycle of anticipation yields to disappointment, and then to an appointment with the doctor. Thus begins the "infertility work-up"—a potentially long, expensive, and draining experience—one that can take its toll on even the most stable relationship.

The basics of human reproduction

Like a computer, reproduction requires not only an intricate mechanism but the "software" to control it. Both must be in working order if a pregnancy is to be established. The mechanism consists of the reproductive organs; the software is the set of hormones, regulated by portions of the brain, that program events leading to fertilization.

The simpler design belongs to the male. The primary features of male anatomy—the testes, epididymis, vas deferens, and penis (*see illustration*)—are geared to one goal: producing healthy, energetic sperm and getting them into the proper location to fertilize an egg. But simplicity doesn't guarantee success: In 40% of infertility cases the problem can be traced to the man alone; in another 40%, the difficulty appears to be solely the woman's, and in the remaining

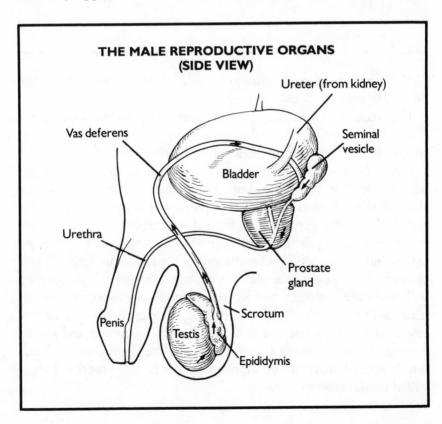

THE MALE REPRODUCTIVE ORGANS
(SIDE VIEW)

Ureter (from kidney)

Vas deferens

Seminal vesicle

Bladder

Urethra

Prostate gland

Scrotum

Penis

Testis

Epididymis

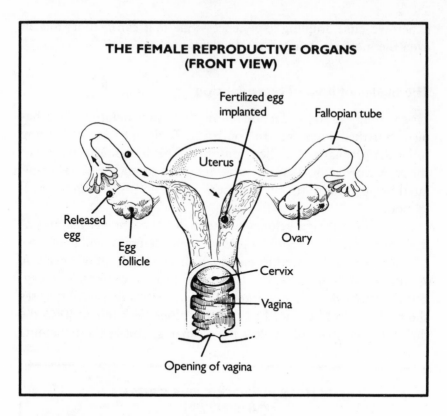

**THE FEMALE REPRODUCTIVE ORGANS
(FRONT VIEW)**

Fertilized egg
implanted

Fallopian tube

Uterus

Released
egg

Egg
follicle

Ovary

Cervix

Vagina

Opening of vagina

20% both partners contribute to the difficulty with conception—or no explanation is found.

The woman's reproductive system has more complicated design features than the man's, and it requires much more elaborate control of its timing. A mature egg is produced monthly by one of the two ovaries, under supervision of 4 principal hormones. Once released, the egg begins a short but somewhat perilous voyage through the fallopian tube to reach the uterus (*see illustration*). If it encounters viable sperm on its way, it will probably be fertilized.

Sperm, entering through the vagina, swim upstream through the cervix and uterus (a little like salmon) to the fallopian tubes. There, only one from among the millions of sperm that began the journey will penetrate the egg's surface and enter to combine the father's genes with the mother's. Thus fertilized, the egg continues its progress to the uterus. There it finds a point of attachment and stimulates the mother's tissue to provide a suitable connection through which nourishment can be supplied for the next 9 months. This is called *implantation*.

Damage to the woman's reproductive structures or poorly synchronized production of hormones can interfere with this process.

Hormones and the menstrual cycle

Hormones are signal molecules produced in various places, such as the brain, ovaries, and testes. The hormones that, to a large extent, control production of sperm and eggs are called *gonadotropins*. They originate in the pituitary gland, a pea-sized extension of the brain located an inch or so behind the bridge of the nose. Men and women produce the same two pituitary hormones. The sexes differ, though, in that each produces a different set of *gonadal* hormones in response to stimulation by the pituitary gonadotropins: testosterone in the male, estrogen and progesterone in the woman.

The first half of a menstrual cycle is governed by *follicle stimulating hormone* (FSH) from the pituitary, which stimulates development of an ovum and, meanwhile, tells the ovary to produce estrogen. At about day 12 of the cycle, FSH levels wane, and a second pituitary hormone, *luteinizing hormone* (LH), takes over. This hormonal shift switches the ovary from a "production" to a "release" mode. The mature egg is now permitted to pop out of the ovary. Simultaneously, the *follicle*, a group of cells that surrounded the ripening egg, is triggered to release progesterone. During this phase, the follicle is called the *corpus luteum* (or "yellow body," after the color it acquires from its high content of hormonal material).

With estrogen, progesterone encourages the lining of the uterus to prepare a lush, thick blanket of blood vessels in preparation for arrival of the fertilized egg. About 2 weeks after the corpus luteum is formed, it stops making progesterone. If an embryo has implanted, the *placenta* (an organ that develops during pregnancy to serve as a way to transfer nutrients and waste products between the fetus and the mother) rapidly begins producing its own progesterone. Otherwise, menstruation (loss of the uterine lining) begins. Then, after several days, the cycle resumes.

It's not surprising that this elaborate system of "do this, do that" signals doesn't work every time. Indeed, it's remarkable that 15% of couples trying to conceive do so in the first month, 63% within 6 months, and 80% by a year. With these statistics in mind, the standard recommendation is to wait a year before assuming that fertility is impaired.

Beginning the infertility work-up

The medical evaluation starts by focusing on the most common causes of infertility. A thorough medical history and physical examination of both partners will often provide a strong clue as to the source of the problem. With a little luck, it may turn out to be something as uncomplicated as bad timing.

Timing of intercourse

There is a relatively narrow window of opportunity in each cycle when the egg may be fertilized, so it is important to establish that intercourse takes place at the appropriate time. Intercourse does not have to occur precisely on the day of ovulation, however. Once sperm are safely inside the cervix, uterus, or fallopian tubes, they can survive up to 72 hours while waiting for the egg to emerge. So intercourse a few days before ovulation will still expose the egg to sperm. In a 28-day cycle, this means that the time between days 12 and 15 is approximately the fertile part of the cycle.

For women whose cycles are longer or shorter than 28 days, timing intercourse can be more of a challenge. A widely used method to identify the fertile interval is charting the *basal body temperature,* or BBT. (A special, sensitive thermometer for measuring BBT can be purchased from pharmacies.) Temperature is recorded first thing every morning, before any activity, such as making love, getting up, or going to the bathroom.

Just before ovulation, the BBT will usually dip slightly. Then just after ovulation, the BBT will rise about half a degree Fahrenheit and maintain that approximate temperature until just before menstruation, when it falls again. All these changes result from fluctuations in hormone levels, and they have the irritating feature that they are most obvious *after* ovulation. Thus, using them to detect ovulation is a little like being told, "Watch me and get off the bus at the stop before I do."

However, at the end of several cycles, a woman and her doctor can look back over the temperature charts and make reasonable guesses as to when ovulation took place during those months, and thus predict future cycles. These are indeed guesses, because BBT is not an infallible guide. Many physicians urge patients not to keep BBT charts longer than a few months, to avoid adding unneeded psychological pressures to an already tense situation.

Male factors

The medical evaluation of the male partner focuses on sperm production and delivery. The physician first checks the testes for potential abnormalities; then semen, produced by masturbation, is analyzed. Microscopic examination of the ejaculate can reveal the number, shape, and motion of sperm, the volume of the semen, and its chemical composition.

The number of sperm may be low (a condition called *oligospermia*) or they may be abnormal in shape or motion. The cause of these abnormalities can be low hormone levels, injuries, or infections affecting the testes or their surrounding structures. One of the more treatable causes is a *varicocele,* an enlarged vein in the scrotum, which can apply excessive heat and pressure to the sperm-producing apparatus. Surgical removal can improve sperm levels and function in approximately 70% of cases. (Overheating of the testes is sometimes attributed to tight underwear. Whether this is the case or not, the shift to boxer shorts is one of the least expensive and least difficult things to try.) Occasionally, a low sperm count can represent a reversible drug reaction.

Some physicians caution against too-frequent lovemaking (more often than once every 36 hours), on the grounds that the number of healthy sperm in each ejaculate is reduced. Others point to evidence that fertility is positively correlated with frequency of intercourse. Given that the experts cannot agree, it's probably best for partners to follow their own inclination, as long as it leads them to have intercourse at least a couple of times during the week preceding ovulation. Lovemaking more often than this is certainly not essential to conception.

Artificial insemination

When the sperm count is consistently low, one remedy is to collect samples of the husband's semen over the course of several days and then instill the whole amount at the cervical opening. For this procedure, called *artificial insemination by partner,* the husband must masturbate to provide the semen. Instillation into the cervix is an office procedure performed as near as possible to the time of ovulation. It is usually painless. If the semen is thought to lack factors required for normal sperm function, it may be processed so as to improve the chances of conception.

Artificial insemination can also be used when sperm have

difficulty penetrating the mucus surrounding the cervix (*see below*). In this situation, a catheter is inserted all the way through the cervix, and sperm are released directly into the uterus. Intrauterine insemination can cause mild discomfort, and attempts over the course of many months are usually required.

Artificial insemination of a woman with her partner's sperm should not be confused with artificial insemination using sperm from an anonymous donor. The latter can be used if the partner's sperm prove incapable of establishing pregnancy. (In this case, the reason for using artificial insemination is not biological but social.) A potential hazard of using donor sperm is the transmission of viral illness, including AIDS. However, semen can be screened, like blood, for presence of the AIDS virus.

Female factors

Evaluation of the infertile woman is complex because the anatomy of conception is elaborate and because the hormonal changes that program the necessary events are intricately timed. As a first step the physician checks to see that ovulation, endometrial development, and cervical mucus production—all of them under the tight control of reproductive hormones—are occurring normally. A second focus of the investigation centers on possible structural abnormalities of the ovaries, fallopian tubes, or uterus that could prevent pregnancy.

Hormones, eggs, endometrium

Although ultrasound can be used to detect production and release of the egg, the test is expensive, inconvenient, and not generally available. So the more common approach is to biopsy the endometrial tissue between days 23 and 28 of the menstrual cycle. If ovulation has occurred, the tissue will show changes characteristic of progesterone stimulation. Progesterone can also be directly measured in the blood.

Simple absence of the 4 reproductive hormones is uncommon. More likely is a failure of the various surges to be properly synchronized. Medication can then be given to bring hormonal events into phase. One commonly used drug, clomiphene citrate (Clomid), is an estrogen-like medication that seems to provoke the pituitary gland to put out FSH, which tells the ovary to start maturing an egg.

If LH fails to appear at the right moment, eggs cannot escape from the follicle. In this case, another version of LH, *human chorionic gonadotropin* (HCG), can be given in conjunction with clomiphene. The timing of both clomiphene and HCG administration is absolutely critical.

If clomiphene treatment has been unsuccessful, *human menopausal gonadotropin* (HMG) may be tried. This very powerful substance is a mixture of the pituitary hormones LH and FSH, derived from menopausal women, who excrete large amounts of both hormones in their urine. Sold as Pergonal and given by injection, this drug can be very effective, but it must be closely monitored with blood or urine tests to prevent multiple births.

Body weight can have a profound effect on ovulation. The production of adequate amounts of estrogen depends on the presence of a certain amount of fat. If a woman is physically very active and too lean, she may not ovulate. The first step in restoring ovulation is to reduce physical activity and permit weight gain. On the other hand, being *over*weight can be part of a complex of problems associated with infertility, and in some such cases weight loss permits conception to occur.

The cervix: open or closed?

The cervix, through which sperm must pass to enter the uterus, spends most of its time producing a mucus barrier to invading bacteria. But during the ovulatory phase, sperm cells must be permitted to pass if fertilization is to occur. So for a few days each month the cervix normally alters the barrier properties of the mucus that it produces. Chemical changes now make the mucus hospitable to sperm. They are able to swim freely through the cervix and enter the uterus. Mucus that is too acid, too thick, or laden with antibodies to sperm becomes a barrier to entry.

If a sample of cervical mucus is microscopically examined at midcycle, and within hours of intercourse (a process called *postcoital testing*), an incompatibility between the sperm and mucus may be identified. Sperm will appear motionless or sluggish, or will be swimming around in circles rather than in straight lines. An abnormal test must be repeatedly observed over several months to establish that a problem exists. Then it is necessary to decide whether antibodies or hormones are responsible. Hormones may be adjusted, for example with clomiphene. An antibody problem may be overcome through experimental drug treatments, in vitro fertilization (*see below*), or artificial insemination into the uterus (bypassing the cervix).

Although postcoital analysis is one of the oldest ways to investigate infertility, it has become much more sophisticated in recent years. Physicians who are experienced with it, particularly those who specialize in infertility problems, will usually recommend the test early on in an infertility work-up. Postcoital testing is painless, but it does have to be repeated for several months to have any validity, and many couples find this disruption of a normal sex life to be emotionally trying.

Structure and function

Normal findings on the physical examination do not eliminate the possibility that structural abnormalities of the ovaries, fallopian tubes, or uterus are preventing a successful pregnancy. Scar tissue (from pelvic infections or previous surgery) can block a tube or prevent it from capturing the egg after it leaves the ovary. Fibroids, polyps, or scar tissue in the uterus can interfere with implantation of the embryo. Adhesions of a tube to the abdominal wall can reduce the tube's mobility and prevent "pick up" of the egg. Endometriosis is a condition in which cells of the type that line the uterus appear where they shouldn't—around the ovaries, the tubes, or the outer lining of other pelvic organs. Endometriosis is sometimes associated with reduced fertility. Three procedures can be used to check for structural abnormalities.

The *hysterosalpingogram* is an x-ray technique used to explore the interior of the uterus and fallopian tubes. A catheter is introduced into the uterus, and an x-ray contrast agent (often erroneously called a "dye") is then instilled. This agent permits the interior of the uterus and the fallopian tubes to be seen on x-rays, and it can reveal a site where normal passage of the egg may be blocked. Sometimes, by breaking down minor blockages, this procedure is also therapeutic.

Laparoscopy is a surgical procedure performed under general anesthesia. The physician makes a small incision beneath the navel and inserts a slender, tube-like viewing instrument (a laparoscope). Carbon dioxide is then pumped into the abdomen so as to create space for maneuvering the instrument. After the gynecologist has a good look at the reproductive organs, *tubal lavage* usually follows. In this procedure, a pigmented fluid is pumped into the uterus and its flow through the tubes is directly observed.

If minor adhesions of a tube to the abdominal wall are discovered, they can often be detached during laparoscopy. But scar tissue blocking a tube, or abnormal growths (such as ovarian cysts or uterine fibroids), require further surgery at a later time.

Delicate microsurgical techniques are rapidly improving the likelihood that a woman with blocked tubes can be helped. But there are no certainties, and anyone considering abdominal surgery for an infertility problem might wish to obtain a second opinion before proceeding.

The "test-tube" solution

Until recently, there were no further options for those couples whose abnormality had failed to respond to treatment (hormonal manipulation, surgery, artificial insemination), or those in whom no treatable abnormality had been identified. However, in recent years the technique of *in vitro fertilization* and *embryo transfer* (IVF-ET) has become a potential, if not always realistic, solution.

First, hormones are given which stimulate the ovary to produce ripe (that is, fertilizable) eggs. Then the tip of a laparoscope is brought near the ovary, and as many eggs as can be seen are extracted and removed to a glass dish. There, sperm and eggs are combined under strictly controlled conditions. After 2–4 days, any fertilized eggs are inserted into the uterus. With occasional exceptions, no more than one of these embryos develops. Often, none of them does.

In the best of hands, only about 30% of couples succeed in establishing a pregnancy with IVF-ET, and in many cases several attempts are required. Each is time-consuming (at least 10 days), expensive ($5,000 per attempt), and somewhat risky (ovarian rupture, infection, bleeding, complications of the anesthesia). Not all couples are candidates for the procedure. At a minimum, the woman must be capable of ovulating, and her partner must be able to produce sperm. Thus, IVF-ET is mainly useful when blocked or destroyed fallopian tubes are the cause of infertility. The technique is occasionally used in other situations, though. For example, IVF-ET has been successful in a few cases where antibodies in the cervical mucus are preventing pregnancy, or when the man has a very low sperm count.

EPILOGUE Some couples travel a long, difficult, and expensive route only to learn that conception is not possible for them. Often, there is no clear reason. Invariably, the quest for a baby leads to some soul-searching as to what having a child means to that particular pair of people. When they recognize that there is no longer a realistic hope of conceiving, many couples decide that the desire to parent is as important to them as the quest to pass along their genes. They may then consider adoption—another long and expensive process, but also a potentially rewarding one.

Special Problems of Women

The health care of women often is compromised by some confusion about what kind of doctor can best take care of specific "female" problems. The answer to that question sometimes depends on the availability of specialty care in a given area. Many women find their primary care physician (family doctor or internist) more than adequate for most problems related to the female genital or reproductive organs. Others, however, find that specialists—obstetrician-gynecologists—provide more informed and efficient care for problems that are unique to women. (Not surprisingly, more women physicians are entering this specialty as patients increasingly indicate a preference for a female obstetrician-gynecologist.) As always, when a specific problem arises, the individual needs to ask her primary care physician if he or she feels competent to deal with it— and then to assess the results of consultation on a given problem.

Pregnancy: age and outcome

Many people believe that delaying pregnancy into the thirties and forties is potentially dangerous. Yet, more and more women are postponing childbirth to the fourth or fifth decade of their lives, often in order to complete their education or establish a career. Along with this trend, expert opinion on the risks of pregnancy later in life is beginning to change.

There are several ways to categorize the health risks to a newborn. The baby may be premature, may be abnormally small for the date of delivery, may have a congenital abnormality, or may become ill or die around the time of birth. How do the infants of older mothers fare in these various categories?

Prematurity and small size

Adequate studies are relatively few, but there is, indeed, some evidence that as a mother's age increases, her baby is more likely to be premature. Whatever the duration of the pregnancy, the child may also be smaller than the average. With prematurity and small size (especially weight below 1,500 grams, or 3.3 pounds), the rate of survival in newborns is reduced. The tendency for babies to be born either premature or "small for gestational age" appears to result not from the mother's age as such but from the presence of medical conditions that are more common at later ages, among them diabetes and high blood pressure. Much the same applies to miscarriage, fetal distress at birth, stillbirth, and early death of the infant: although each of these occurs more commonly at later ages, it is not age so much as the increased risk for age-related medical problems that appear to be the culprit. So the general statistics may not apply to the older mother who is otherwise healthy. The obstetrician can also use such techniques as ultrasound to follow the fetus's growth and plan the safest possible delivery.

Birth defects

There has been so much publicity about the birth defects in babies born to women over 35 years that the risk has become a major worry of mothers planning or expecting babies later in life. True, the likelihood of bearing a child with an abnormality increases with age, but there is, in reality, no magic age separating "low risk" from "high risk." The age of 35 has some practical meaning, however, because at that age and beyond, the risk of amniocentesis (tapping and examining the fluid surrounding the fetus) becomes less than the risk of giving birth to a baby with Down's syndrome (the correct term for "mongolism"). The probability that the fetus will have this condition increases by about 30% every year for mothers over 30. Specifically, the chance is 4 in 1,000 for mothers between 35 and 39, goes up to 12 in 1,000 between 40 and 44, and becomes 40 per 1,000 after the age of 45—according to one study. Down's syndrome is just one of several disorders that become more frequent with the mother's increasing age. Some other birth defects, such as spina bifida, are about equally common at all maternal ages. The father's age may also have some influence on the frequency of birth defects, but it does not appear to influence the probability of Down's syndrome.

The net effect, as reflected in a large study conducted in Atlanta, is that there are 15 major birth defects in every 1,000 babies born to mothers under the age of 35, 17 at ages 35–39, 31 at ages 40–44, and 76 after 45. These odds for mothers over 40 may sound poor; however, fetuses with major defects can often be identified with amniocentesis and other methods of prenatal diagnosis. If abortion is then an acceptable alternative to the parents, the pregnancy may be terminated. As a rule, diagnosis through amniocentesis cannot be completed before about the midpoint of pregnancy; thus, abortion also takes place relatively late. Current research on a new technique, *chorionic villus sampling,* indicates that it should be applicable earlier in pregnancy.

Prenatal diagnosis and selective abortion are cumbersome techniques. They can also be emotionally trying and are not universally acceptable. However, they are quite effective at diminishing the probability of birth defects. It has been estimated that the risk can be reduced by almost one-third for women 35–39, and by about 60% above the age of 45. Thus, the woman between 35 and 44 can reduce the risk of an abnormal birth to about the same level as it is for a woman of 34 (*see illustration*). After 45, however, this level is no longer attainable.

The mother's health

Of course, not all the risks of childbirth are experienced by the infant. Despite dramatic improvements in care, the mother may also have trouble with pregnancy and delivery. Here again, the rule seems to be that age is less important than health. Thus, age should be regarded as a reason to monitor the mother's health very carefully but not as an absolute barrier to childbearing.

The most common problem that older women experience is a difficult delivery, according to a study conducted at the Beth Israel Hospital in Boston. First-time mothers over 35 were more than twice as likely as mothers under 20 to experience prolonged labor; this difference lessened if the older mother had had previous de-

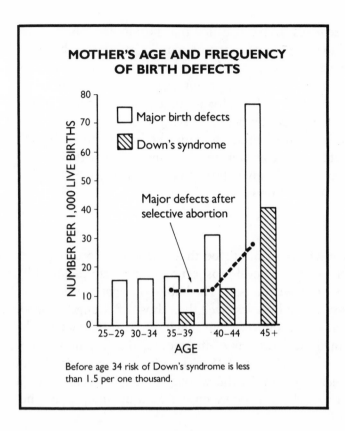

MOTHER'S AGE AND FREQUENCY OF BIRTH DEFECTS

□ Major birth defects

▨ Down's syndrome

Major defects after selective abortion

NUMBER PER 1,000 LIVE BIRTHS

AGE: 25–29, 30–34, 35–39, 40–44, 45+

Before age 34 risk of Down's syndrome is less than 1.5 per one thousand.

liveries. Thus, the first-time older mother is more likely to receive drugs during labor or to require cesarean delivery, and she should be forewarned of this possibility.

There is also considerable evidence that the later a woman has her first pregnancy, the more likely she is to develop breast cancer. There may also be a slight increase in the risk of choriocarcinoma (a rare tumor of the placenta), and perhaps of ovarian cancer. Otherwise, the mother's age seems to have little effect on the occurrence of cancer. The take-home message is that women who delay childbirth, or who remain childless, should be mindful of recommendations for early detection of cancer.

Fertility

There is yet another gamble to consider in delaying pregnancy: the risk that fertility will decline and make conception impossible. It used to be thought that fertility remains relatively high until around age 35, but recent research has called that notion into question. A study reported in 1982 found that a woman's fertility may begin its decline after the age of 30. Many factors besides age come into play in determining a couple's fertility. But age does appear to be an important factor, and if difficulty is anticipated, starting earlier rather than later may be the better strategy.

Another, perhaps incidental, factor is the likelihood of having twins, which are more common in older mothers (as they are in women who have already given birth to twins or in couples with a history of twins in the family).

In sum

The current consensus seems to be that a healthy woman in her thirties or forties enjoys a good prospect of giving birth to a healthy infant and remaining well herself. The babies of older mothers, as a statistical group, fare a little less well than those of younger women during pregnancy or at delivery, but much of this difference can be attributed to medical problems of the mother that are more common at later ages. Past the age of 45, risks to mother and baby begin to climb significantly. But on the whole, there is no reason for a woman to feel that she absolutely must take a pregnant pause before she hits 35.

Premenstrual syndrome (PMS)

"It's like being on drugs," explains one woman of her experiences with premenstrual syndrome (PMS). "I feel completely out of control. The only good thing is that I don't have to keep a calendar because I always know when my period is coming on."

Because her symptoms appear so regularly before each menstrual period, this woman probably has premenstrual syndrome, as opposed to some other recurring form of distress. PMS is easier to define by the timing of the symptoms than by the symptoms themselves. Although any one woman will usually experience only a few of the discomforts of PMS, more than 150 complaints have been attributed to this condition. Some of the common ones are fatigue, headache, mood swings, crying spells, depression, tension, bloating, breast swelling and tenderness, junk-food binges, constipation, joint pain, and clumsiness. From this short list, it is evident that some of the items are physical and others emotional. No one knows the precise way that the somatic and psychological symptoms are related to each other, but few doubt that they are interconnected.

PMS, to one degree or another, will beset an estimated 40% of women during their reproductive years. Some individuals notice symptoms but are not troubled by them. For others, however, the effects are more disturbing. According to a recent estimate, 5–6 million women experience symptoms severe enough to disrupt their personal and work routines. For example, PMS might be sufficiently distressing in one woman that she misses an important business meeting. In another, the syndrome might precipitate a suicide attempt or other aggressive act. In the British courts several years ago, three women successfully pleaded "diminished responsibility" for violent actions they attributed to PMS.

Evidence versus anecdote

If symptoms of PMS are hard enough to pin down, effective therapies are even more in dispute. One reason is that the evidence underlying most of the popular treatments is suggestive rather than scientific. It takes the form of reports that a treatment was tried on some women and they responded well to it. In reading such reports, we can be glad for the patients who seemed to benefit, but without evidence for an untreated comparison group, we cannot be sure that the intervention really was effective.

The few PMS studies that have been properly controlled to avoid distorted observation have generally been too small and too brief to be conclusive. Because the symptoms of PMS can be so dissimilar from one woman to the next, definitive research requires many subjects to compensate for individual quirks. And each woman needs to be followed from cycle to cycle to make sure that the severity of symptoms is not spontaneously diminishing (as would be expected if women came into the study at a time when discomfort was at its maximum). Yet the paucity of reliable data on treatment of PMS has not prevented people from making large claims for one or another "cure."

Some practical advice is in order, however. The first step in treating PMS is to recognize that the syndrome begins as a real problem due to biological events. The simple awareness that it is not "all in their heads" is all many women need to feel they can take the recurring symptoms in stride, much as they do menstruation itself. The reason that placebos work so well for PMS (*see below*) is probably, in large part, because they serve to acknowledge the reality of the problem and thus help to make it less frustrating.

Before the start of any kind of treatment, a woman who suspects that she is suffering from PMS would do well to keep a symptom diary for several months. This is a list of physical and emotional variables on which a woman grades herself every day. Which items are chosen for the record depends on the individual's previous experience. Other information to be included would be timing of menstruation and also any significant events in her life. The diary will tell the person keeping it whether her symptoms are actually related to her menstrual cycle or rather are correlating with something else—perhaps the stresses of work or family. It also helps to identify the symptoms causing the greatest difficulty. Here again, the sense of control that comes from precisely identifying and quantifying problems related to PMS may be sufficient to relieve the distress and make it manageable without further treatment.

Home remedies

If this process of objectifying the problem is not sufficient, the woman with PMS can move into even less certain territory. She may begin by trying modifications in lifestyle. Whether or not they are fully supported by research, such changes are probably about as effective in alleviating PMS as many of the medical therapies being advocated. Exercise, stress management techniques, or cutting down on caffeine and sugar have been among the more popular recommendations. Reducing salt intake is frequently suggested, and some women swear by it. An odd but very common suggestion is to eat vegetables such as cucumbers and parsley, which are claimed to act as diuretics. Herbal teas likewise get a plug from time to time (but beware of overdosing, as many herbs taken in large quantities prove to have serious drug-like effects). Likewise, vitamin B6 has been rumored to help combat PMS, but again, this treatment may cause harm. Many cases of multiple-sclerosis-like symptoms have now been reported in women taking vitamin B6. In all cases, these home remedies for PMS have received support from testimonials, but no solid research backs them up.

Medical approaches

Medical therapies are hardly on firmer ground. Nevertheless, if a woman is severely troubled by what appears to be PMS, she may

• Painful periods •

Many women with unusually painful cramping during their periods (dysmenorrhea) have higher levels of body chemicals known as prostaglandins in their menstrual discharge than do women with less intense cramping. This knowledge has led to the widespread use of anti-prostaglandin drugs (such as Motrin and Ponstel) for the relief of these symptoms. These drugs, long used for their anti-inflammatory effect in arthritis, can often provide substantial relief when taken at the beginning of a period and continued for several days.

benefit from seeking a physician's advice. (Beware of grandiose claims; there is plenty of room in this field for quackery.)

The first step should be a thorough physical examination to rule out specific endocrine disorders or other health difficulties that might also be cyclic. Problems such as endometriosis (abnormally located uterine tissue), tension or migraine headaches, or serious depression can fluctuate with the menstrual cycle. Whether or not one chooses to label them PMS, these conditions can be specifically treated. Likewise, if bloating is a significant premenstrual complaint, it can be treated with diuretics; swollen and uncomfortable breasts may also respond to drug therapy.

The most popular medical treatments of PMS have been based on the theory that the symptoms have something to do with the fluctuating hormone levels of the menstrual cycle. Thus, progesterone supplements and, more recently, anti-prostaglandin drugs—proven to be effective against menstrual cramps (*see box*)—have been widely recommended. A number of women with PMS have reported getting relief from these agents, but the evidence is not compelling. It is important to bear in mind that placebo treatments for PMS usually have about a 50% success rate—higher than 30%, which is the usual finding with placebos. Indeed, one study compared the effect of lithium (a psychoactive drug), a diuretic, and a placebo. This carefully designed test found that the placebo was most effective; next came the diuretic; and lithium trailed in last place.

Psychotherapy has also not been stringently evaluated for its effectiveness in PMS. However, counseling would probably help at least some women handle the emotional distress that is often associated with this condition, and thus have their lives less disrupted by their symptoms.

Currently, no one can say what PMS is, what causes it, or how best to treat it. PMS is, however, an identifiable medical syndrome affecting some women some of the time; it is not a condition that disqualifies all females from normal life. J. M. Davidson of Stanford University puts the problem in perspective: "Although crime, accident and suicide rates are higher in women during the premenstruum, it is noteworthy that these rates are still lower than those seen in the noncycling male subject."

Lumpy breasts

"Fibrocystic disease," as this condition has often been called, is a misleading and frightening term meaning little more than "lumpy breasts without cancer." Half of all women have lumpy breasts. And 90% of all women whose breast tissue has been studied at autopsy have had microscopic features that could be fibrocystic disease. Why should a condition that is both common and harmless be labeled a disease—or even an abnormality?

Lumpy breasts in themselves are not medically serious. But there is a common, and erroneous, belief that having "fibrocystic disease" increases a woman's risk of developing breast cancer as much as 4 times. On that basis, when fibrocystic disease is present, some surgeons suggest "preventive" mastectomies—making an incision, scooping out the breast tissue, and putting in a silicone replacement. This operation is inappropriate in this instance for two reasons. First, it is not truly needed. And, second, even if it were, it is unlikely to accomplish what it claims since not all of the breast tissue can be removed. The remaining breast tissue is at the same risk of developing cancer as before. Furthermore, the inserted silicone implant makes breast examination much more difficult. Many experts feel that it is only because the patients are not at high risk to begin with that this operation appears to be successful.

Hyperplasia

It *is* true that breast tissue often contains certain features that may be forerunners of cancer. And these features are included under the general term fibrocystic disease. But a better term is "hyperplasia"

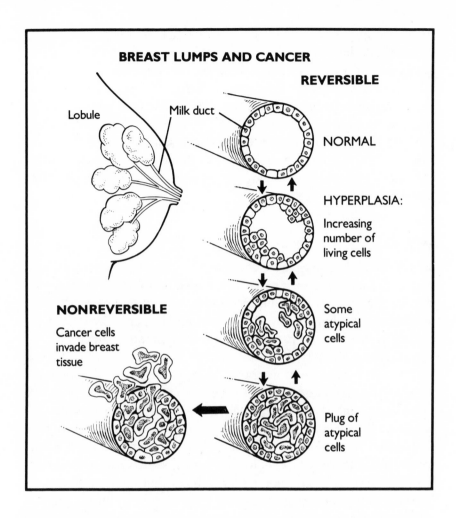

BREAST LUMPS AND CANCER

REVERSIBLE

Lobule

Milk duct

NORMAL

HYPERPLASIA:

Increasing
number of
living cells

NONREVERSIBLE

Cancer cells
invade breast
tissue

Some
atypical
cells

Plug of
atypical
cells

(which is just a Greek work for "overgrowth"). In this situation, cells lining the milk ducts change their appearance, begin to multiply, and build up in a cluster inside the duct (*see illustration*). As the condition progresses, these cells may increase in size while becoming even more irregular in appearance. Eventually the abnormal cells may plug the duct and then go on to break out of it—at which point they have turned into an invasive cancer.

In the early stages, hyperplasia does not produce a lump that can be felt. And hyperplasia does not inevitably lead to cancer. The whole process appears to be reversible up to a point, which probably comes as the invasive stage is reached. Thus, when a breast is biopsied, the finding of hyperplasia can be difficult to interpret.

From autopsy findings, we can predict that as many as 30% of women will develop hyperplasia, but the majority of them will *not* get cancer. Yet many of them undergo mastectomies as though the condition *were* cancer. This approach distorts breast cancer treatment statistics by including women who did not have cancer to begin with among the "cures."

Hyperplasia is an indication that the risk of breast cancer is higher than average, but it is not the first step on a road leading inevitably to malignancy. Individuals with evidence of hyperplasia should be carefully followed.

Biopsies

Breast cancer becomes more common the older a woman gets. Especially after menopause, a newly discovered lump should be regarded as potentially cancerous until proven otherwise. Before menopause, most lumps are benign, but a biopsy should be performed whenever there is a suspicion of risk. Mammography cannot replace a biopsy in evaluating a newly discovered lump.

The usual area that warrants biopsy is called a "dominant" lump—one that stands out in the general lumpiness of a breast and persists through the menstrual cycle. Obviously, many biopsies will prove to be normal. That's fine; you want to do many more than "necessary" to be sure you find the occasional cancer. Before menopause, there are so many confusing structures in the breast that 12 biopsies are done for every cancer that is discovered.

Dominant lumps, which raise the issue of doing a biopsy, may be of four different types:

FIBROADENOMAS Fibroadenomas are smooth, round, solid, and freely movable. They are often described as feeling like "a marble within the breast tissue." They are most common in the late teens and early twenties and are essentially benign, but they should be removed to be certain of the diagnosis. Fibroadenomas do not go away by themselves, and they may enlarge during pregnancy and lactation.

PSEUDOLUMPS Pseudolumps are an unusually distinct area in otherwise lumpy breast tissue. They may fluctuate in size with the menstrual cycle; often they are sore or tender. This is the most common type of lump in the thirties. Biopsies show variations of normal breast tissue, but they are often needed to be certain of the diagnosis.

CYSTS Cysts are firm, fluid-filled sacs. They often do not have a smooth feel. Frequently they are painful, and they may appear overnight. They are most common in the forties, are benign, and can be diagnosed and treated by removing the fluid with a needle.

CANCERS Cancers are hard and, as a rule, not tender; they may be movable or fixed to skin or underlying tissue. They are the most common dominant lump in postmenopausal women; thus, any newly detected lump in this age group should be biopsied promptly.

For many decades, research papers have purported to show an increased rate of cancer among women with fibrocystic disease. However, the researchers really were not writing about all women with lumpy-feeling breasts but only those who underwent breast biopsy. This is a crucial distinction. Doctors do not biopsy every woman with a questionable area in a breast; they tend to select women who are at increased risk for other reasons (say those with a history of breast cancer in the immediate family, or those who have lumps with a suspicious form or texture). Thus, the biopsied women will indeed have a higher rate of cancer. They were at higher risk to begin with; that's why the biopsy was done.

In other words, the outcome of the biopsy studies has been distorted by the choice of subjects to be biopsied (a problem technically known as "selection bias"). As a result, in these studies even the women whose biopsies were normal proved to be at an increased risk of developing breast cancer. This was not, however, because the biopsy procedure in some mysterious way "caused" the cancer, as is shown by the fact that the tumor was as likely to appear in the opposite breast as in the one that was biopsied.

Treatment

Aside from concern about cancer, lumpy breasts may pose a real problem of pain and discomfort. Several treatments have been proposed, the most common being to eliminate caffeine and related substances (methylxanthines) from the diet.

Since the original study that supported this idea, other and better trials have not demonstrated a significant caffeine connection. If the caffeine theory had only produced another placebo treatment for breast discomfort, it would not be of concern. But, unfortunately, a lot of women have come to think that an occasional cup of coffee will give them fibrocystic disease, which will then lead to breast cancer. This is simply untrue.

A more plausible theory is that breast lumpiness and the associated discomfort is related to fluctuations in levels of various hormones. If so, then a way to treat the conditions would be simply to override these fluctuations. A version of male hormone known as danazol can be used; the result is no lumps, no pain, no periods— and possibly hair on your chin. It also costs about $200 a month, and when the drug is stopped, the lumps and discomfort come back again. It may be feasible to devise a hormonal treatment that works in a less blunderbuss fashion, but a lot needs to be learned before such a therapy is possible. But when there's no discomfort, why treat a nondisease at all? A drug treatment for lumpy breasts may well produce more serious consequences than the condition itself.

Estrogen and menopause

The average American woman now lives to the age of 77. This means that at least a third of her life goes on after menopause. With the quantity of life so dramatically increased, quality becomes an even more important issue. Symptoms that occur during menopause or subsequently may be sufficiently unpleasant or disabling to warrant treatment.

Menopause is the phase in a woman's life when menstruation ceases because the ovaries no longer produce enough estrogen, their principal hormone, to keep cycles going. Hot flashes are the most dramatic response to this change in estrogen level. The term "hot flash" is fairly descriptive: an abrupt sensation of warmth is followed by sweating and a chilly feeling. About 75% of menopausal women have them, and about a quarter of these women are made sufficiently uncomfortable to seek treatment.

Menopause may also bring about changes in the vagina—dryness and thinning of the lining—which lead to pain during intercourse. These symptoms, if they appear, are usually delayed by approximately 3 months after the onset of menopause. A common response is to diminish the frequency of intercourse; the vagina then shrinks, and further attempts at intercourse may also produce bleeding. This problem (technically termed *vaginal atrophy*) is both common and correctable. In the past, physicians were disinclined to discuss it with their patients. But now that the importance of an active sex life in older people has been recognized, vaginal atrophy is more likely to be talked about and treated. Pain on urination may also occur in postmenopausal women. Like the vagina, the opening of the urethra is sensitive to estrogens. After menopause, the mucous membrane in this area may also become thinner, drier, and hypersensitive. Urination then becomes painful.

All these symptoms can usually be treated with estrogen replacement.

Other benefits

Osteoporosis is one of the most important health problems affecting older women. By the age of 90, some 20% of women will have suffered a hip fracture (as compared with 7% of men). At that age, as many as 20% of women with the injury do not survive more than 3 months. Though not as deadly, collapses of the vertebrae, known as *spinal compression fractures,* are also very frequent and take their toll in pain and disfigurement. Collapsed vertebrae are the cause of the stooped posture sometimes referred to as "dowager's hump."

An accumulating body of evidence strongly suggests that women who start taking estrogen within 3 years after menopause, and continue taking it for at least 6 years, reduce their rate of hip and spine fractures by half (*see "Osteoporosis," below*). However, carefully controlled studies remain to be done—as well as a lot of basic research to clarify the effect of estrogen on the formation and strength of bones.

Women may experience emotional distress at menopause. By and large, though, the numbers have been overstated; most women cope well with this transition in their lives. For the few who do become significantly depressed and need help, estrogen is not an adequate therapy, despite the claims sometimes made for it. On the other hand, estrogen can be helpful to women who have severe hot flashes, especially at night, and lose sleep as a result. The loss of sleep can be very taxing, and estrogen replacement, by providing a good night's sleep, can improve mood considerably.

The use of estrogen for "more youthful skin" is sometimes promoted. However, there is no good evidence that it reduces wrinkling, though it will increase the thickness of skin.

Estrogen risks

Although women have less atherosclerosis and fewer heart attacks than men, heart attacks are still their leading cause of death. If estrogen contributes to the development of atherosclerosis, it might be ill advised as a long-term treatment. Scientific opinion on this subject has fluctuated dramatically in the past 30 years. In the 1950s, available studies suggested that estrogen actually prevented heart disease, but then in the 1970s birth-control pills containing fairly high doses of estrogen were implicated as a possible cause of death from heart attacks. In 1976, the Boston Collaborative Drug Study came up with results indicating that modest doses of estrogen had no effect either way. Studies released since 1980 have brought us back to the assertion that estrogen may actually retard development of atherosclerosis. At present, there just isn't enough information to support a firm recommendation with respect to estrogen and heart disease. On the other hand, estrogen replacement given to postmenopausal women does not increase the rate of strokes or abnormal blood clotting (thrombophlebitis or pulmonary emboli), at least not in women with no known tendency to develop these conditions.

Cancer is the second most common cause of death, and the questions about estrogen are somewhat more troubling in this area. In particular, the risk of endometrial cancer in women receiving estrogen is 2–8 times the average. The endometrium (the lining of the uterus) is exposed to estrogen from puberty until menopause. The reason cancer doesn't develop in this period is that progesterone (another female hormone, also produced by the ovary) counteracts the effects of estrogen. Thus, *progestin* (synthetic progesterone) should be given with estrogen supplements, because, as research has shown, doing so minimizes the risk that an endometrial cancer will develop. In any case, most endometrial cancers grow very slowly, and a diagnosis can be made before spread occurs. Nevertheless, any woman receiving estrogen should watch for vaginal bleeding and, if it occurs, see a physician immediately. Those women who have undergone a hysterectomy, of course, need not worry about endometrial cancer as a complication of estrogen replacement.

Although some studies have implicated estrogen use in the development of breast cancer, most have not. However, estrogen should not be used if a woman has already had breast cancer.

Other risks associated with estrogen replacement are, on the whole, minor. Gallstones are about 2.5 times more likely to occur. Estrogen may also interfere with liver function. And, in susceptible patients, high blood pressure or high blood sugar may result from taking oral estrogen.

Who should take estrogen?

It's easier to say who shouldn't. Women with a history of endometrial or breast cancer, blood clots, strokes, coronary artery disease, severe migraine, liver disease, or unexplained vaginal bleeding should not be considered candidates for estrogen replacement. In the case of women who have had strokes, blood clots, coronary artery disease, or breast cancer, treatment is discouraged only because the evidence is inconsistent or there are theoretical risks.

Treatment decisions should otherwise be made case by case, and patients should be fully aware of the risks—which are not high, but are not altogether negligible. Women who go through menopause early, either naturally or because their ovaries have been surgically removed, are at higher than average risk of developing osteoporosis, and they develop vaginal atrophy earlier than usual. In these cases, the benefits probably outweigh the risks. For women going through menopause in their fifties, severe hot flashes or a strong family history of osteoporosis are good reasons to consider treatment.

The major area of controversy centers on the situation of a woman who has no symptoms but *might* be at risk of osteoporosis. Should she be treated? The risk of osteoporosis is increased not only in women with a family history but in thin, fair-haired smokers. The extent and progress of osteoporosis can be assessed by a device known as a *bone densitometer,* or with a CT scan, and it's conceivable that useful information can come from screening for early signs of the disease. But the technology is still in its infancy, and is very expensive. There are at present no universally accepted guidelines.

How much estrogen is needed depends on the reason for giving it. When hot flashes or vaginal dryness are the problem, the lowest dose that controls the symptoms should be used. If estrogen is being given to prevent osteoporosis, it appears that the lowest effective dose is 0.625 milligrams a day of "conjugated estrogen," a commonly prescribed form. Sufficient amounts of supplemental calcium intake could halve this minimal dose level, according to one study. No matter what the reason for giving estrogen, it should always be given with progestin to reduce the risk of endometrial cancer.

Estrogen is most often given by mouth, although there are creams that can be applied directly to the vagina. In either case, the estrogen is readily absorbed into the blood stream. The Food and Drug Administration has approved a skin patch that supplies estrogen in a form identical to that produced by the ovaries. Delivered this way, estrogen does not increase blood pressure, and it may have some other advantages.

It's not yet possible to write up a set of simple rules for estrogen replacement. The decision should be an individualized one, based on thorough, thoughtful, and frank discussion between the physician and patient.

Osteoporosis

Curved spines, broken hips, and fractured wrists are common and disabling occurrences among the elderly. For example, 25% of women over age 60 have spinal compression fractures due to osteoporosis. Although fragile bones with frequent fractures are problems of older people, especially women, the process that weakens bones actually begins early in middle age. Bones get their strength from a structure of flexible protein fibers combined with hard calcium phosphate crystals. Throughout life, bone is remodeled by cells that add a little to it and take a little away. Up to the age of 35 or so, the yearly result is a net increase in bulk and strength of bones. After that age, very gradually, more bone is removed than deposited, so that a net loss occurs in both sexes, but at a faster rate in females. At any age a woman has lighter bones than a man of the same weight. For the first 5 or 6 years after menopause, she loses bone at a faster rate than usual. Three factors—less bone to begin with, a greater rate of loss during middle age, and the postmenopausal loss—make women particularly vulnerable to fractures in old age.

The commonly occurring form of bone loss is termed *osteoporosis* (bone thinning). Bone protein and calcium are both reduced in this condition. Its cause is not known; indeed, there may not be a single cause. Inadequate calcium and vitamin D in the diet, hormonal changes, insufficient exercise, and possibly reduced exposure to sunlight may all contribute.

Another condition, *osteomalacia* (bone softening), is also seen in older adults. In this disease, the bone protein is deficient in calcium. Osteomalacia can be treated with vitamin D (which some people are unable to absorb in normal amounts). Osteoporosis and osteomalacia may be present simultaneously, and the two conditions can work independently to weaken bone.

After decades of bone loss, fractures can occur very easily. Most commonly, one or more vertebrae of the spine collapse slightly in the forward, weight-bearing part. If enough vertebrae are affected, a curvature or hunchback deformity results. Back pain can also become a problem. Broken wrists (often incurred in a fall) are the next most frequent type of fracture. Hip fractures are the third most common and the most serious.

Treatment

It is important to bear in mind that the process leading to fractures usually begins 30–40 years before the first break occurs. It is impossible to repair a condition overnight when it has taken decades to develop.

When a vertebra collapses, as a rule there is little to be done other than to provide pain-relieving drugs. If pain is severe, a brace or corset may be helpful. Broken hips can be treated by replacing the broken bone with a metallic prosthesis, or by reinforcing the bone with screws and plates. Other fractures may be handled in the traditional way by cast immobilization, but healing is slow for the same reason that the bone is weak to begin with.

Several methods for strengthening abnormally weak bones are used. None of them is ideal, especially when treatment is begun late.

ESTROGEN   Estrogen (a female hormone) is often given to older women with osteoporosis. This therapy is valuable for some, but it is no panacea.

On the other hand, there is now widespread agreement that women can *prevent* or retard bone thinning by taking estrogens during the first half-dozen years after menopause. Women who have had a hysterectomy (and therefore are not at risk for endometrial cancer) and those women who are at special risk for osteoporosis because of a sedentary lifestyle or diseases such as arthritis should be considered for estrogen therapy—with the realization that periodic check-ups may be essential to detect any side effects that might result. Combining progestins with estrogens reduces the risk of the treatments' contributing to endometrial cancer.

CALCIUM   Calcium and vitamin D supplements are frequently a part of treatment. When used appropriately, these supplements can slow the rate at which bone is lost, but they will not necessarily lead to formation of new bone (unless osteomalacia is also present).

The bad news is that high calcium taken at the time of menopause, all by itself, probably doesn't prevent bone thinning. Calcium is most rapidly lost from bones during menopause and for a few years afterward, so any effort to prevent osteoporosis must be effective at this time of life. The hope has been that increasing dietary calcium would, by itself, do the trick. In the past few years, this hope has almost become gospel. But several reports provide evidence that calcium alone at the time of menopause has little effect on bone loss from the spine.

▪ Calcium in food ▪	
Food	*Mg of calcium*
An 8-ounce glass of milk or cup of yogurt	300
3 ounces of sardines	300
Oyster stew	300
A cup of enriched macaroni and cheese	300
A cup of New England clam chowder (made with milk)	240
Half a cup of canned salmon	170
An ounce of cheddar cheese	160
Half a cup of cooked greens (collard, dandelion, kale, mustard)	75–150
A stalk of broccoli	150
Half a cup of baked custard	140
Half a cup of cottage cheese	120
A slice of pizza	100
A slice of pumpernickel	30
A slice of French bread	9
3 ounces of beefsteak	9

In one study, conducted in Denmark, bone density of post-menopausal women was measured by a very precise technique. Fourteen women maintained a daily intake of 2,000 mg of calcium for 2 years—but lost about as much mineral from their skeletons as 11 others who received a placebo. By contrast, another 11 women who were given estrogen therapy without supplemental calcium kept their bone mass. Several women receiving estrogen left the study, however, because of unpleasant side effects (such as uterine bleeding, migraine headaches, itching from the estrogen patches applied).

Meanwhile, a group of postmenopausal women in San Francisco were participating in a somewhat similar study of calcium supplements and estrogen. This study provides good news. Women given *only* calcium supplements lost 10.5% of the mineral from their vertebrae during the first 2 years after menopause—not significantly different from the loss in untreated subjects, 9.0%. But women receiving estrogen *plus* calcium showed no loss in the mass of their spinal bones. And only 0.3 milligrams a day of the estrogen preparation—half the usual dose—was required to achieve this level of protection. Similar trends of smaller magnitude were observed in other bones.

So, although vigorous calcium supplementation by itself is not effective, it may permit a reduced dose of estrogen and thus, presumably, a lowered risk of adverse effects. Also, calcium may play a greater role in protecting the hip and upper arm from fractures.

While the hazards of calcium supplementation are low, it is hard to escape the conclusion that calcium has been oversold as a weapon against osteoporosis. The emphasis has clearly shifted to estrogen replacement for preventing bone loss during and after menopause. It remains to be seen whether taking extra calcium earlier in life will help maintain higher levels of calcium in bones, and thus provide greater reserve when menopausal loss begins. On the whole, it is advisable for women to maintain adequate calcium intake, 750–1,000 milligrams a day, throughout adult life, and too many women fall short of this intake.

FLUORIDE Fluoride, when given in relatively large doses, causes bone to "fill in." But this new bone is not normal in structure, and it is not yet certain whether it improves resistance to fractures. Because fluoride can have serious side effects, patients must be closely monitored.

A study from Finland suggests that fluoridation of the local water supply may help to reduce the rate of fractures in older people. The rates of hip fractures in residents of two very similar Finnish towns were compared. The people of Kuopio have been drinking fluoridated water since 1959, whereas the water supply of Jyväskylä has never been fluoridated and contains only trace amounts of the substance. In the period 1967–1978, fracture rates were much lower among those drinking the fluoridated water of Kuopio. For women, the protection became apparent after the age of 70; at earlier ages it was not observed. Men were protected at all ages.

The modest amount of fluoride involved—1 part per million—typically reduces rates of tooth decay in children by about two-thirds. The new study suggests that this same level of fluoridation is capable of diminishing the number of hip fractures in older women by about a third, and in men by about half.

OTHER NEW TREATMENTS   Work still in the research stage suggests that certain hormones, especially variants of the basic vitamin D molecule, can be used in some patients to shift the balance back from bone loss to bone formation. These approaches suggest the possibility of controlling the remodeling process, at least to the extent of encouraging new bone formation when it is needed.

Prevention and screening

If treatment once osteoporosis exists is uncertain or inadequate, long-term prevention is even more in doubt. It is very difficult to produce good data on the effects of various strategies 20 or 30 years down the road when it counts—at the time of menopause. However, the kinds of prevention tactics usually advised—adequate calcium intake and weight-bearing exercise—are low risk and therefore usually worth doing, even if just to hedge a bet.

Far more controversial and potentially costly is the issue of whether or not all women—or even so-called high-risk women—should have tests which allegedly determine whether or not a person's bones are at higher than usual risk for osteoporosis. There is a movement afoot—fueled in part by entrepreneurial instincts—to recommend widespread screening using a relatively simple technique known as *single photon absorptiometry*. This test measures bone density at the wrist and can be done in the doctor's office. However, the test is being criticized on at least two counts:

- First, osteoporosis experts question the correlation between wrist-bone densities and those that really count—densities of back and hip bones. The prevailing opinion is that there is very little predictive correlation—which would make the single photon test rather worthless.
- And since bone testing would not change the prevention strategy for women in general—or even the advice to consider estrogen at the time of menopause—critics question the value of doing screening tests at any cost.

There are two tests which *can* accurately measure bone density in the hip or spine—CT scans and dual photon absorptiometry. However, both these tests require expensive equipment. Most experts feel they should be reserved for research studies and selected women at especially high risk for osteoporosis.

IN SUMMARY   Osteoporosis is a common condition in postmenopausal women. However, most women will not experience serious consequences, and therefore all women should not live in dread that this condition will surely ruin their elderly years. It would seem prudent, though, to begin early in life those lifestyle practices that *might* help reduce the risk for some women. That means daily calcium in the range of 1,000 milligrams and exercise that puts some stress on the bones. At this time, routine screening tests are not recommended by most experts. And, finally, all women should talk with their doctor or clinic about the advisability of taking estrogen when menopause begins.

Vaginitis

Vaginitis is one of the most prevalent afflictions of womankind. Although the condition is rarely serious in a strictly medical sense, it usually produces both physical and emotional discomfort. Moreover, several forms of vaginitis can be transmitted sexually. For these reasons, accurate diagnosis and prompt treatment of vaginitis is warranted.

The term vaginitis as it is commonly used refers to a group of infections that lead to irritation and inflammation of the lower genital tract (*see illustration, p. 268*)—the vulva (or outer area), the vagina itself, and the cervix (the ring of tissue joining the vagina to the uterus). Strictly speaking, "vaginitis" should be reserved for infections of the vaginal canal itself, whereas "cervicitis" should be applied to infections of the cervix. Practically speaking, symptoms of the two conditions are easy to confuse, and symptoms of the various types of vaginitis are generally similar. Nevertheless, it is essential for the physician to make fine distinctions, as the success of treatment depends on identifying the specific disorder.

One of the cardinal symptoms of vaginitis is an increase of vaginal discharge above the woman's typical level. The discharge of vaginitis can be white, gray, yellowish, or occasionally blood-tinged instead of clear or slightly milky, as is usually the case. Copious vaginal secretion is normal in some individuals (especially at midcycle, around the time of ovulation). In one survey 10% of women complaining of vaginitis simply had an above-average quantity of otherwise normal secretions. Itching around the vulva is a common but by no means universal symptom of vaginitis. Sometimes urination is painful, though not necessarily because the urinary tract is involved. Rather, urine touching the irritated tissue causes a burning sensation. Intercourse may be painful. "Spotting" (a bloody discharge seen between periods) may also indicate vaginal infection, though it is probably more common when the cervix is involved.

General principles

Although douching may seem like a reasonable form of first aid, douching within 24 hours before a visit to the physician can interfere with the examination and interpretation of results. At the examination, the doctor, nurse clinician, or other trained assistant needs to examine a sample of the discharge under a microscope. Along with direct examination of the vagina, this is the single most important step in identifying the cause of the infection. A diagnosis based only on asking about symptoms or simply looking at the discharge has a good chance of being wrong. In some cases, even the microscope fails to reveal the germ that is responsible; then other diagnostic techniques, such as cultures, are in order.

There are three principal causes of vaginitis. The most common, in one series of some 25,000 patients, was bacterial infections (33% of cases). Candida, a yeast, was responsible for a further 20%, and trichomonas, a protozoan, for about 10%. In about a quarter of cases, the vagina itself was not infected; rather it was the cervix. Of these various conditions, all but candida infections are thought to be acquired primarily by sexual contact, although other factors may play a role in susceptibility.

Bacterial vaginitis

There really is no accepted term for this condition, which has long been inappropriately called "non-specific vaginitis." Currently the most popular label is hemophilus or gardnerella vaginitis. Both names refer to the same bacterium, which has frequently been implicated as the main cause of this condition (and recently had its name changed, hence the two terms). New findings indicate that another type of bacterium, as well as gardnerella, must be present to cause the symptoms, so we have opted for the term "bacterial" vaginitis.

The hallmark of bacterial vaginitis is increased discharge, which is usually described as having a "foul" or "fishy" odor and a milk-like consistency. Symptoms of irritation (itching, burning, or pain) are not always present. Women who are sexually active seem to run an increased risk of bacterial vaginitis. The role played by male sexual partners is not altogether clear, but it appears that a man can carry the bacteria and transmit them to any woman with whom he has sexual relations. A monogamous sexual partner may also re-infect a woman with bacterial vaginitis if both are not treated at the same time.

The most effective treatment for this type of vaginitis appears to be the drug metronidazole (Flagyl). It was originally marketed for trichomonas infections (*see below*), but it is also active against certain bacteria, including those that cause bacterial vaginitis. Metronidazole seems to work best when given several times a day for a week. The drug is not recommended for use during pregnancy. There are no clear guidelines for treating male partners.

Other therapies have been used or proposed for bacterial vaginitis, but their effectiveness has not been clearly established. One alternative is ampicillin (to which some people are allergic). For a long time, topical creams containing sulfa drugs (triple sulfa) were virtually the standard treatment, but there is some question as to whether they work at all.

Candida

The earliest sign of a candida infection (also sometimes called "monilia" or yeast infection) is usually itching around the vulva. Later on, soreness, pain during or after intercourse, and burning on urination may develop. There may be no noticeable discharge, but if one is present, the material is likely to be white, thick in texture, and odorless.

Candida is a yeast or fungus. When it is present in vaginal secretions, it can usually be found with a microscope, but sometimes culturing techniques are necessary. This organism is so common that up to 15% of adult women carry it without symptoms. Candida has a pesky tendency to recur in some women; predisposing factors include diabetes, prolonged use of antibiotics, pregnancy, or the use of oral contraceptives. Sexual transmission plays a less important role than with other forms of vaginitis.

For many years the standard treatment for candida has been nystatin (Mycostatin) suppositories. However, creams and suppositories containing miconazole or clotrimazole, two newer antifungal agents, appear to be more effective. Treatment should continue for a full week. Now virtually obsolete as a treatment for candida is the dark blue dye known as gentian violet. Although it is effective, this approach has never been popular because it stains clothing and bedding.

Trichomonas

Trichomonas vaginalis (often nicknamed "trich") is a protozoan (a one-celled organism somewhat like an ameba). It can produce no symptoms at all, or it can cause pain, discharge, and itching. In symptom-free individuals, the infection may be identified during a routine examination or on the Pap smear. The discharge of trichomonas vaginitis is sometimes described as "foamy," but this is not a definitive sign. As with all types of vaginitis, accurate diagnosis requires examining a sample of the discharge with a microscope. Trichomonas appears to be sexually transmitted, and "ping-pong" reinfection between sexual partners is frequent. However, sexual transmission is not always the case, and the organism may be found in young girls.

The most effective medication is metronidazole. A single, 2-gram dose given at the time of the diagnosis will eradicate 95% of infections. Even better results are possible if the drug is given in smaller doses, several times a day for a week, provided the patient strictly follows this schedule. Whether to treat an asymptomatic patient is a judgment that has to be made by the physician along with the patient. Treatment of the male sexual partner appears to be useful, as it prevents reinfection.

Prevention and home remedies

Recommendations for preventing or treating vaginitis with certain simple measures are abundant, but are not well supported by careful research. Perhaps the most frequent suggestion is to wear cotton underpants that "breathe," instead of nylon or other fabrics. No known harm can come from following this advice, but how helpful it may be is not clear.

Douching is a common practice, but it probably does not reduce the risk of vaginal infection. Indeed, washing away the normal secretions and bacterial inhabitants of the vagina may allow infectious germs to set up shop. Douching solutions themselves can produce chemical irritation and inflammation.

A "natural" therapy, often mentioned in self-care books, is to put yogurt into the vagina. The rationale is that yogurt contains lactobacillus, the type of bacterium that is most common in the vagina. Lactobacilli help to keep other organisms in check as well as to maintain the normal, slight acidity of the vaginal secretions. Yogurt instillation is probably not harmful as a rule, but there is no research to prove that it is beneficial.

Occasionally, the suggestion to avoid sugar is made, but again there is no solid evidence that this or anything else in the diet normally makes a difference in susceptibility to vaginitis. On the other hand, abnormal metabolism of carbohydrates (as in diabetes) may lead to an increase in the sugar content of vaginal secretions. Since both candida and trichomonas are organisms that depend on sugar for their nourishment, poorly controlled diabetes may increase the risk of vaginitis caused by these two invaders.

Cervicitis

Many women with an abnormal discharge do not actually have vaginitis. Instead, they have an infection of the cervix (the neck of the uterus protruding into the vagina). Spotting of blood between periods or after intercourse may occur. Usually there is no vaginal soreness, itching, or burning, but there may be a crampy discomfort during intercourse. Cervicitis has 4 main causes: gonococcus, chlamydia, trichomonas, and herpes. All of these are thought to be sexually transmitted. How the condition is treated depends on which of these organisms is present.

Atrophic vaginitis

In females with a low level of estrogen (mainly postmenopausal women, but also nursing mothers and preadolescent girls), the lining surface of the vagina becomes relatively thin and dry. This is a normal state of affairs and need not be associated with any problems. However, the thinned vaginal lining can become mildly infected, usually with bacteria that would not affect a vagina that is fully stimulated by estrogen. The symptoms then may include discharge, itching or burning, or spotting. Again, accurate diagnosis is important to rule out other possible problems and to identify the cause of the vaginitis. Then specific treatment should be given to eliminate the offending organism. Sometimes, estrogen-containing cream applied to the vagina will help to speed healing.

Vaginal ulcers

A few women develop ulcers—areas where the surface lining breaks down—in the vagina. Usually, such ulcers lead to slight, persistent bleeding between periods. They may be caused by tampons, diaphragms, trauma, tumors, or infection (syphilis or herpes). Again, consultation with a doctor is needed.

Urinary tract infections

As long as urine remains within the body, it is normally free of bacteria. When urine does contain bacteria, the person is said to have a urinary tract infection (UTI). UTIs can range from a silent infection (no symptoms) to a distressing illness. Although these common conditions generally are simple to treat and rarely cause lasting harm, they have an exasperating tendency to recur.

Who and how

Infections of the urinary tract occur mainly in women. An estimated 10–20% of all women will suffer a UTI at least once in their

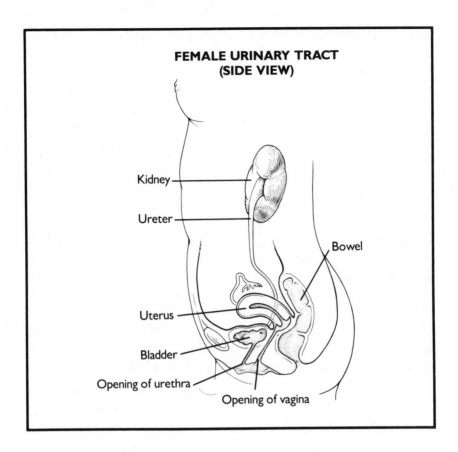

**FEMALE URINARY TRACT
(SIDE VIEW)**

Kidney

Ureter

Bowel

Uterus

Bladder

Opening of urethra

Opening of vagina

lives. UTIs are also common in older men with enlarged prostates and among persons with structural abnormalities of the urinary tract.

The arrangement of a women's anatomy poses an easy pathway for infection (*see illustration*). First, bacteria from the bowel spread across the skin to the lower vagina. From there, they may travel up the urethra (the tube carrying urine out of the body) and into the bladder. If the bacteria multiply in the urine but cause no symptoms, the patient is said to have asymptomatic bacteriuria. If they infect the bladder wall, the result is cystitis; common symptoms include burning pain during urination, frequent urination, the feeling of an urgent need to urinate, and the urge to urinate during the night. Most UTIs go no further than the bladder, but some extend upward into the kidney and thus cause *pyelonephritis*. The symptoms of pyelonephritis include back pain, chills and fever, nausea and vomiting, plus the symptoms of cystitis. In women, episodes of UTI may follow sexual intercourse, which seems to promote the movement of bacteria into the urinary system. Indeed, "honeymoon cystitis" is a well-recognized condition, and UTIs are said to be rare in nuns.

Diagnosis

By definition, a UTI is present when the urine contains a significant number of bacteria. Thus, the diagnosis is made by obtaining a sample of urine and examining it by microscope and by growth culture. The specimen should be carefully collected, so that it is not contaminated by bacteria from skin or other sources.

Once a UTI has been diagnosed, other tests may be ordered. For example, x-ray dye studies of the urinary tract (so-called IVPs or intravenous pyelograms) can be very useful in searching for malformations, stones, obstructions, and other correctable problems predisposing the patient to infection. Physicians often recommend an IVP for males or young girls who suffer even a single UTI and for adult women who have repeated infections. Sometimes a fiberoptic tube (cystoscope), which is inserted into the bladder through the urethra, may be used to directly inspect the bladder lining.

Treatment

Drugs active against bacteria are the mainstay of treatment for UTIs. When to use them (and for how long) depends on who is infected and how extensively.

ASYMPTOMATIC BACTERIURIA This term refers to the presence of bacteria in the urine without associated symptoms. Most authorities agree that this condition should be routinely tested for and treated in pregnant women because of the potential for pyelonephritis. In addition, many physicians favor treating asymptomatic bacteriuria in children, in whom it may tend to interfere with the development of the kidneys. What to do about asymptomatic bacteriuria in the rest of the population, however, remains uncertain; the prevalent view appears to be that the condition is very unlikely to cause lasting damage and thus is not worth routinely testing for.

CYSTITIS Cystitis often may clear up by itself. But because the infection can persist and spread, treatment is usually advisable. Traditionally, patients with cystitis are treated with anti-bacterial agents for about a week. Recent findings, however, indicate that a single large dose of appropriate antibiotics can cure many infections that are limited to the bladder. Advantages of such brief treatment include convenience, low cost, and decreased risk of side effects.

PYELONEPHRITIS Because bacteria are more difficult to eradicate from the kidney than from the bladder, a patient with pyelonephritis generally receives an antibacterial drug for 10–14 days.

Recurrent UTIs

For reasons that remain largely unknown, some women are prone to repeated UTIs. Although these infections rarely pose a significant risk of lasting kidney damage, they cause much discomfort, inconvenience, and expense. Preventing and managing recurrent UTIs often require a woman to modify aspects of her lifestyle and adapt to a suitable drug program. Communication and cooperation between the patient and health care providers are especially important.

The woman who tends to develop UTIs may find it worthwhile to adjust her habits to help keep bacteria from spreading up the urethra and growing in the bladder. Being careful to wipe only from front to back after bowel movements is one recommended (but never verified) measure. And although avoiding sexual activity is rarely an acceptable approach, cleansing oneself beforehand may be worthwhile. In addition, drinking plenty of fluids and urinating frequently may aid in flushing bacteria out of the bladder. Although cranberry juice is popularly alleged to help prevent UTIs, it seems no more effective than other liquids. Likewise, specific foods and drinks generally need not be avoided.

Some physicians continue to recommend urinating shortly after intercourse, although findings from at least one study indicate that doing so does not decrease the frequency of recurrent UTIs. Some speculate that in the woman prone to UTIs, tampons may be preferable to sanitary napkins, but others say the reverse. In addition, various forms of birth control—including oral contraceptives, the diaphragm, and foam—have been cited as possibly predisposing certain women to UTIs. In short, modifying such factors may be a matter of trial and error. If a measure seems to work and is not too burdensome, it's probably worth continuing.

At least three types of drug programs may be used to treat or control recurrent UTIs. First, each new episode may simply be treated as it occurs. Second, those women in whom infections tend to follow sexual activity may be instructed to take a single dose of an antibacterial drug after intercourse. And third, a patient may take a low dose of an antibacterial drug regularly. The appropriate choice among these should be based on careful consideration of a number of items, including the expense and possible risks of the medication and the frequency, discomfort, and bother of the UTIs. It is usually important to know the type of bacterium responsible for recurring symptoms and whether anatomical abnormalities are present before settling on any given drug program.

Over the years, physicians have dilated and otherwise manipulated the urethras of countless women in attempts to prevent recurrent UTIs. Today, however, most experts seems to agree that except in special circumstances, such procedures merely cause pain and cost money. Unless a specific structural abnormality of the urinary tract is found, surgery is rarely indicated.

UTIs are common and often distressing. But with proper treatment, they rarely pose lasting risk to kidney function and health. Recurrent UTIs are a frustrating problem for many women, but hygiene practices and antibacterial drugs can help keep them under good control.

Special Problems of Men

For some reason, the medical profession has been slow to recognize the special medical problems of men. Women have obstetricians and gynecologists who specialize in their health care. There is no direct equivalent of the gynecologist for men. Instead, men with disorders of their urinary or genital organs must find medical advice and treatment from urologists, endocrinologists, psychiatrists, and other professionals who happen to have an interest in disorders of the male reproductive organs. Two of the most common disorders are impotence and prostate problems.

Impotence and erectile dysfunction

Difficulty with erections is common and often alarming, but frequently treatable. Narrowly defined, *impotence* means the inability to have an erection. *Erectile dysfunction* is becoming a preferred term, and can be defined as the failure to achieve and maintain erections during more than 1 out of 4 attempts at intercourse. The figure is somewhat arbitrary, but it emphasizes that most men have occasional difficulty with erections as part of a normal sexual life. A pronounced decrease in formerly normal sexual functioning, however, is an important symptom deserving medical evaluation.

The normal adult erection is produced by a change in the circulation of blood in the penis. Blood flowing through small arteries enters the penis faster than it leaves. The accumulating blood swells the penis to its erect size. This subtle control over blood flow is maintained by two sets of tiny muscles that encircle the entering and exiting vessels. They, in turn, are supervised by a complex set of nerves which are part of the involuntary nervous system. The male hormone testosterone, which is produced by the testicles, is needed to keep this system working properly.

Thus, broadly speaking, erectile dysfunction can be caused by three types of problems: (1) insufficient blood supply to the penis (as may occur with severe disease of the arteries), (2) malfunctioning of the nervous system (which may be anything from an emotional difficulty to a specific injury of nerves), or (3) abnormal amounts of hormone.

One or two episodes of impotence hardly qualify for medical attention. It is reasonable for a man who experiences impotence more often than a quarter of the time to wait up to 2 or 3 months to see whether the problem resolves of its own accord. Most spells of impotence will be shorter than that, and the delay does not risk permanent harm. Discussing the situation with one's sexual partner may resolve temporary difficulties. But if the condition persists longer than 3 months, it is certainly time to get help.

Many men worry about the effect of aging on potency and wonder what to expect. From Kinsey's studies it would seem that the peak of sexual activity for males comes around the age of 20. Potency, however, changes little until after the age of 50 or so. Thereafter, potency may gradually and partially decline: the penis may become less erect, loss of erection before orgasm may be more frequent, more intense stimulation may be needed, and the interval between orgasms may become longer. All these effects are partial, normal, and extremely variable. Although some decrease in potency is expected with advancing age, it does not necessarily occur, and in a normal male the capacity for an erection should persist at least into the seventies. Thus, an abrupt or complete change in an earlier pattern should be carefully and sympathetically investigated, not written off to "age."

Common causes

Most often, impotence results from a problem affecting the set of nerve connections that control erection. An illness such as diabetes may damage the nerves, but drugs are probably the most common cause of malfunctioning nerves leading to impotence. Drugs that lower blood pressure, anti-depressants, sleeping pills, and tranquilizers all are common causes. Alcohol is a self-administered drug that may produce impotence before other signs of damage appear. A variety of other agents, either taken by prescription or self-administered, can have the same effect.

The only way to prove a drug is causing impotence is to stop using it and see what happens. Obviously, before a patient stops taking any prescribed drug, he should discuss the problem with his doctor. In the case of high blood pressure, the wide variety of available drugs means that it is usually possible to substitute another effective medication for the offending one and thus keep adequate control of pressure. Fortunately, drug effects are reversed when the agent is stopped.

Psychological factors play an important role in impotence, and they have been much discussed in popular articles and books. Beyond brief episodes of anxiety and fatigue, there may be prolonged difficulties arising from guilt, marital stress, or depression. In particular, depression is often not recognized, as it may be relatively subtle and cause only one or two obvious signs (such as constipation, loss of appetite, sleep disturbance, or impotence). Frequently, a judiciously prescribed anti-depressant drug can restore potency, but sometimes, ironically, the drug itself causes impotence. Psychological factors can also play an aggravating role in any type of erectile dysfunction. Fear of failure, embarrassment, and worry about the problem can all compound an organic or other medical cause of dysfunction.

Disease of the pituitary or testis can produce a deficiency in the hormones needed to maintain the male reproductive system in working order. Recent reports have emphasized that such abnormalities may be more common than supposed. A low level of testosterone is the principal hormonal cause of impotence. Another hormone, prolactin, produced by the pituitary gland, may interfere with erection if present in excess.

Sometimes with severe vascular disease, blood flow to the penis becomes too slow to permit erection. Usually there will be other evidence of insufficient circulation (such as leg pains on walking). This condition can sometimes be corrected with surgery to the narrowed arteries.

Treatment

The treatment of erectile dysfunction is much improved over what it was 10–20 years ago. Increasing candor about sexual matters has made patients less reluctant to seek help, and more open discussion within the medical profession has improved sensitivity to the problem and understanding of it.

A man affected by impotence should talk with a doctor. They should discuss possible causes—emotional factors, including the possibility of an underlying depression; drugs, including alcohol; and so forth. It is generally reasonable for the physician to take a blood sample and check for levels of the two hormones that affect potency (the older method of measuring urinary hormones is not accurate). An endocrinologist (specialist in hormone disorders) can help interpret the results. Hormonal abnormalities can be treated with either medication or, sometimes, surgery. Poor blood flow, if identified as the problem, can sometimes be improved with vascular surgery. More recently, injection of medication directly into the penis to increase blood flow has become a recognized form of therapy. Persistent psychological difficulties may call for consultation with a psychiatrist or other counselor. The newer forms of sex therapy are still controversial. The approaches seem reasonable and promising, but it has been difficult to prove they work as claimed.

If the complex apparatus that controls erections has been permanently damaged by illness or injury, it is now possible with surgery to insert an implant in the penis. Some implants maintain a permanent state of erection while others utilize a device that can be inflated or deflated from a reservoir implanted under the skin. The device permits intercourse, but does not restore the capacity for orgasm if this has been lost. Most major hospital urology departments now include specialists in such surgery.

Sex after a heart attack

Depression commonly follows a heart attack, but it doesn't really take shape until discharge from the hospital. After they arrive home, patients are chronically tired and easily fatigued, and they often spend large blocks of time alone, reflecting on what has happened to them. They tend to assume the worst: that they will never fully recover. Under the circumstances, decreased libido (feelings of sexual desire) is understandable. For most patients—about 85%—this state of affairs passes within 3 months and never becomes a major problem. For the remainder, impotence severe enough to require further treatment does occur. It's important to recognize this development early in its course. If a patient has not resumed his usual sex life within 6 months, it is unlikely that he will ever do so.

In the early 1970s, researchers in Cleveland were able to document that the average amount of energy expended while having sex was equivalent to climbing one flight of stairs. This research was done with couples who had stable, long-term relationships, and it pertains to a situation very different from the "Garfield syndrome"—named after John Garfield, an actor who died, presumably of a heart attack, during intercourse with a mistress. A widely quoted Japanese study has provided some more information on that phenomenon. The investigators obtained and analyzed the autopsy records of 5,000 people who had died suddenly. Of this group, 34 had died during intercourse, and of the 34, 30 were with someone other than their spouse, and the partner was, on average, 18 years younger. Moreover, all had blood alcohol levels either close to or in the range of intoxication. These results are not conclusive but suggest that extramarital affairs, especially when they involve a younger partner, produce more, and potentially lethal, stress.

The position adopted during sex appears to make no difference in the level of stress placed on the heart. There was a time when patients recovering from a heart attack were instructed to assume the underneath position or, if that wasn't feasible, to have sex while lying on their side. These precautions were unnecessary, and luckily so, for position turns out to be one form of behavior that is highly resistant to modification.

In general, the effects of heart attacks on sexuality have been exaggerated. The people most likely to resume regular sexual activity after their illness are those who were most active before it. Some decline in frequency of intercourse is routinely observed after the age of 40, though, and the shock of a major illness may serve to bring this decline into focus. Then a medical event, for example a heart attack, is labeled as the cause of the change. Even if a heart attack is not directly responsible for diminished sex drive or potency, it may be indirectly responsible, because of the medications (to lower blood pressure, prevent palpitations, or control angina) required afterward. These medications can often be changed to reduce or eliminate such side effects.

Fatigue is to be expected during any recovery process, and it is unrealistic for patients to expect an immediate return to their normal sexual patterns. It may be helpful for the first 2–3 weeks for a couple to limit themselves to foreplay and abstain from intercourse, not because it's dangerous but because it takes the pressure off both the partner and the patient to perform. Masturbation is also perfectly safe and may ease the transition back to partnered sex. After 3 weeks there are usually no restrictions, though this schedule may be modified in some cases of severe illness. If problems with sexual feeling or performance remain after 3 months, then special attention and possible treatment are required. However, these cases are uncommon, and the large majority of patients return to their normal sex life.

Prostate ailments

First, a spelling lesson. We humans, accidentally or otherwise, may assume a pro*strate* position, but we don't have a gland named after it. Male members of the race do, however, have a pro*state* gland. And this walnut-sized gland all too often spells trouble as men grow older.

The prostate's potential for trouble is directly related to its position in life (*see illustration*). The prostate gland surrounds the urethra—the tube that emerges from the bladder and carries urine, via the penis, to the outside world. Little imagination is needed to understand how infection or enlargement of the prostate can interfere with the act of urination. However, the prostate gland is also close to the front wall of the rectum, making much of the gland accessible to the physician's finger during a rectal examination, so that it is relatively easy for the physician to evaluate the condition of the prostate.

The prostate also surrounds the duct through which sperm pass

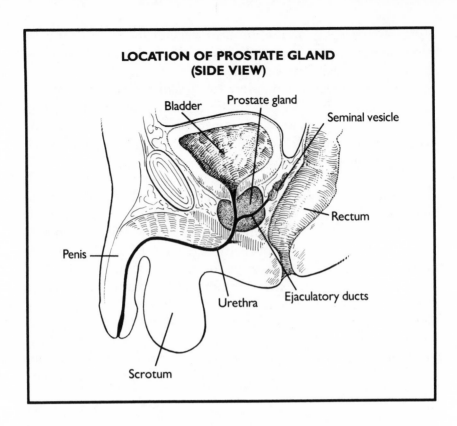

LOCATION OF PROSTATE GLAND (SIDE VIEW)

Bladder
Prostate gland
Seminal vesicle
Rectum
Penis
Ejaculatory ducts
Urethra
Scrotum

on their way into the urethra. During ejaculation, the prostate gland squeezes fluid into the urethra to aid in the transport and nourishment of sperm. Given this strategic location, one might expect the prostate to perform essential functions. But, in fact, apart from its contribution to semen, the gland's major role seems to be to cause trouble. This essay will survey two of the three major disorders associated with the prostate gland. The third, prostate cancer, is discussed in Chapter 7.

Benign prostatic enlargement

The exact reasons for enlargement of the prostate gland are unclear. Presumably they are related to hormonal changes associated with aging. About 10% of males aged 40 already have some degree of enlargement, and by age 60 prostate enlargement is almost universal.

When the prostate increases in size, it may impinge on the urethra, thereby narrowing the passageway for urine flow. This, in turn, causes a set of symptoms known as *prostatism*—difficulty in starting the flow of urine, decreased force of the urinary stream, dribbling of urine after voiding is felt to be completed, and increased frequency of urination, especially during the night (*nocturia*). Prostatism usually develops gradually but may, in advanced states, produce a sudden and complete blockage to the flow of urine—obviously requiring emergency treatment. Even lesser stages of blockage can lead to serious infections of the urinary tract caused by the back-up of urine.

Benign enlargement is caused by an overgrowth of glands associated with the urethra but located inside the prostate gland. The usual form of surgery to alleviate the blockage is a *transurethral resection* (TUR). The excessive tissue is extracted via a tube inserted into the penis, through which an electrical cutting device removes the central portion of the gland. Thus, much of the original prostate gland, which was pushed to the outside, remains after surgery. The prostate must be checked periodically for further growth or the development of cancer.

The decision for surgical removal and the type of surgery to be done depend ultimately on the level of discomfort of the patient and the judgment of a competent urologist. Whether there are symptoms or not, surgical removal may be necessary because of an associated urinary tract infection that threatens kidney damage or changes in the bladder, which is forced to work extra hard to expel urine through the penis. Most surgical procedures done for benign enlargement do not result in any degree of impotence. They may, however, cause retrograde ejaculation—meaning that semen is passed back into the bladder during intercourse. At present, there are no therapies scientifically proven to cause shrinkage of the prostate gland.

Infection

Fortunate is the male who makes it through life without at least one bout of prostatitis. Unfortunately, some men also become the victims of so-called chronic prostatitis—recurring, low-grade infections which are difficult to treat and which, while not life-threatening, cause considerable discomfort and annoyance.

Acute prostatitis is characterized by the rather abrupt onset of fever, pain at the base of the penis, and painful urination. Uncontrolled dripping of cloudy fluid from the urethra may also occur (a problem associated with some venereal diseases as well). Usually, an infecting bacterial organism can be identified from urine specimens and the infection treated with antibiotics. In older men, prostate infections may be associated with gland enlargement, which may require surgery. When there is persistent inflammation of the prostate, it may be necessary to use x-ray dye studies or direct inspection via the penis (through a cystoscope) to rule out underlying anatomical problems.

Chronic prostatitis is usually a more difficult problem. Often no bacteria can be identified as the certain cause. In recent years, newly identified forms of microbial life—some requiring special antibiotics—have been implicated in chronic prostatitis. But, quite frankly, physicians frequently resort to somewhat blind trials of various antibiotics in the hope that one will alleviate the symptoms.

Some experts who believe that emotions can play a role in chronic prostatitis may use tranquilizers as well. Caffeine, decreased sexual activity, prolonged sitting, and many other factors have been associated in popular myth with prostate infections, but scientific evidence does not support these as significant causes.

6

Stress and Strain: Emotional Problems, Sleep Disturbances, Headaches, and Back Pain

We confess that this chapter contains a somewhat odd assortment of topics—ranging from suicidal thoughts to hemorrhoids. We offer no apology, but perhaps a wry nod to the human condition. Discomfort and misery are discomfort and misery, whether the source is lowly or profound. The subjects covered here are capable of immobilizing otherwise healthy people. An acute reactive depression, a run of sleepless nights, the excruciating pain of a bad back, the nausea and then ache of a migraine—all can render us helpless until relief is found.

These conditions have another important feature in common: for most, treatment and prevention can be medical, nonmedical, or a combination of the two. Pains, aches, and anguish are sometimes amenable to a purely biochemical treatment. But in the best of circumstances, drug therapy has severe limitations. The effectiveness of all known sleeping pills diminishes rapidly with each night they are used; pain medications also lose their effectiveness and in the process may become addicting; anti-anxiety drugs can give blessed relief for a few days or weeks but when mixed with alcohol are potentially lethal. When treatment is nonmedical, it may be something people can do quite simply for themselves. Sometimes, the help of another kind of professional is required.

In focusing principally on the medical aspects of these problems, we do not imply that medical treatment is necessarily the most important approach, or the first-line therapy. Here, as elsewhere, we see our purpose as explaining this aspect of self-care. We would like our readers to have a clear sense of their medical options, to be able to ask pointed questions of the professionals who treat them, and to assess the replies.

Emotional Problems

Good health is necessary, but not sufficient, for full enjoyment of life. When stress, anxiety, or depression take over, feeling really well becomes impossible.

There is a growing awareness that emotional and physical problems are located at various addresses on a two-way street. To take a banal but important example, anxiety and diarrhea are often companions—and it may be hard to know not only which is causing the other but which came first. Another type of emotional distress, grief or bereavement, appears to increase physical illness and even death among those affected. On the other hand, many conditions termed "mental" illness appear to have a biochemical cause and respond well to relatively specific medications.

Stress

The term *stress* is difficult to use with any precision because so many meanings have become attached to it. In physiological terms, the definition is relatively well established. In response to certain kinds of challenge, heart rate rises, blood pressure soars, breathing becomes rapid and shallow, and muscle tension increases. These go along with measurable shifts in hormone levels and activity of the nervous system. As preparation for "fight or flight," these changes make biological sense—an observation made as early as 1914 by the physiologist Walter B. Cannon. In the mid-1940s, Hans Selye began to popularize the term "stress" for this pattern of response, and he observed that in contemporary life it could work either for or against us. The stress reaction is highly appropriate when it's observed in a runner at the starting block—and will contribute to a better performance. But when it happens to someone sitting in a stalled subway car, all it does is contribute to the general level of misery.

In the past 40 years, "stress" has come to refer not only to this stereotyped physical response but to the spectrum of social and psychological events that can trigger it. Indeed, we now often use the word as a synonym for feelings of anxiety or tension, and we may also use it to mean "overwork" or even as code when referring to the misbehavior of employers, colleagues, or family.

To some degree, this broadening of the term is understandable. It

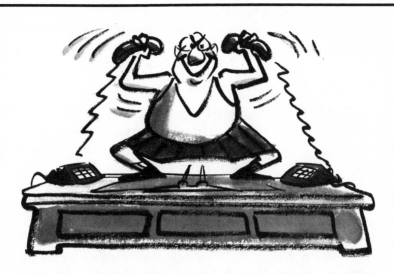

Stress is no easier to deal with than to define, though we often know when we feel it. Regular exercise sometimes helps: it can give you a sense of control over your body, a feeling of accomplishment, or a means to release pent-up frustration. And it never hurts to stand back and reevaluate your priorities; if something has to give, better for you to choose it than wait for it to choose you.

reflects a certain reality of civilized life. Neither flight nor fighting is possible or desirable in a variety of situations that potentially stimulate the stress response. The nasty office memo, for example, arouses a state of smoldering frustration that we instinctively, and accurately, sense does us no good. On the other hand, exploding with expressions of anger may not improve the situation at all, both because it can stimulate further physiological reactions and because it can make the social situation untenable. So, as some experts have suggested, "stress" has come to be used in place of a somewhat more precise term, "frustration."

Stress and disease

Because the stress response couples physiological to emotional responses, it seems probable that stress can translate frustration into physical illness. But the precise mechanisms by which this occurs are not known. In some situations, as with tension headaches or upset stomachs, the connections appear fairly clear. On the other hand, both headaches and belly aches can occur with no emotional provocation whatever. The chain of causation is even less clear when it comes to more chronic and serious conditions such as heart disease, hypertension, and cancer.

HEART DISEASE If animals are subjected to repeated or prolonged stress (unavoidable electric shocks or separation from mates), they develop heart disease. How this observation bears upon the human experience is not all that clear. In the 1950s, two cardiologists popularized the concept of a "Type A" personality—the person who is competitive, time-conscious, and never able to feel approval except from the latest achievement. This personality has been widely accepted as a predictor of coronary heart disease—but not without dissent. Various personality scales are used to assess the presence of Type A traits. They seem to work for some investigators but not for others. It may also be the case that there really are two types of "fast-paced" or "hard-driven" people. Studies of management hierarchies suggest that those who rise to the top and experience real success in their lives may suffer little or not at all from their personality type. At a lower level in management, where frustration may be greater, risk of heart attack may be higher. Some authorities have suggested that the pressure of working in a situation where one has little sense of control may be more "stressful" than the sense of high-risk, high-rolling autonomy. Currently, it appears exceedingly difficult to look at a particular person and say for sure whether his personality type or behavior is contributing to heart disease.

HIGH BLOOD PRESSURE It's not clear whether emotional factors make an important contribution to chronic high blood pressure. The medical term "hypertension" is partly responsible for the widespread popular belief that tension and high blood pressure are linked, but the word doesn't imply anything about this relationship. On the other hand, behavioral scientists have shown quite clearly that meditation techniques (popularized as the "relaxation response" by Dr. Herbert Benson) can help to lower moderately elevated levels of blood pressure. These techniques, which can sometimes be self-taught but may work even better after a few sessions with an expert, are a valuable component of the approach to lowering blood pressure without medication.

CANCER For some years, reports that destructive emotions contribute to the progress of cancer, or even cause it, have been in circulation. One popular version of this theory holds that such emotions weaken the immune surveillance mechanisms that normally hold cancer in check. A logical extension of this theory is the claim that developing more healthy emotions can help retard the progress of cancer.

These theories deserve further study, but they must be regarded as tenuous at best. Anyone, with or without cancer, can benefit from increased emotional health. That would be reason enough to offer emotional support and help to cancer patients. But the flip side of the coin—suggesting that cancer patients have somehow brought on their disease through inadequate emotional responses—is unjustified by any valid evidence, and it smacks of "blaming the victim."

OTHER DISEASES The list of diseases that have been linked to stress is almost endless. It includes asthma, allergies, rheumatoid arthritis, ulcers, ulcerative colitis, and migraine headaches, among many others. There's an important distinction that needs to be made. Any of these chronic illnesses can be made harder to bear by a stress-laden situation, or by an emotionally inadequate response on the part of the patient. On the other hand, it is no longer possible to credit older theories that specific emotional experiences or reactions actually cause these various diseases. On the whole, it seems most likely that stress plays a nonspecific role in disease, by throwing off the body's natural ability to heal itself.

Stress management

Although the idea that stress alone causes many diseases is not very plausible, stress management appears nevertheless to be worthwhile—as long as expectations are tempered with realism. Some of the general principles of stress management are these:

- *Avoid equating "pace" with "stress."* To label a hectic pace or schedule as dangerously stressful may just contribute another level of inappropriate anxiety. As emphasized by many stress researchers, the person who works long hours and leads a busy life may be far less frustrated than the person trapped in a seemingly less harried position, but one that gives no sense either of release or accomplishment. And for some, being deprived of a fast pace may be the frustration that is most difficult to tolerate.

- *Consider the role of regular exercise in reducing apparent stress.* Although exercise produces a stress-like response, by raising heart rate and levels of stress-related hormones, the experience of exercise has profoundly different consequences for the body. The shot of adrenaline that comes during exercise is much less likely, for example, to produce an abnormal heart rhythm than the equivalent surge experienced as a result of pain, frustration, or anger. Regular exercise may contribute to an overall sense of relaxation—reflected in a lowered tendency to show the signs of a fight or flight response. The psychological value of physical activity includes a sense of control over one's own body, the experience of accomplishment, and an opportunity to step outside daily routine for a period resembling meditation. Exercise may also have rather specific effects that combat emotional problems. A popular, if not fully substantiated, theory is that exercise increases the level of endorphins, natural chemicals in the brain that seem to play a role in enhancing our sense of well-being and relieving anxiety. It is rather widely believed that exercise has antidepressant effects.
- *Periodically re-evaluate priorities.* Trite advice, perhaps—but there is strong experimental and clinical evidence suggesting that the sense of "helplessness and hopelessness" is among the most destructive experiences one can have. To the extent that we create this sense in ourselves, by making rigid assumptions about ourselves and the world, we probably sabotage our opportunities to substitute fulfillment for frustration.

Anxiety

Anxiety is another one of those terms that is more easily understood than defined. In general, anxiety is a condition resembling fear, but without an appropriate threat (such as a charging lion) to be afraid of. Short of the lion, though, many people find generalized areas to be anxious about, and a variety of ways to express their worries. These form the basis of the standard classification system for anxiety disorders, which includes: agoraphobia (fear of public places), panic disorder, simple phobia (for example, fear of snakes), social phobia, obsessive-compulsive disorder, post-traumatic stress disorder, and generalized anxiety disorder.

Three types of anxiety disorder are both common and often relieved in a rather specific way by medication. This is not to imply that medication should be given without counseling, but only to point out that there are effective drugs that can be used to accomplish specific purposes.

Generalized anxiety

Sometimes, anxiety appears to be so diffuse that no particular situation or event seems to provoke it. Through psychotherapy, an underlying cause may be identified, but in the meantime it may be exceedingly difficult for the affected person to function. When, if ever, is anti-anxiety medication appropriate in this situation? Until the 1950s, the answer to this question had to be weighed with the recognition that the only available medications, the barbiturates, had two potentially catastrophic side effects—easy overdose and easy addiction. Then, in the mid-1950s, new compounds, first meprobamate (Miltown and Equanil), then the benzodiazepines (Valium, Librium, and others), led to a revolution in the treatment of anxiety. These compounds—called collectively the "minor tranquilizers"—were less sedating, less addictive, and less toxic. Recently the FDA has approved a yet newer chemical type of anti-anxiety agent, buspirone, that reputedly causes even less sedation or functional impairment than the earlier drugs.

The benzodiazepines proved to be far more effective and safe than anything that came before. Not surprisingly, patients and physicians turned to them quickly—rather too quickly, in the judgment of many medical and social critics. The pendulum currently is pointing to the following generalizations about these drugs:

- They do indeed have a potential for both physical and psychological addiction.
- The risk is minimal if the drugs are used in low doses and for short periods—weeks as opposed to months or years. But some people are unusually sensitive to their effects; even a low dose will have potentially dangerous effects in this population.
- The danger is minimal when anti-anxiety drugs are used alone in low dosage, but rapidly increases when they are combined with other drugs, especially alcohol.

On balance, these drugs are best used for the relief of anxiety that is tied to an obvious cause and that promises to be self-limited: loss of a job, death or illness of a loved one, and so on. But they should be used for the long term only after other approaches to disabling anxiety have been tried—and then only under very careful medical supervision.

Performance anxiety

This form of anxiety is very close to straightforward fear—there is indeed something real to worry about, but the level of worry is out of proportion to the threat. Moreover, the symptoms themselves may become disabling: if someone about to give a speech gets a dry mouth from stage fright, the chance of performing well is radically diminished.

For this type of anxiety, drugs known as *beta-blockers* (Inderal and others) can be quite effective. These drugs prevent some of the typical expressions of an adrenaline surge: rapid heart beat, sweaty palms, tremulousness, dry mouth, rapid and shallow breathing. By blocking these physical signs of emotional distress, beta-blockers make the moment *feel* less distressing, whatever the actual situation may be. Since awareness of these physical reactions feeds back into the sense of distress, blocking them can be very helpful. And in some studies of musicians, those taking beta-blockers were judged to have performed better than those who were not—by critics unaware of who was taking the medication.

Beta-blockers can be obtained only by prescription. Not everyone can tolerate them, though most people have no adverse effects from the single low dose prescribed for situational anxiety. However, anyone who plans to rely on a beta-blocker to get through a tense situation should give it a trial dose before the big day, just to make sure that it will be tolerated.

Panic disorder

A more complicated and controversial type of anxiety is the panic attack, which has been the subject of a theoretical and therapeutic revolution in the past decade. Victims of this disorder describe sudden and severe attacks of panic that come on out of the blue. Typical symptoms can include a pounding heart, dizziness, disorientation, difficulty breathing, a sense of lost control, and a great need to escape from one's immediate surroundings. Episodes may last minutes to hours. In time, a secondary anxiety builds up around anticipation of the next attack.

This dread easily and understandably becomes translated into fear of being in public when the next attack occurs, and thus leads to *agoraphobia* (avoidance of public places). Agoraphobia is a relatively common problem, affecting between 2–5% of the general population, especially women between ages 15 and 35. The problem is now considered to be more biological than psychological in its origin. The evidence includes the following observations:

- The disorder runs in families and is more likely to be shared by identical than by fraternal twins.
- Panic attacks can sometimes be triggered by a specific biochemical challenge, such as an injection of sodium lactate (which is normally released by overworked muscles or those with an inadequate blood supply).
- Rather specific kinds of medication can prevent many panic attacks, whereas a variety of medications known to diminish anxiety are ineffective in this situation.
- Traditional forms of psychotherapy have a dismal record in treating panic disorders.

The tranquilizer alprazolam and the antidepressant imipramine are the two drugs most favored for treatment of panic disorder, and many specialists begin with one or another of them. Even when they work—and they don't always—these drugs must be given in adequate doses for relatively long periods of time.

The object of drug therapy is to relieve the patient of the secondary anxiety that an attack will come on in a potentially embarrassing situation. Social rehabilitation can then begin, with a return to public places and activities. When attacks in public places seem to be under control, behavior therapy aimed at helping the patient to identify and overcome situations that might provoke the panic reaction can be undertaken. Although there is a continuing dispute between people who favor drugs and those who favor behavioral control of panic, the weight of the evidence suggests that drug therapy followed by behavioral modification of avoidance behavior is the appropriate sequence to try.

Depression

Depression can be used to cover a multitude of experiences, from the transitory blahs of Monday morning to the profound blues that follow an emotional loss. Depression at times also may be a fundamentally biochemical abnormality without obvious provoking causes. For reasons that are not at all clear, the diagnosis of depression is on the rise, and some authorities believe this reflects a real increase in the occurrence of this condition.

Severe depression is not always an easy diagnosis to make; it can masquerade in many guises. Often the only indication is the emergence of physical symptoms: loss of appetite, weight, sleep, or sex drive. Sometimes there is no obvious mood change, but just a gradual withdrawal and diminution in activity; this is typical of depression affecting many elderly people. The difficulty is compounded by the reluctance of both doctors and patients to use a label they perceive as psychiatric and therefore somehow disparaging. Also, there is no simple biological or psychological test for depression; the diagnosis must be based on the whole clinical picture, and very often certain other conditions that may mimic depression, such as hypothyroidism, must be ruled out.

Signs and symptoms

The clinical signs that support a diagnosis of depression include a variety of changes in basic body functions:

- *Eating and weight.* Most persons with a serious depression will show weight loss with diminished appetite. (Some people complain that they "overeat" in response to relatively milder depression. Such people appear to be mainly chronic dieters, who "give in" to food as a way to comfort themselves during periods of emotional upset.) Documented weight loss is a valuable clue that serious depression may be present.
- *Sleep.* Awakening early in the morning, well before the habitual time, is a classic sign of depression. Typically, the person is unable to go back to sleep because of depressive ruminations. Difficulty getting to sleep, though less characteristic, also occurs.
- *Libido.* Diminished sexual desire may be the most obvious clue in some people—but it may also be missed if the change was gradual or has been attributed to other factors, such as age or overwork.
- *Physical complaints.* A marked increase in physical complaints, such as headache or fatigue, characterizes people who find it difficult to speak directly in terms of emotional difficulty.
- *Psychological aspects.* These include a diminished ability to have fun (which may be rather explicitly stated), a sense of worthless-

ness, an inability to see beyond the present, reduced ability to take the initiative (say to make a telephone call), social withdrawal, and thoughts of suicide.

- *Precipitating events.* The loss of a family member is one of the most typical of these, but other forms of loss—of a job, a body part, a function—are also very common causes. Here, a distinction must be made between the appropriate grieving, which may continue for a period of months to years, and depression, which is a self-perpetuating and self-defeating pattern of response.

Dealing with depression

Many cases of mild depression—perhaps most—require nothing more formal in the way of treatment than the personal support of family and friends. But sustained suffering or disturbed ability to work, to play, and to participate in family or social activities warrants professional help. What kind of professional help is a difficult question to answer in our complicated society. There are many options.

PSYCHOTHERAPY Pure psychotherapy ranges from traditional analytic approaches to a variety of therapies that have been designed specifically to deal with depression. In the latter form of treatment, considerable attention is paid to the thought patterns of depression, which can work to defeat any opportunity to feel better. The patient may be instructed in ways to block self-defeating notions and substitute more effective ideas, for example.

DRUGS Effective drugs for the treatment of depression also exist. The fact is that depression tends to be a self-sustaining frame of mind, with withdrawal leading to reduced social support and pleasure, thus leading to more withdrawal, and so on. If this cycle can be interrupted with medication, a return to more normal patterns of thinking may permit a restructuring of attitudes that makes life possible, in time, without depression and without the medication.

The most commonly used drugs for pure depression are the so-called *tricyclics* (after their chemical appearance). Familiar trade names include Elavil, Sinequan, and Tofranil. Newer drugs are being introduced, but they are not as well studied. These drugs differ in various ways, but on the whole they are more alike than different. Most require a matter of weeks to become fully effective, and often a higher dose is needed than originally prescribed.

Many experts have charged that physicians who aren't familiar with these drugs prescribe them in doses that are too low and for periods that are too short—then erroneously conclude that the medication can't help. As a rule, these drugs are not effective below a dose that produces some side effects, such as dry mouth or a slight hesitancy in urination. Guesswork about proper doses can be reduced, because blood tests can measure the actual level.

For some people, an entirely different type of drug, lithium carbonate, can be very effective. However, this agent appears to be most helpful in the disorder known as *bipolar disease*. This condition is typified by a swing from such manic behaviors as talking nonstop, making grandiose plans, or going on spending sprees, to withdrawing and feeling severely depressed. Lithium can help both to blunt the upswing and to reduce the severity of the depression.

"SHOCK" TREATMENT Finally, *electroconvulsive therapy* (ECT), also known as "electric shock" therapy, can be used to treat severe depression, although it remains controversial. The controversy stems from concerns about the side effects—mainly memory loss—and from social opposition.

There is little question about the effectiveness of ECT as a treatment for depression. Most psychiatric authorities hold that ECT is often more effective than drugs in the treatment of very severe depressions. A panel of experts convened by the National Institutes of Health stated in 1985, "It should be emphasized that for certain patients with very specific and narrow indications, ECT may be the only effective treatment available. In certain circumstances of acute risk to life or of medical status incompatible with the use of other effective treatments, ECT may be the first treatment [that should be used]."

The clearest indication for using ECT is when the potential for suicide is high. Suicide is far from rare; it is the tenth leading cause of death in this country and the second in the age group from 15 to 34. The risk that a depressed person will take his or her own life must be weighed against the possible side effects of ECT treatment.

As performed today, ECT is very safe. Short-acting anesthetics, muscle relaxants, and oxygen are given to prevent injury from physical convulsions during the application. Relatively low voltages can be used, and the electrodes can be applied in ways that minimize side effects.

The SAD phenomenon

One form of depression seems not to result either from a triggering situation or from an internal biochemical shift. Known as *seasonal affective disorder* (SAD), this type of depression seems to arise from inadequate exposure to light. Sensitive people are evidently dependent on the stimulus of daylight, or nearly equivalent light, for the production of certain brain chemicals that keep them energized. In winter, especially in temperate latitudes nearer to the poles, these people can become dejected for no apparent reason.

There has been some success in treating this condition both with a drug, fenfluramine, and with exposure to bright lights. It is not clear that treatment with just any light is adequate; a special variety whose spectrum is somewhat similar to sunlight may be more beneficial. Exposure early in the morning seems to be the most effective in producing relief, although phototherapy also works at other times of day.

The use of psychotherapy

For many kinds of emotional distress, in which the person feels a sense of being unable to function or to cope with the normal demands of life, or in which a specific symptom, such as an anxiety or a behavior, is troubling, psychotherapy can often be effective. The number of "talking" therapies is myriad, and would take much more space to describe than we have available here. Folklore about the different types is also abundant. Choosing from such a range of therapies would be daunting if any of us really were to start from scratch. Most of us don't. Rather, we work through the available networks, getting recommendations from friends, physicians, school personnel, and so on.

It is exceedingly difficult, at present, to find clear guidance as to which theoretical orientation is best in any given situation. There is some reason to believe that a therapist's explicit theoretical position may be less important than his or her professional style.

Psychotherapy seems to work best when the therapist and client feel a mutual affinity, which includes some degree of shared values and a sense of rapport. There are relationships that just don't click, and it's not worth spending a lot of time trying to analyze why. A candidate for psychotherapy is well advised to judge within the first

2 or 3 sessions whether he or she feels able to work with a particular therapist. If not, looking for another one is probably the next step to take. It can be difficult in a time of extreme emotional discomfort to take an independent position and say to oneself, "This isn't working," and move on. But passively assuming that the therapist is automatically the one to make all the decisions and evaluate the relationship is not a productive point of view.

After a few sessions, when a relationship has formed between the therapist and the client, evaluating whether to continue or not becomes more complicated. Negative feelings may be an expression of the very problem that therapy is intended to treat. On the other hand, a sense that no progress is being made may be entirely valid. It is perfectly reasonable, and productive, to discuss with the therapist how progress will be evaluated and to set, in advance, a time when it will be discussed. But to ask a therapist for precise promises as to how long the treatment will take, or what the outcome will be, is unrealistic.

Sleep Disturbances

It is sometimes said that Napoleon slept only a few hours a night—implying that the rest of us could go out and conquer the world if only we spent less time sleeping. However, the record for time awake probably belongs to an Australian woman who routinely slept only about one hour a night but otherwise was not an unusual person. People often complain about the time they must spend sleeping, as though it deprived them of opportunities to do other, more interesting things. Yet there are some indications that dreams contribute to creativity. In any event, sleeping is, as it always has been, the way most of us will spend about a third of our lives.

The act of sleeping may seem familiar, but almost everything about it is puzzling.

- Few needs are felt more intensely than the "need" to sleep, yet nobody really knows why sleep is biologically necessary.
- Sleeplessness makes most people feel thoroughly miserable. Surprisingly, though, no diseases are known to result purely from lack of sleep.

- The sleeper is often thought to be "out of it"—but a great deal of mental activity goes on during sleep.
- The "deepest" sleep is the phase during which people are most likely to move around, talk, or even walk; by contrast, the body is most relaxed precisely when dreaming is most active.
- Substances that make us sleepy often make sleep less restorative.

Even though sleeplessness does not, by itself, produce illness, nobody can deny that feeling well and being effective require adequate amounts of restful sleep. Sleepy people are also at relatively high risk of having or causing accidents; to that extent, lack of a good night's sleep is potentially lethal.

The nature of sleep

The brain does not just shut down during sleep. On the contrary, being asleep involves a lot of mental activity, which has its own organization. Nerve cells located deep in the brain are responsible for managing sleep, and one of their major roles is to disconnect mental interaction with the outside world. Sensory input is markedly reduced (but not necessarily eliminated) and signals to the muscles are diminished.

For practical purposes, there are two major types of sleep, which tend to alternate through the night.

The type that is associated with vivid dreaming is called REM, for rapid eye movement (which occurs at this time). As dreams flash across the mental screen during REM sleep, the nervous system essentially segregates the brain from the rest of the body. Muscles go limp, breathing becomes steady and regular. This feature of REM sleep—virtual paralysis—probably permits the brain to dream while protecting the body from reacting to the content of the dream.

One aspect of bodily function, however, is not eliminated during REM sleep. Both men and women show signs of sexual arousal during every period of REM sleep. Indeed, the erectile response is so reliable that it can be used as one way to evaluate whether a man complaining of impotence has a physical problem or a psychological one: physical impotence is likely if erections do not occur during REM sleep.

The other type of sleep, not very helpfully called "non-REM," is what we associate with a "deep, dreamless" state. Both adjectives are misleading, however. A person who is awakened from non-REM sleep is likely to report that some kind of mental activity was going on—perhaps with the familiar statement, "I wasn't really sleeping; I was just thinking," though the subject matter of the thoughts may be hard to state. Or some very ordinary train of thought may be described: "I was thinking about the work I have to do tomorrow." Mental activity in this phase of sleep seems to lack the visual intensity, the extravagance, or the illogical character of REM thoughts.

During non-REM sleep, people typically move around—readjusting their bodies, taking pressure off an arm or a leg that has been slept on. This is an absolutely normal feature of sleep—indeed, no one truly "sleeps like a log." You may wake up in the same position as when you fell asleep—but there's been a lot of travel time in between.

The normal night begins with a rapid descent into the deepest stage of non-REM sleep. After an hour or so, a REM period (or "dream") begins. It lasts for 20–30 minutes, and is then followed by a return to non-REM sleep. This sequence is repeated 2 or 3 times a night, with the cycles getting a little shorter. Finally, after a last hour or so of non-REM sleep, arousal begins.

The average amount of time spent sleeping varies quite a bit from person to person. Some people require 9 or 10 hours of sleep; others do well with 5 hours. The difference between the two extremes is accounted for mainly by the time spent in REM sleep. Those who sleep longer spend almost all of their "extra" time in this stage of sleep.

The amount of sleep any one person requires may well be under genetic influence, and it is a trait that is relatively resistant to modification. However, there has been at least one experiment in which volunteers agreed to go through a period of gradually reducing their sleep time. During the study, the subjects managed to cut out an hour or more from their habitual sleep time without reporting any discomfort; for years afterward, some of them continued to sleep less than before.

The preferred time for sleep seems to be somewhat more fixed. Although most people choose the period between about 11 at night and 7 in the morning for sleep, there are "larks" and "owls" who function best very early in the morning or late at night, respectively, and who do not take kindly to having their sleep—wake cycle shifted to another time of day.

A good life's sleep

At least part of the psychological comfort of sleep comes from the sense that it is a reliable, unchanging part of life. The fact that sleep takes us away from thoughts about work and worries is what makes it pleasant. So waking up in the middle of the night is often viewed as a particularly unpleasant intrusion, an abnormality that needs to be corrected.

Waking up during the night is far from abnormal, however, and it becomes progressively more common with age (*see illustration*). After infancy, most children, once they're asleep, stay asleep. Except perhaps for a few minutes here and there, they're out for the night—and the night typically lasts 8 or 9 hours. The amount of time spent sleeping increases during adolescence, for reasons that are not known.

Time spent sleeping diminishes somewhat during young adulthood. On the whole, the sense of passing an unbroken night persists, even though, in reality, most people at this age wake up for a few minutes from time to time. These periods of wakefulness are usually too short to be registered, and by morning they are forgotten.

But with age, the pattern of normal sleep changes. The total time spent sleeping is likely to diminish from 7 or 8 hours to something between 5 and 7. And sleep no longer occurs as an unbroken period; it becomes a sequence of naps lasting an hour or so. Between naps, the person may wake fully enough to be aware of his or her surroundings, and to remember being awake when the night is over. The periods of wakefulness become more frequent and longer as morning approaches, so the memory of a "restless" night is likely to focus on the last couple of hours of alternate dozing, dreaming, and thinking.

In itself, this pattern of sleeping is normal and should not be regarded as a problem. The felt lack of sleep does not impair performance during the day, and need not be associated with daytime drowsiness. People who dislike the sense of being in bed but not really sleeping can sometimes adjust by planning to sleep shorter nights—going to bed later and getting up somewhat earlier.

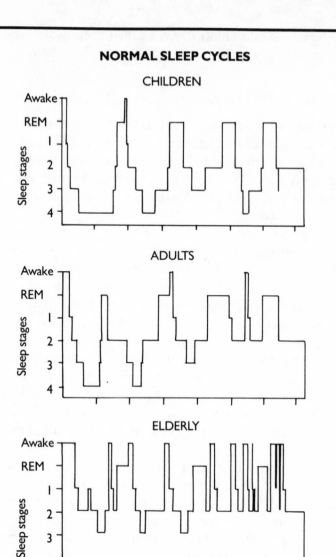

NORMAL SLEEP CYCLES

CHILDREN

ADULTS

ELDERLY

Hours of sleep

People in all three age groups get about the same amount of REM sleep, but the time spent awake during the night markedly increases with age. The time spent in stage-4 sleep (the "deepest" of the four stages into which non-REM sleep can be divided on the basis of distinct changes in brain-wave patterns) decreases with age. The significance of these different stages of non-REM sleep is not clear.

Sleep insurance

Given the amount of time we spend sleeping, a modest investment of effort to review and revise sleeping conditions would seem well spent. People who aren't sleeping well may find the source of their problem in the following checklist.

THE BEDROOM Light, temperature, ventilation, humidity, noise—most of these are potentially correctable factors, though apartment and city dwellers may find that noise is outside their control. Various types of preformed and moldable wax ear plugs can be purchased—although this strategy seems like a poor compromise at best. Many people adapt to routine levels of noise—failing to register the passing of airplanes or noisy vehicles at a conscious level—but there is evidence from EEG studies that sleep in a noisy environment is never as complete as in one that is quiet, even when people think they have adjusted. The fact that people are still "listening" to sounds in the environment is exemplified by the fact that some will awaken when the expected sound is *not* heard.

THE BED Soft, hard, large, small—there are so many differences in taste that a uniform prescription for the type of bed one should choose hardly seems possible. The point is for the restless sleeper to evaluate his or her usual bed to see whether it could be contributing to the problem.

People with physical disorders that interfere with sleep may be able to modify their beds in ways that relieve discomfort and favor sleep. For example, those who are prone to developing cramps in their feet or legs may find help by relieving the pressure of bed coverings with a simple support for the covers, placed at the foot of the bed. People with heartburn—the discomfort of stomach acid rising into the esophagus—may be helped if they slightly raise the head of their bed. Specific orthopedic problems may require more elaborate modifications.

BEDTIME The restfulness of sleep is only partly a matter of how much one gets. A critical factor is *when* it occurs. People who change their habitual times for going to sleep and getting up are bound to have trouble. Even the shift from week to weekend and back produces detectable abnormalities of the sleep cycle and of daytime functioning. An elaborate system of controls, depending both on the nervous system and on certain hormones, programs the body for waking and sleeping functions at roughly predictable times of day. One of the first steps in correcting mild insomnia is to establish a perfectly regular schedule, including weekends.

THE ALARM CLOCK An alarm clock can be an aid to sound sleep. Alarm clocks are probably not, strictly speaking, necessities. Most people have the ability to pre-program themselves to wake up spontaneously at any particular time (more evidence that the brain is thoroughly active during sleep). However, most people who do this, unless the habit is very strongly ingrained, will be more vigilant in the course of the night, wakening from time to time, checking the clock to make sure they haven't overslept. Setting an alarm clock is a way to reassure oneself that the time to get up has not arrived and thus to diminish unnecessary vigilance prior to the final awakening.

By contrast, anyone who must rely on an alarm clock to waken— and can only drag out of bed if a noisy alarm is placed on the other side of the room—isn't getting enough sleep. This use of an alarm is an invitation to misery. People who are getting enough sleep should waken spontaneously, more or less at the time they need to.

DRUGS Many drugs, most notably alcohol and caffeine, have the potential to disrupt sleep. Anyone who is having difficulty with insomnia should minimize his or her intake of both these drugs. Consumption of caffeinated beverages should be limited, and restricted to the hours before noon. Consumption of alcohol probably should not exceed the two-drink-a-day limit, and drinks after dinner should be avoided.

DINNER It may seem too obvious to mention that some foods, particularly spicy ones, may interfere with sleep. But any checklist of factors contributing to insomnia should include a quick review of problem foods.

EXERCISE Timed right, which means in the late afternoon or early evening, a period of brisk exercise almost automatically improves sleep. Jogging right before bed probably isn't as effective, both because it's stimulating and possibly because it may throw off the normal temperature cycle that is part of the way the body organizes its day–night functions. Morning exercise may make an afternoon nap very desirable but contribute little to the ease of sleeping at night.

COMPANY People always sleep better—as measured by the EEG—when they sleep alone. There's a marked tendency for regular bed partners to synchronize their sleep cycles and minimize whatever disruption occurs, but such synchrony is never perfect. Sex adds a dimension of complexity as well. If partners are aroused at different times, or if conflict over the timing and performance of sex is an aspect of the relationship, sleep is likely to suffer. The only solution is probably a negotiated settlement. Bed partners should be prepared to discuss the effect they have on each other's sleep.

CONDITIONING People are much more complicated than pigeons, but the two species have some things in common. One of them is susceptibility to conditioned learning—the formation of habitual responses to certain stimuli. If bed and bedroom come to be associated with activities other than sex and sleep, distraction is almost inevitable. Although the most efficient use of space in a house or apartment may indicate that a work space should be combined with the bedroom, the hazard is that associations to work will butt in to stimulate arousal when sleep might otherwise be forthcoming. People whose sleep is troubled by intrusive thoughts and worries should make it a flat policy to use their bedrooms only for sleeping and sexual activity—and may even want to relocate the latter if sleep is excessively fragile.

Slumber aids

Basic sleep patterns are relatively difficult to alter. But disruptions that are transient, or create a lot of discomfort, can often be handled fairly simply.

Prescription

Sleeping pills are not, as a rule, the route to go. Sleep medications help people fall asleep 20 minutes faster, or so, and they often prolong sleep by half an hour or more. But the full effect only lasts for a few days, then people start getting used to them. After a few weeks, sleep medications become virtually ineffective, in that the person taking them is back to the same sleep pattern as before. But by now the drugs may seem essential, because dependency has been established. What this means is that the person now needs a pill simply to get the same, unsatisfying, amount of sleep as before the drug was started.

Essentially all sleeping pills produce a slight hangover, which is detectable as impairment of performance during the following day. The effect may be minimal, but it is consistently measurable when studied. Even the so-called short-acting drugs have a lingering effect, though the person who has taken one may not feel groggy.

Sleeping pills have certain valid uses. People who are going through a period of severe emotional stress, with identifiable causes, may be helped through a couple of rough nights with medication. Such stresses may include hospitalization, bereavement, or events in life that are anxiety-provoking but recognizable as temporary. Drugs with a very short duration of action have been reported to help people adjust to jet lag. And people with chronic insomnia sometimes benefit from *occasionally* using a pill, if only to protect them from panic at the thought that they will never again experience a solid night's sleep.

There are many conditions—medical and situational—that make the use of sleeping pills dangerous or unwise. Medical reasons include pregnancy and nursing, lung diseases, and sometimes kidney disease. Advancing age makes pills both less effective and more dangerous. Alcohol and sleeping pills often make a lethal combination; use of one should preclude the other. Anyone who may need to be alert at night—say to take care of a child or to perform a task—should avoid sleeping pills, and so should people who get up during the night to go to the bathroom. For that matter, anyone who needs to perform well the following day may do better after a night of fitful sleep than after taking a sleeping pill, because the medication hangover may interfere with ability more than the loss of sleep would.

The sleeping pills currently most prescribed are relatives of the familiar tranquilizer Valium, a class of drugs known as the *benzodiazepines*. These range from the very short-acting, which are mainly given when difficulty falling asleep is the complaint, to the longer-acting variants, which may help people who waken early in the morning. Unlike barbiturates, which were widely used in the past, these newer drugs don't lend themselves to lethal overdoses; to that extent, they are considered "safe." However, like the barbiturates, they mix very poorly with alcohol.

Barbiturates (such as Seconal and Nembutal) are prescribed much less frequently now than 15 or 20 years ago. As a result, there are many fewer deaths from overdose. Barbiturates were never all that satisfactory as sleeping medications because of their tendency to produce hangovers and to disrupt the normal pattern of sleep. Barbiturates rather rapidly produce addiction, as do some of the miscellany of other sleeping medications that served as alternatives before the benzodiazepines came into common use.

Nonprescription

Various nonprescription drugs, drinks, or foods sometimes serve as alternatives for people who don't want to take a prescription sleeping pill.

The main over-the-counter (OTC) drugs marketed as sleep promoting—such preparations as Nytol and Sominex—are *antihistamines*. When these drugs are used for allergies and colds, sleepiness is regarded as an undesirable side effect. On the other side of the coin, the drowsiness has been exploited both by manufacturers, who have packaged antihistamines as OTC sleep medications, and by people who have discovered for themselves that these drugs can work as a "mild" sleeping pill. Antihistamines are most effective in people who don't take them regularly, because tolerance to the drowsiness they produce does develop after a few days. And they are somewhat safer in relatively young people. Older people in particular may react rather badly to antihistamines—with confusion, dizziness, visual effects, and other distressing responses.

The amino acid L-*tryptophan* has enjoyed a lot of publicity as an aid to falling asleep, and can be purchased in tablet form from health food stores and drugstores. Tryptophan, which is normally present in the diet, enters the brain, where it favors formation of serotonin, a substance that is involved in the normal mechanisms of sleep induction. To be at all effective, half a gram to a gram of L-tryptophan should be taken with a few crackers or some sugar on an otherwise empty stomach. Eating some pure, rapidly absorbed carbohydrate promotes secretion of insulin, which, in turn, helps the L-tryptophan to be taken up by the brain. There is no reason to think that using L-tryptophan as a "natural" alternative to sleeping pills is effective for any but the mildest difficulty in falling asleep. And although L-tryptophan is touted as natural, the safety of taking repeated, high doses of the pure substance has not been established.

Alcohol is one of the least effective sleep medications on the open market. Although it usually induces drowsiness, within hours after an alcoholic drink is taken a kind of withdrawal syndrome develops and disrupts sleep. What begins as a kind of dopey slumber easily turns into a night of tossing and turning. Getting up to take another drink might relieve this problem—at the price of setting up a pattern perilously close to alcoholism. Unfortunately, this seems to be precisely the pattern that is followed by many people who rely on alcohol for sleep. People who have difficulty sleeping are well advised to minimize their alcohol intake in general and to drink nothing after the dinner hour.

Insomnia

Sleeplessness has many causes, but *insomnia,* as the term is commonly used, refers to a poorly understood situation in which people habitually have difficulty falling asleep and staying asleep *when it is time to go to bed.* In front of a television set, sleep may come rapidly and comfortably, but when the covers are turned back, vigilance takes over.

It has been suggested that there are two main components to this type of insomnia. One of them is a high level of anxiety. As soon as the distractions of the day are removed, obsessive and unpleasant thoughts begin to intrude. The other component is probably a set of learned responses related to bedtime. One such response is the expectation that falling asleep will be difficult and fraught with discomfort. As this expectation becomes established, going to sleep acquires some of the features of performance anxiety. Asking oneself, "Will I be good enough to master the task of falling to sleep?" is hardly conducive to relaxation. Many treatment programs for insomnia are based on the assumption that learned associations to the bedroom, bedtime, and the act of going to bed are part of the problem. For example, it is said that many insomniacs have little difficulty going to sleep in hotel rooms, guest rooms, or on the living room couch.

Although there's some dispute about these two components of "learned" insomnia, they seem plausible, and many behavioral recommendations for combating insomnia are based on them. For example, a common recommendation is that bed and bedroom should be associated only with successful sleep. If the insomniac can't fall asleep after a specified period of time, rather than lying in bed to dither and obsess, he or she should get up, go to another place, and pursue a relaxing activity until sleepiness is felt, then return to bed. This routine should be repeated as often as necessary to establish the belief that, once in bed, the person will fall asleep. This kind of behavior therapy, called *stimulus control,* may help retrain the insomniac to expect only sleep in the bedroom, and to associate bedtime only with going to sleep. For hardcore insomniacs, however, these methods may not be particularly successful.

Certain treatable conditions sometimes manifest themselves primarily as insomnia; once the underlying disorder is treated, the insomnia goes away. Depression quite commonly leads to disordered sleep patterns, with early-morning awakening as the most conspicuous abnormality. Psychotherapy or antidepressant medication can restore normal sleep. When the hot flashes of menopause interrupt sleep, estrogen replacement therapy can relieve this symptom and make sleep more restful.

Sleep demons

A variety of odd conditions that interfere with sleep go under the generalized term *parasomnias.* These can be as mild as little jerks that sometimes occur during the phase of drowsiness before deep sleep begins, or they can be seriously disruptive, if not to one's own sleep, to that of a bed partner. The "restless legs syndrome" is one of the more troublesome parasomnias, and it becomes more prevalent with age. Related complaints include head banging (usually in small boys), tooth grinding (bruxism), sleep headaches (in the migraine/cluster family), and various abnormal movements occurring during sleep.

The cause of these many disturbances is not known. They are not a sign of either epilepsy or mental illness. They do seem to run in families, and they may reflect a peculiar lapse in the ability of the brain to organize sleep. Perhaps the abnormal movements are successfully suppressed during consciousness but break through as drowsiness takes over. Yet, most of the parasomnias also become worse with anxiety, and caffeine can exacerbate them.

Restless legs syndrome may be a good deal more common than is often assumed. Some investigators have found the symptoms in around 10% of normal subjects they studied. At rest, or as sleep begins, the person with restless legs syndrome develops an uncomfortable sensation, usually in the area between knee and ankle, but sometimes involving the feet, the thighs, or even an arm. The sensation is difficult to describe, but is often characterized as creeping or crawling (like worms or ants in the muscles) and seems to come from deep within the leg, not the skin. It virtually forces the victim to change position or get up and walk around in the hope of relieving it. Movement is "voluntary," in the sense that it can be suppressed for a while, but usually the sensation is so uncomfortable that the sense of needing to do something about it is irresistible.

Often there is no explanation for restless legs syndrome, but it sometimes is associated with iron deficiency, and a check for this cause of anemia is warranted. Drug treatment has generally been unsatisfactory, although clonazepam, a drug used to treat epilepsy, sometimes helps. Because tolerance develops, the drug may have to be used only a few days a week, or only 2–3 weeks out of the month, with drug "vacations" in between. A recent report indicates that L-dopa, in levels much lower than those used to treat Parkinson's disease, can be quite effective. L-dopa usually is given with another drug, carbidopa, that helps reduce side effects. Some patients get relief by keeping their legs cold at night; a smaller number resort to heat.

Bruxism, or tooth grinding at night, seems to be a feature of people who do precise, demanding work; it is associated with tension; and it may run in families. Dentists are most likely to make the diagnosis. Treatment may include both sleeping with a guard to protect the dental enamel and counseling to work on the tensions expressed this way.

Other parasomnias are less common. They range from peculiar movement disorders (such as tensing of the torso) to unexpected episodes of aggression in otherwise mild-mannered people. The theme running through all of these disorders is a failure of the motor system to fully relax during sleep and "disconnect" from thought processes.

Narcolepsy

Once regarded as something of a clinical rarity, narcolepsy is now recognized to be a relatively common, and potentially very disabling, condition that affects around one person in a thousand. This condition is not a disorder of sleep at night. It takes the form of sudden sleep attacks occurring unpredictably during the day. These may last as long as half an hour or pass off in a matter of seconds.

They are more common during quiet moments, but can also be provoked by stimulation, such as laughing, a feeling of anger, or being startled.

Narcolepsy can be quite dangerous when it is accompanied by a tendency to go suddenly limp when the sleep attack begins. This condition, termed *cataplexy,* affects about three-quarters of people with narcolepsy.

Sometimes, the narcoleptic continues to function—carrying on with tasks, conversations, and the like—but in an uncharacteristically mechanical fashion. When the episode is over, there will be no memory of these activities or events.

Narcolepsy can be seen as a disorder of the mechanism governing REM sleep. The brain centers that manage this phase of normal sleep seem to be unusually active or irritable. They turn themselves on all of a sudden, leading to altered consciousness on one hand, and paralysis on the other. This interpretation is supported by the fact that REM sleep tends to appear earlier than normal in nighttime sleep.

Despite the sound of its name and some of its clinical features, narcolepsy has no connection with epilepsy. It is a unique disorder, which runs in families and probably reflects a combination of genetic and environmental factors.

Narcolepsy can usually be recognized on the basis of descriptions given by the victim and relatives or friends. Evaluation of sleep in a sleep laboratory may help pin down the diagnosis. Various drugs have been used to help mitigate this condition. The stimulant methylphenidate (Ritalin) is most commonly used, and it works quite well. If cataplexy is a prominent feature of the sleep attacks, one of the antidepressant drugs may be needed. (Here, as in many other situations, the fact that these drugs are primarily used to combat depression is incidental; they have other important effects on the brain's activity.)

Sleep apnea

Some people stop breathing for alarmingly long periods of time at night, say longer than 10 seconds. If this occurs more than 30 times during a typical night's sleep, the diagnosis of sleep apnea (nonbreathing) is made. Most of the people affected are men in their mid-40s or older. They tend to be overweight and to have hypertension. Sleep apnea is potentially a life-threatening condition because blood oxygen levels fall during the breathless period. If coronary artery disease is also present, as is not unlikely, the lack of oxygen may trigger a heart attack.

As a rule, sleep apnea is not at first identified as a disorder of sleep. Falling asleep is easy, though some people may complain of disruptions later in the night. However, a bed partner or roommate is likely to report periods of ominous silence followed by loud, raspy snoring and gasping sounds.

The main complaints have to do with daytime drowsiness or sleep attacks and irritability. Careful assessment may show that attention span is reduced, thinking is slowed, and recent memory is impaired. Psychological distress is often apparent and is presumably both a result of the disorder and an exacerbating factor.

As with most of the other sleep disorders, the real cause of sleep apnea is not known. There are, broadly speaking, two types. The *obstructive* type seems to be associated with distorted passageways for breathing—an inability of the muscles to keep the upper airways open. Some evidence suggests that the area where the back of the nose and mouth connect to the trachea (the *pharynx*) may be abnormally small in people affected by obstructive sleep apnea. Much less common is *central* sleep apnea, which is not associated with snorting, gasping, or snoring. The best explanation of this condition is that brain mechanisms controlling normal respiration tend to switch off during sleep. They allow a build-up of carbon dioxide to much higher than normal levels before switching on again.

Diagnosis of sleep apnea requires both painstaking discussion with other people in the victim's life, especially those who sleep near him (or, less commonly, her). A few nights in a sleep laboratory may be needed to verify a history suggestive of sleep apnea and to establish the type.

The disorder can be quite devastating, both to the patient and to family and associates—especially if it has gone on for a while without being recognized. Treatment should, therefore, include careful explanations and counseling.

Various measures can be taken to relieve obstructive sleep apnea. Weight loss is invariably recommended, but it is often difficult to achieve and is not always that helpful. Associated medical conditions, such as high blood pressure, heart or lung problems, and hormonal abnormalities must be treated and may help with the problem. Various anatomical approaches to keeping the upper airway open are the next line of treatment. Mechanical aids may be tried, but they are often not very acceptable to the patient and they work inconsistently. Surgery on the upper airway is a possibility, especially if there are obvious abnormalities contributing to closure of the airway, but the results are not predictable and complications are possible. A relatively simple surgical procedure is to create a direct opening to the trachea (a *tracheostomy*) in the lower neck. The tracheostomy bypasses the blocked airway further up and permits unobstructed breathing throughout the night. The tracheostomy can be plugged during the day to permit normal speech and breathing. This surgery is not free of complications, and it can have a major effect on the patient's body image, so it is not a procedure to be undertaken lightly.

Treatment of obstructive sleep apnea should probably begin with mechanical devices, which don't involve permanent changes in the body. If, as is all too common, these devices don't work, a surgical procedure may have to be tried.

Headaches

Most headaches are annoyances that disappear on their own. When they don't, a mild pain reliever or a relaxation break is usually enough to handle the discomfort. Sometimes, though, headaches become disabling. And, rarely, they are the earliest sign of serious trouble.

As common as headaches are, surprisingly little is known about what causes them. The very term "tension headache," used to describe the garden variety, is ambiguous. Does it refer to tension in the muscles at the back of the neck and scalp, which are known to tighten in response to stress? Or does it refer to emotional tension, supposedly responsible for the headache? The fact is that high levels of stress do not necessarily accompany tension headaches. So it is inaccurate, and perhaps unjust, to assume that everyone who suffers from tension headaches is severely stressed, or failing to cope with stress. Indeed, the headaches themselves may be the main source of emotional tension.

So-called tension headaches

When tension headaches interfere with daily activities, medical help is often sought. By this stage, a variety of pain relievers, including aspirin and acetaminophen, have been tried without consistent benefit. Narcotic medications, especially those with codeine, may be very effective, but they also carry the risk of overuse leading to addiction. Techniques to achieve rest and relaxation are often beneficial; biofeedback and acupuncture both have their advocates (and a track record of occasional success). In some cases, very sensitive spots ("trigger points") can be located at the back of the head. Injection of these scalp regions with a local anesthetic may help to stop the pain.

Before the diagnosis of tension headaches is accepted, some other conditions ought to be considered as a possible cause of the problem.

A very common cause of headache is caffeine withdrawal. Many people get unpleasant headaches between 18 and 36 hours after their last cup of coffee. Headaches of this type are apt to occur on weekends, when the first cup of coffee of the day is delayed. The headache is both diagnosed and treated by drinking a cup of coffee. People who are vulnerable to such headaches may wish to taper off their consumption of caffeine.

When sinusitis is the cause of headaches, other symptoms are often, but not always, present. These include nasal congestion and postnasal drip, production of greenish mucus, local tenderness of the face, and occasionally toothache. Antibiotics along with a decongestant will usually bring relief, but they must be taken for several weeks. Hot compresses on the forehead and cheeks may also help the infection to resolve.

Occasionally, a toothache will masquerade as a headache. This diagnosis may be a difficult one to establish. But once made, it leads to effective treatment.

When headaches regularly occur after close work, such as reading or sewing, the possibility of eyestrain should be investigated by an ophthalmologist or optometrist. People who already wear glasses or contact lenses should have their prescription checked. Sometimes, however, the problem is not in the eyes so much as in the work environment. Improving the design of the work station to provide adequate light and reduce glare may markedly lessen eyestrain, especially among people who work at video display terminals. Opportunities to rest the eyes from close work should be scheduled into the daily routine, whether or not headaches are a problem.

The diagnosis of temporomandibular (jaw) joint disease is in vogue these days. TMJ disease is a great deal less common than the diagnosis, and it is likely that only a tiny fraction of patients with headaches have anything seriously wrong with this joint. Surgery to correct purported abnormalities of the TMJ should be undertaken only after careful deliberation, supported by a second, and perhaps even a third, medical opinion.

Migraine

Migraine headaches are sometimes difficult to distinguish from tension headaches. In fact, many people appear to suffer from both conditions. It is a misconception that migraine headaches have to be severe—many are mild, and many tension headaches are quite as severe as the worst migraine. One clue that a headache may be a migraine is its location; typically, though not always, a migraine is felt on one side of the head, often behind the eye. Unlike tension headaches, migraine headaches can wake a person from sound sleep.

The exact cause of migraines is not known. The most popular theory relates the symptoms to changes in arteries near the surface of the brain. In many cases migraine headaches begin with spasm in one of these arteries. Reduced blood flow then produces the initial forms of discomfort—often hours before pain occurs. Nausea and vomiting are common, hence the old designation, "sick headache." Other advance warnings include flashing lights or lines (scintillations), appearance of a blind spot (scotoma), dizziness, or just an indescribable feeling that "It's coming!" These symptoms are called the *prodrome*. This form of migraine attack can occur even when no headache follows; this tends to happen more commonly in later life and is sometimes confused with a transient ischemic attack, a warning sign of stroke (*see Chapter 7*). It's important to bear this possibility in mind for two reasons: expensive and sometimes risky tests can be avoided, and the episodes may respond to treatments that work for regular migraine.

After a period of spasm, the arteries participating in a migraine attack may dilate excessively. The result is pain, usually throbbing, which is attributed to distention of sensitive tissue near the artery. During the headache, and even at other times, the migraine patient is made more uncomfortable than usual by bright lights (photophobia) and loud noises (sonophobia). The sufferer is apt to look for a quiet dark place, but this tendency is not distinctive; similar refuge is sought by people with tension headaches or other kinds of pain.

Susceptibility to migraine often runs in families. There's also a curious connection to motion sickness. Many adults with migraine recall that they were often car-sick as children. Women with migraine often have more difficulty just before and during menstruation than at other times. During pregnancy, the headache pattern often changes. Most often headaches worsen, but some women with migraine are amazingly headache-free during pregnancy.

In addition to "classic" migraine, several other distinctive types of headache are considered to be in the migraine family, and all are treated in much the same way as migraine.

- *Cluster headaches,* which mainly affect men, are severe migraines that occur very frequently for days or weeks at a time, usually at the same time of day. They are often associated with a teary eye and runny nose on the side of the headache.
- *"Ice pick" headaches* are experienced as sudden severe stabs of pain at a single point on the surface of the head, as though struck by an ice pick.
- *Benign orgasmic headaches* occur especially in men. For a period of days or weeks, a severe headache is triggered each time sexual orgasm is reached. Then the phase passes, and all is well, though the problem may recur.
- *Postmenopausal migraine,* as the name implies, refers to severe headaches affecting women after menopause. This disorder may occur in women who never before tended to have migraine or other forms of headache.
- *Post-traumatic headaches* may occur in some people even after a very minor head injury without loss of consciousness. Such headaches can persist for up to a year after the trauma. They have many of the characteristics of migraine and are probably a variant of this condition.

In a small fraction of migraine patients, neurological symptoms go beyond the common tendency to have visual scintillations. There may be tingling, numbness, or weakness of part or all of one side of the body, or difficulty with speech may develop. *Very* rarely, the neurological deficits can become permanent.

As is true of tension headaches, physical or emotional stress may precipitate migraine, but migraine also has the peculiar tendency to be set off by relaxation. Sunday is the day of the week many people are most likely to have a migraine attack. (Since alcohol often triggers migraine headaches, Saturday night drinking may help bring on the Sunday headache.)

Acute migraine attacks are treated with a variety of pain relievers; often narcotics are needed for the most severe headaches. Some people report being helped by drinking black, undecaffeinated coffee. The patient who knows a migraine is coming on may be able to abort it by taking a medication containing ergot alkaloids (Cafergot, Migral, and others); these drugs are not as effective after the headache arrives. They should never be taken in the first trimester of pregnancy.

Newer kinds of drugs are being used to prevent attacks from occurring, but they must be taken on a daily basis. Beta-blocking agents (commonly used to treat angina, high blood pressure, and disorders of the heart's rhythm) can be very helpful. Calcium-channel blockers, used for many of the same heart conditions, are also being tried for migraine, but results are not yet clear and consistent. The use of antidepressant drugs is being explored, because it is known that this type of medication can bring pain relief to people who are not depressed.

Migraine sufferers should make the effort to be aware of any habits and activities that provoke attacks. Many people have been greatly helped by eliminating particular foods, discontinuing alcohol, or avoiding bright lights and glare. Some women have found that hormone pills (especially estrogens) precipitate or worsen migraine, and a reduction in dosage or discontinuation of the medication may alleviate their attacks. A subgroup of women who use birth-control pills, smoke cigarettes, and have migraine appear to be at special risk for developing a stroke during a migraine attack— another reason to stop smoking.

Headaches demanding medical attention

Most people who develop an especially severe headache wonder whether their symptom is a warning of serious trouble and whether to call a doctor. Could it be a brain tumor, a blood clot, or meningitis?

Although it is difficult to give absolute guidelines, here are some situations that demand early medical attention:

- A severe headache accompanied by fever and a stiff neck that resists being flexed forward means meningitis until proven otherwise. A medical assessment should not be delayed.
- Any headache accompanied by impairment of function, such as difficulty with speech, paralysis, imbalance, double vision, could be caused by bleeding, a clot, an abscess, or another process impinging on a portion of the brain.
- Sudden excruciating head pain, sometimes referred to as a *thunderclap headache,* deserves an immediate check for bleeding into the head, a possibility that can be assessed with a CT scan.
- A headache that slowly but inexorably worsens over days or weeks, especially if it is felt in one particular region of the head, may signal a blood clot or tumor and should be investigated.
- Pain at the temple in people over the age of 60 raises the question of cranial arteritis, a treatable condition which, if ignored, may lead to blindness. A simple blood test, the erythrocyte sedimentation rate (*see Chapter 8*), can be used to screen for this ailment.
- A headache, especially at the back of the head, that is worse in the early morning and gets better as the day goes on can be a sign of elevated blood pressure. This feature contrasts with tension headache, which is more common late in the day. High blood pressure does not cause headache nearly as often as most people think—in fact, dangerously high blood pressure often occurs in people who feel fine. But when new headaches make an appearance, the blood pressure should be checked—it's easy to do, and the returns can be high.

Back Pain

The human back is composed of a vulnerable column of individual bones (24 of them), known as vertebrae, which are held together by ligaments and muscles—and separated from each other by cushion-like discs (*see illustration*). Passing down through a continuum of central spaces in the vertebrae is the spinal cord. And emerging

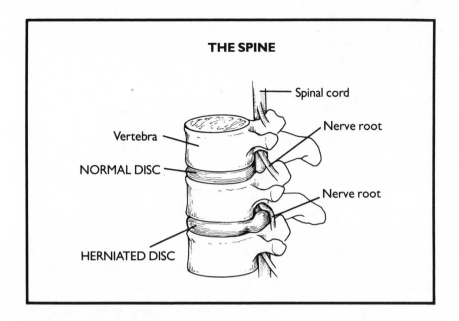

THE SPINE

Spinal cord

Nerve root

Vertebra

NORMAL DISC

Nerve root

HERNIATED DISC

from the spinal cord and coursing out between the vertebrae at all levels of the neck and back are spinal nerves which carry messages to and from all parts of the body. Talk about potential for trouble! Indeed, surveys indicate that 4 out of 5 people suffer back pain sometime in their life, and that back symptoms cause more visits to the doctor than any other ailment.

Unfortunately, the magnitude of the problem far outweighs precise knowledge about causes and treatment. In 80–90% of cases, doctors will never know the exact underlying cause. That's the bad news. The good news is that most individuals will get much better within several weeks, no matter what the cause or what they do about it. Thus, the precise diagnosis of a back problem is often not worth the time and money it would require.

Possible causes

When a patient comes to a doctor complaining of back pain, it is important for the physician to consider a variety of fairly uncommon but often serious possibilities, such as a benign or malignant tumor, local or widespread infection, or a generalized arthritic condition. Back pain that occurs at rest, especially during the night, or that causes a person to constantly shift position should raise the possibility of a tumor or an abscess in or near the spine. It is not our intention to review the many generalized diseases associated with back pain. Rather, we will focus on the much more common problems of the back associated with local structural derangements. One convenient way to think about such back problems is to group them as follows:

MUSCLE OR LIGAMENT STRAIN Most back pain is probably caused by the over-stretching of some of the many muscles and ligaments that hold our back bones together. Too much stretch can result in small tears of sensitive tissues. Often the exact site of tenderness can be pinpointed by an examining finger—which might also be able to outline actual muscle spasm. The standard answer to these back problems remains tincture of time, body positioning to avoid continued strain on the injured area, and temporary use of pain medicines and muscle relaxants as necessary.

BONE DEFECTS Standard x-ray studies are usually required to make a diagnosis in this category. Often, *congenital defects* in vertebral structure are found to be the cause of back pain that comes on for the first time in late adolescence or early adulthood. Another problem that has been receiving increasing attention is *lumbar spine stenosis* (LSS). This condition, which occurs in later life, is due to compression of the lower spinal nerves by the overgrowth of bone and other tissue into the spinal canal. Typical symptoms include not only back pain but pain, numbness, weakness, or heaviness in one or both legs during walking or standing erect—symptoms which can be relieved by bending at the waist to take pressure off affected nerve tissue. A common cause of back pain in older women is actual collapse of vertebrae as a consequence of bone thinning (*osteoporosis*).

DISC DISEASE This specific form of back problem accounts for 10–15% of all back pain. When it is suspected, a diagnosis may be worth pursuing.

Each of the discs which separate the spinal vertebrae has a soft, jelly-like center and a fibrous outer casing. Rapid protrusion of the soft center through the outer casing—so-called *herniation* of the disc (*see illustration, page 349*)—may be caused by sudden jerking movements, heavy lifting, or otherwise awkward positions. When the protruding material presses against an adjacent nerve root emerging from the spinal canal, pain will follow the pathway of the exiting nerve. Classical *sciatica,* a pain extending from the back of the thigh down the outer part of the lower leg and foot, is caused by squeezing of nerve tissue by a herniated disc.

A diagnosis of disc disease can often be made on the basis of a physical exam (responses to lifting a patient's leg from the supine position, as well as changed reflexes), but special imaging techniques are necessary before any invasive treatment can be planned. Most people with disc disease will get better with time and the same conservative treatments used for other back ailments—bedrest, pain relievers, muscle relaxants, local heat (and in severe cases possibly a trial of traction). However, surgery is more likely to be needed for disc protrusion than for any other back problem.

Diagnosing an aching back

In the vast majority of back-pain episodes, there is no need to pursue a precise diagnosis, since treatment would not be changed by doing so. However, when back pain is unusually severe, or progressive, or even when it is a first-time episode, a diagnostic evaluation is appropriate. As always, a good history—the story of how and when symptoms developed—should be taken and a physical examination should be performed. This exam should involve a fairly careful assessment of movement, sensation, and reflexes in the legs. Indeed, the hallmark of disc disease is that it involves the legs more than the back. One or more of the following tests may be indicated by the exam:

LABORATORY TESTS   If there is any concern that back pain may be due to a malignancy, infection, or metabolic problem, such tests as a blood count, sedimentation rate, urinalysis, and certain blood chemistries will usually be obtained (*see Chapter 8*).

BACK X-RAYS   These are among the more abused tests in medicine—ordered too often and too repetitively. However, when a back problem deserves sorting out, back x-rays are usually the first test ordered, mostly to check for structural or disease problems in the vertebrae. Back x-rays are not reliably useful for so-called "alignment" problems—a very subjective judgment at best—or for disc disease; soft tissues such as discs do not show up on regular x-rays. And repeated x-rays for each new episode of back pain are seldom justified. Many experts now use only two views, front and side, to assess the relevant anatomy, and dispense with the traditional multiple-angle "back series."

MYELOGRAM   This time-honored procedure consists of injecting a contrast material—sometimes called a dye—into the space surrounding the spinal cord, followed by x-rays. This will permit the visualization of a protruding disc or an obstructing tumor that would not be demonstrated by regular x-rays. Many back surgeons still insist on this test as the gold standard for diagnosing disc disease. Modern techniques have reduced the discomfort and risks of this procedure.

CT SCAN   This computerized imaging technique (produced from multiple x-ray pictures) is being increasingly used to diagnose disc disease. It has several advantages compared with a myelogram:

- No needle has to be stuck into a confined neurological space and no foreign substance is injected.
- The CT scan provides more information than just the outline of the spinal cord.
- It avoids the rather common after-effect of a myelogram, namely a headache that can be severe for hours or even longer.

Because of all these advantages, many experts are predicting that the CT scan will replace the myelogram as a diagnostic test—though some insist that both techniques will be used, since the different images provide complementary rather than duplicated information.

MAGNETIC RESONANCE IMAGING (MRI)   Not surprisingly, this latest imaging technique—which has the advantage of not using radiation—is being applied to back problems. It is too early to tell the exact role the technique will play in diagnosis, but it may have an important one.

Interventions

When time and conservative measures do not bring adequate relief from back problems, other approaches may be considered.

MANIPULATION   Even advocates of manipulative treatment acknowledge that scientific support is hard to come by. Those studies that have been attempted show short-term relief at best—something that often happens with time alone.

EXERCISE PROGRAMS Most experts believe that exercises to strengthen the muscles of the back and abdomen can be useful in keeping the back in proper position and in avoiding strain injuries. However, exactly which exercises are best for a given individual is often a matter of trial and error. Any exercise that causes pain should be avoided.

LEARNING PROGRAMS The recent explosion of "back schools" is testimony to the growing belief that people can prevent back problems by learning proper standing, sitting, lifting, and sleeping techniques. (The YMCA has a widely available, convenient, and low-cost program called "The Y's Way to a Healthy Back.") There has also been a corresponding growth in products such as special chairs and support devices for people with back problems. Most of these approaches still seem to require trial and error to find what works best in an individual case.

Surgery and its substitutes

Since it was first attempted in 1934, the surgical procedure to remove a protruding disc has had its ups and downs in terms of medical and public reputation. There is a growing consensus that surgery should be a treatment of last resort—and that too much back surgery has been done in the past. However, the questions of when disc surgery should be done, and whether alternatives should be considered, are still not clearly answered. The alternatives currently available are:

CHYMOPAPAIN INJECTION This much-publicized procedure was formally approved in November 1982 by the FDA—after many years of approved use in Canada and other countries. During the following year, thousands of American spinal surgeons were trained during one-day courses in the use of chymopapain, a substance injected directly into the disc to theoretically dissolve disc substance and thereby reduce protrusion. The number of such procedures done during 1983–84 rose dramatically.

Then in the spring of 1984, the principle distributor of chymopapain sent a letter to doctors warning of possible complications. Since that time—and because of legal pressure and medical skepticism—the use of chymopapain injections for disc disease has dropped dramatically. Only 10,000–15,000 were done in 1986. Many spinal surgeons argue that chymopapain injection can still be a valuable alternative in certain patients who need disc removal but who cannot tolerate—or will not choose—surgery. However, in this country, most neurosurgeons and many orthopedic surgeons have abandoned the procedure.

SUCTION DISKECTOMY This latest wrinkle in the removal of protruding disc material involves the insertion of a screw-driver-sized probe through a small incision in the skin into the disc—much in the manner that the smaller needle used for chymopapain injection is inserted into the disc under x-ray guidance. However, in the case of suction, no dissolving material is injected; instead, mechanical suction is applied to the probe to literally suck out the offending portion of the disc. This procedure still must be regarded as experimental.

Many spinal surgeons feel that neither of the above alternatives to disc surgery is as safe and sensible as the direct visualization of the spinal anatomy afforded by surgery. They argue that only when the exact anatomical problem can be seen in direct view can the most appropriate action be taken—sometimes removing the entire disc, but more often removing only the part that is causing actual pressure on a spinal nerve.

Other Nagging Ailments

Hemorrhoids

Some things never change. Hemorrhoids continue to hurt, and even though most of medicine has entered the Buck Rogers era, the treatment of hemorrhoids remains basically horse-and-buggy.

Hemorrhoids form in a cushion of blood vessels located just inside the anal canal. If these veins are put under pressure, they become engorged with blood. If the pressure is recurrent or sustained, the wall of one or more of the vessels becomes stretched, and the result is what we call a hemorrhoid (*see illustration*). Straining during defecation—because of constipation or hard bowel movements—is the most common cause of elevated pressure in this area, and thus of hemorrhoids. Pregnancy is another common cause.

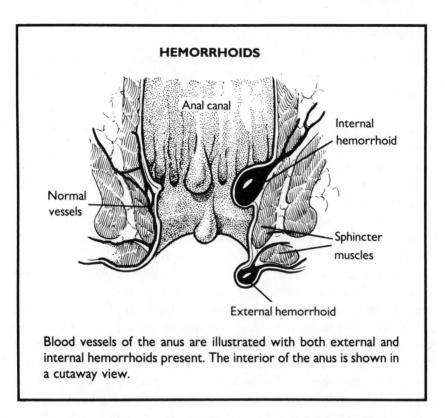

HEMORRHOIDS

Anal canal

Internal hemorrhoid

Normal vessels

Sphincter muscles

External hemorrhoid

Blood vessels of the anus are illustrated with both external and internal hemorrhoids present. The interior of the anus is shown in a cutaway view.

The distended vessel is fragile and thus tends to ooze blood. Bleeding or itching are, for most people, the first sign that a hemorrhoid has developed. Distention or distortion of the vein also slows the flow of blood within it, and this favors formation of a clot. Clotting makes the hemorrhoid swell further; pain, which may be quite severe, is the result. Such a *thrombosed* hemorrhoid may or may not be easily visible. If it is external, that is, outside the anal sphincter (the circle of muscles that controls defecation), it can be seen or felt as a round, tender bump. Hemorrhoids inside the sphincter are less easily observed. However, if an internal hemorrhoid protrudes into the anal canal, it may create the sensation that a bowel movement is needed, or has been incomplete.

The symptoms of pain and itching can be mimicked by a crack in the skin surrounding the anus, a *fissure*. The cause of a fissure is much the same: increased rectal pressure and hard bowel movements stretch the sphincter and abrade the mucous membrane. Home treatment of anal fissures is similar to that for hemorrhoids.

Home care

Sitting in a warm bath several times a day and using stool softeners usually suffice to relieve the discomfort of a thrombosed hemorrhoid. The associated anal itching or burning comes from skin breakdown which is exacerbated by inadequate clearing of fecal matter. Gentle washing or use of over-the-counter anal wipes can help to cleanse and soothe the area. Suppositories, creams, and ointments promoted for treatment of hemorrhoids are not clearly helpful, and some of them may cause allergic reactions of their own, or have other adverse effects. It's probably better not to use them. Occasionally, home treatment isn't adequate to clear up an acutely painful, thrombosed hemorrhoid. In that case, a surgeon can provide rapid relief by opening the vessel and removing the clot.

Regular evacuation of soft stools minimizes the pressure applied to the veins, thus allowing them to shrink. Soft, regular bowel movements are, therefore, both the best treatment for hemorrhoids and the best prevention. Any agent that attracts water into the bowel and adds bulk to the stool will serve this purpose. High-fiber diets and fiber-based laxatives, which work this way, are the mainstay of home therapy for hemorrhoids. Exercise and ample fluid intake also help. If a hemorrhoid gives repeated trouble despite simple preventive measures, further treatment may be needed.

Doctor care

The general principle underlying treatment of hemorrhoids is that no one needs all the veins in this area; there are plenty of others. So treatment is a matter of doing something to close off blood flow through the distended vessel, either by removing it or by inducing scar tissue to form so that it will not reopen.

Internal hemorrhoids are commonly "banded." A tiny rubber band is slipped, like a noose, around the swollen vessel and allowed to tighten in place. After about a week, the hemorrhoid falls off, painlessly. An alternative is to inject a scar-promoting chemical into the involved veins; known as *sclerotherapy,* this procedure seals off the distended veins. Banding and sclerotherapy cannot be used on external hemorrhoids, which are too sensitive to pain.

There is a procedure that can be carried out under local anesthesia to close off external hemorrhoids. An infrared device known as a photocoagulator can be used to burn the tissue. (A laser can be used for the same purpose. This fancier, and currently more expensive, technique has no clear advantage, although some observers report that it is less painful.) When external hemorrhoids resist both home treatment and photocoagulation, the only way to remove them is by a formal surgical procedure in which the veins are tied off and cut out or frozen with a very cold probe.

Once hemorrhoids have formed, the chances are fairly high that more will develop unless stools can be kept soft. Thus, dietary changes and the use of stool softeners are an essential part of therapy, even after surgery.

Hemorrhoids are everyone's idea of a minor medical problem (everyone, that is, who doesn't happen to have a hemorrhoid at the moment). But there is a life-and-death aspect to the subjects. Many rectal cancers are initially misdiagnosed as hemorrhoids because, like hemorrhoids, they often announce themselves with a show of red blood on the stool. Hemorrhoids are, to be sure, a much more common cause of blood observed on the stool. But the diagnosis should be proved, and never assumed. This usually requires, at a minimum, a careful examination of the anus and rectum. Rectal bleeding, when first observed, should be brought to a physician's attention.

Hiccups

The word *hiccup* comes from the sound they make. The alternative spelling "hiccough" apparently arose from a misconception that they were the result of some kind of breathing reflex, similar to a small cough. Not so.

Why hiccups exist is not known. They serve no useful purpose. Unlike a sneeze or a cough, they don't clear the respiratory tract. Unlike a gag, the hiccup doesn't protect the windpipe from accidentally inhaling solid or liquid food. Hiccups just occur and, for no known reason, affect men 4 times as often as women.

Hiccups come in two major categories, depending on how long they last. Most commonly, a bout lasts for minutes to hours. This type of hiccupping is associated with distention of the stomach, drinking alcohol or carbonated beverages, overeating, taking a cold shower, sudden excitement, emotional stress, or any of numerous other triggering events.

If hiccups last longer than 2 days, they enter the "persistent intractable" category. Such hiccups can just come on out of the blue, or they may be associated with causes that are almost as varied as with garden-variety hiccups. But occasionally the cause of long-term hiccupping is serious. Persistent hiccups have been associated with ulcers, heart attacks, epilepsy, or tumors of the brain stem. Indeed, virtually anything affecting the head, chest, or abdomen can be implicated.

The reason is partly understood. Hiccups are rhythmic contractions of the breathing muscles: the diaphragm (the sheet of muscle separating the chest from the abdomen) and the muscles connecting and bracing the ribs, the intercostals. The whole routine is coordinated by a group of nerves located in the upper end of the spinal cord (*see illustration*). If this hiccup "center" is stimulated, it responds by sending signals down the main nerve that controls the diaphragm, the *phrenic nerve*. This process is a reflex—a little like the knee-jerk—a more-or-less automatic response. Irritation of tissues anywhere in this circuit of nerve signals can trigger hiccups. Thus the source may be in the brain (if it affects the hiccup center), in the chest (where the phrenic nerve is located), or high in the abdomen (where the diaphragm can become involved).

Remedies

For the simple siege of hiccups, your favorite family remedy is probably as effective as any. Holding a spoonful of granulated sugar in your mouth, breathing into a paper bag, holding your breath, sneezing, arranging for a sudden fright, tickling the back of the throat with a cotton swab—take your pick.

Drugs can be used for intractable hiccupping. Most physicians begin with chlorpromazine (which is both an antipsychotic and an antinausea drug, as well as having other actions). Quinidine, a drug that suppresses the muscles' response to stimulation, may then be tried. Drugs effective against epileptic seizures—phenytoin, valproic acid, or carbamazepine—are a third choice. If drugs do not work, and the need for relief becomes desperate, the phrenic nerves can be surgically cut. This is not a procedure to be lightly undertaken, however, as respiratory paralysis can result.

The longest documented bout of hiccups on record lasted for 60 years; relief was attributed to prayers to St. Jude, the patron saint of lost causes.

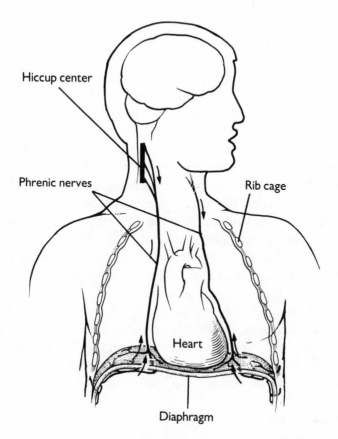

HICCUPS

Hiccup center

Phrenic nerves

Rib cage

Heart

Diaphragm

Signals carried mainly by the phrenic nerves are responsible for hiccups. Messages coming from the area of the diaphragm or heart (*up arrows*) travel to an area of the spinal cord where the "hiccup center" is located. The phrenic nerves also conduct spasmodic impulses (*down arrows*) that make muscles of the diaphragm and chest contract in a hiccup. Irritation at many locations in this circuit is capable of starting an attack.

Gas

Gas in the lower bowel never killed anyone—but that's about the best that can be said for it. Millions of people spend too much time worrying about foods they shouldn't eat, noises they shouldn't make, sphincters they shouldn't trust—all because they are prone to excess gassiness.

The complaint of "too much gas" is one of the leading problems brought to doctors who specialize in bowel diseases. In actuality, people who complain of gas can be referring to any (or all) of three distressing symptoms: excessive belching, the frequent passing of gas from the rectum (flatus), or a general sensation of bloating accompanied by squeaking or groaning noises. Of course, belching, expelling flatus, and experiencing occasional rumbles in the belly are perfectly normal. It's usually the extent to which these occur that disturbs the individual. More fastidious people become exasperated by even a few minor eruptions, whereas others will take no note of them. When the amount of gas in the intestines of patients with long-standing complaints of bloating and gas pockets is actually measured, it does not differ from normal. Thus, in most cases, internal sensations attributed to "too much gas" are probably due to other factors, such as disordered peristalsis of the intestines or unusual sensitivity to normal peristaltic waves. Gas in itself is not dangerous; its main consequence is usually embarrassment and social isolation for the person who can't "turn it off."

Where gas comes from

Five gases make up more than 99% of intestinal gas: oxygen, nitrogen, carbon dioxide, hydrogen, and methane. The first two, oxygen and nitrogen, enter the stomach as swallowed air, with 2 or 3 ml of air accompanying each swallow of food. Swallowed air increases when food is gulped. Carbonated drinks (which contain carbon dioxide) add considerably to gaseousness after eating. Some people swallow air as a nervous habit, totally unaware of what they are doing. The result of all this is excessive belching, meaning the expulsion of stomach gas back up the esophagus and out the mouth—with sound effects at no extra charge.

Hydrogen, carbon dioxide, and methane are the major gases produced in the large intestine. Hydrogen and carbon dioxide are formed by bacteria in the lower bowel (colon) when they ferment undigested food. Beans, for example, contain the complex sugars stachyose and raffinose, which cannot be broken down by the body's digestive enzymes to smaller sugars that can be absorbed. When they enter the colon with its large reservoir of bacteria, bacterial enzymes cause them to ferment, and gas is a product, much as it is when grapes ferment to form champagne. Patients with malabsorption problems due to pancreatic or small intestinal diseases will often complain of excessive gas because unabsorbed food reaches the bacteria in much larger amounts. Persons with a deficiency of the intestinal enzyme lactase cannot absorb lactose normally. It will undergo fermentation after reaching the colon, producing the typical bloating, cramping, and flatus they experience after taking milk or other dairy products. Whereas hydrogen and carbon dioxide form during fermentation, methane is produced differently and will be present even during fasting—but only in one person out of three. Who becomes a methane former is generally determined at an early age (probably mid-childhood) and depends less on genetic influences than environmental ones. Youngsters who grow up in houses where both parents are "methane formers" are very likely to be so themselves, whether they are biological or adopted children. Methane is the magic ingredient that makes flatus burn blue when lit—a well-known phenomenon in college dormitories and military barracks.

None of the gases thus far mentioned give flatus its most disturbing feature—its various odors. These are due to minute amounts of volatile chemicals formed by bacterial metabolism of residual protein and fat. Products responsible for the typical odor of feces, such as skatoles, indoles, ammonia, and hydrogen sulfide, are expelled with the larger quantities of other gases, but they are not the principal culprits in producing "too much gas."

Gas busters

Unfortunately, complete relief from gas problems is seldom achieved, but a number of things can be tried. For excess belching, the goal is to reduce aerophagia (air swallowing) by encouraging slower eating, more complete chewing, and avoidance of fizzy drinks. Controlling anxiety, when this is a factor, can also improve aerophagia, as can reduction in gum-chewing and smoking.

When trapped gas and bloating are the source of distress, remedies that can be tried include the use of simethicone drops (to break up the "big bubbles"), anti-cholinergic drugs, and paradoxically, fizzes to get out that big belch that lies there in waiting. Peppermints—frequently an after-dinner offering at restaurants—have some sound rationale for their use, since they relax the passageway from the stomach to the esophagus and thus make it easier for trapped gas to escape.

Excessive offensive-smelling flatus is, for many, the most disturbing of the functional bowel problems. The most important way to improve the situation is to examine the diet carefully and then make appropriate adjustments. Persons with lactase deficiency, for example, can expel massive amounts of flatus when they drink milk, and this can be reversed by avoiding dairy products. For others such "classic" incitants as beans, broccoli, onions, cauliflower, cabbage, radishes, and raw apples should be removed from the diet because they contain substances that ferment in the colon. There are really no good drugs for flatus control. While activated charcoal may be useful at times, it tends to bind other drugs a person may be taking and thereby prevent their absorption. The chronic use of antibiotics to rid the colon of its normal bacteria is hazardous.

Sometimes, simple behavior goals, such as practicing rectal sphincter control, avoiding crowded elevators after baked beans, and glaring at the next guy when all else fails, can make life easier. If these measures are of no avail, it's worth remembering that in remote sites such as the upper Amazon, there are societies where flatus-passing is not only socially acceptable but even a reason for envy by others. So there may be times when one's travel agent can be more helpful than any doctor.

Night sweats

It's bad enough to wake up in the middle of the night—but waking up with clammy sheets and the phrase "night sweats" running through your head has to be one of life's less pleasant experiences. Night sweats have become associated in the public mind with such diseases as tuberculosis, lymphoma, cancer, and AIDS. It is true that night sweats can be a feature of these conditions, but much more often than not the cause is benign.

To get an idea of how many people experience night sweats, two physicians at Hershey Medical Center in Pennsylvania asked a sample of all patients entering the hospital if they recalled an episode in the previous 3 months. It turned out that 40% of them did—and usually there was no clear connection with a disease. The strongest association was with pregnancy; some 60% of women entering the hospital for delivery reported night sweats.

Of the entire group of patients, about half reported episodes so mild that turning a pillow or moving back the covers was a sufficient remedy. One-quarter of the people were bothered to the point of getting up and washing. The remaining 25% actually needed to change their night clothes. As you might expect, some of these people also reported sweating during the day (it was summer). And a few indicated that night sweating ran in the family.

It should really come as no surprise that night sweats are so common. Of several daily cycles that the body goes through, one of the most important is a slight rising and falling of body temperature, which normally reaches its lowest point in the early hours of the morning. Among the most important ways the body has to dissipate heat and bring down its core temperature is to sweat. So, the warmer you are at bedtime, the more likely it is that you will sweat during the night. Exercising right before bedtime, for example, may lead to sweating a couple of hours afterward. Taking a bedtime dose of aspirin or acetaminophen, both of which act to lower body temperature, seems to be a relatively common cause of night sweats. Alcohol affects temperature regulation, and an evening of drinking can lead to a night of sweating. Obesity also predisposes to night sweats. Anyone with a fever is likely to go through a cycle of rising and falling temperature, with sweating during the cooling-off period. This is a perfectly normal part of having the flu, for example.

The daily temperature cycle, like the cycle of sleepiness and appetite, is controlled by the nervous system and is slowly shifted when time zones are crossed or habits changed. Moreover the various cycles are not all reset at the same rate. So people who alter their daily schedule, or travel to another time zone, are likely to notice themselves getting hungry, sleepy, or sweaty at inconvenient times. Usually, it takes about a day for each hour of time change to readjust these cycles.

The occasional damp forehead felt at night is not a cause for alarm but merely a sign that the body is making a minor adjustment of its thermostat. More conspicuous sweatiness, if there is no fever, may also be normal. But drenching sweats after a chill, sweats that come with a fever, or sweats occurring in a time of unexplained weight loss should prompt a call to the doctor.

7

The Big Three: Heart Disease, Stroke, and Cancer

Most death and disability in industrialized countries can be traced to the three diseases spotlighted in this chapter. But heart disease, stroke, and cancer are the "big three" in another, more positive sense—namely, in the amount of new information that has emerged in recent years on the prevention and early detection of these dreaded diseases.

Since the Second World War, enormous amounts of money have been poured into a series of battles against these three major killers. Improved techniques for the treatment of well-established disease are a very important outcome of this research, and some of the new therapies will be described in the following pages. But of far greater long-term significance is the information that is being developed about the underlying causes of heart disease, stroke, and cancers. New insights on the role of various triggers of abnormal cell growth, for example, may soon give us greater control over our chances of developing cancer. And a better understanding of the initial stages of malignant cell growth will yield more reliable screening methods and more precise interventions.

Heart disease, stroke, and most of the common cancers take many years to develop, and so they usually strike people in middle or old age. Our very ability to understand and control other kinds of disease—particularly the infections that once killed large numbers of children and young adults—has, ironically, left us vulnerable to these illnesses of later life. The current expansion of our biomedical knowledge should make the "big three" much less of a threat to well-being in the decades ahead. And the individual's role in avoiding premature death or disability from one of these illnesses is likely to increase rather than diminish, as we learn more about the interaction of lifestyle and health.

Heart Disease

Heart disease can take many forms, but the most dreaded by far is what is commonly called a *heart attack*. A heart attack occurs when the blood supply to some portion of the heart is reduced to such low levels that cells in the area cannot survive. Heart cells have two functions: to carry the electrical signals that coordinate the heart's rhythmic pumping action, and to contract, thus providing the force needed for the pumping. During a heart attack, as cells suffer from a severe shortage of blood and die, dangerous abnormalities of heart rhythm may occur and the pumping force may be weakened. If only a small area of heart muscle has been damaged, and if the damaged area is not in the main line of conducting tissue, heart function may return to almost normal once healing is complete. But a large area of injury, or injury to more than one area of the heart, makes full recovery less likely.

Often, reversible symptoms precede the permanent damage of a heart attack. These reversible changes are usually due to *ischemia*— a decreased blood supply often caused by a narrowed coronary artery. The characteristic response of any muscle to inadequate blood supply is pain. When the heart muscle is so deprived, the resulting pain is known as *angina*. Once the blood flow falls to a critical level in relation to the demand, the muscle tissue may be irreversibly damaged and die. This event is known as an *infarction*—in the case of the heart, a myocardial infarction. (Because a blood clot, or thrombosis, often forms in an already narrowed coronary artery, a heart attack is also sometimes referred to as a *coronary thrombosis*, or simply a coronary.)

In short, *coronary artery disease* (CAD) is a continuum of disease that ranges from a symptom-free state to an infarction large enough to cause death. In recent years, scientists have discovered a great deal about *atherosclerosis*—the process which usually narrows the coronary arteries.

Atherosclerosis and coronary artery disease

Atherosclerosis (from the Greek *athere* = gruel + *sclerosis* = hardness) underlies most heart attacks and strokes. In a normal artery, blood is strictly confined to the *lumen* (the central channel through which blood flows) by a smooth lining of flattened cells

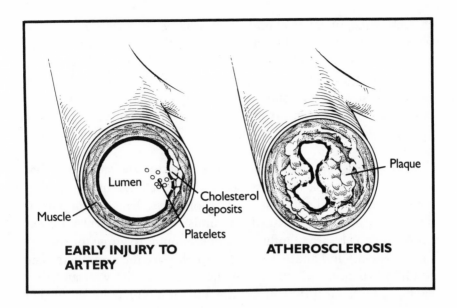

Lumen

Muscle

Cholesterol deposits

Platelets

EARLY INJURY TO ARTERY

Plaque

ATHEROSCLEROSIS

tightly joined to each other (*see illustration*). Virtually nothing penetrates this protective barrier. When kept in good repair, this lining (called the *endothelium*) permits blood to flow without sludging or clotting. Surrounding the lining is a relatively thin sheath of muscle cells. By contracting or relaxing, this muscular sheath controls the diameter of the coronary artery and thus helps regulate the rate at which blood flows through it.

The earliest change in atherosclerosis seems to be some kind of damage to the endothelium of the artery. A frequent cause of damage may simply be wear and tear by excessively rapid or turbulent flow of blood in a particular area. It is certainly true that narrowing occurs most commonly where an artery branches or takes sharp bends. At these spots, blood strikes against the vessel walls with greater force. High blood pressure leads to atherosclerosis in part by increasing stress on the lining of the major blood vessels.

Once the lining of an artery is damaged, blood penetrates into the arterial wall, which normally is shielded from direct exposure to the blood stream. When this happens, *platelets*—little sacs of chemicals in the blood stream that initiate the clotting of blood—gather in the area of injury. Once there, they stick to the injured surface of the endothelium and begin to release chemicals, among them thromboxane, which stimulate other platelets to aggregate in the same neighborhood. Some research indicates that while producing thromboxane, platelets manufacture a by-product which combines with cholesterol in the blood stream and changes its chemical nature so that the muscle cells in the vessel wall avidly take it up. Unfortunately, once the cells have ingested cholesterol, they can dispose of it only very slowly. Consequently, cholesterol accumulates and the cells begin to bloat with accumulated fat. The more cholesterol there is in the blood, the more rapidly this process takes place.

At the same time that platelets are releasing the substance that modifies cholesterol, they also seem to release a factor that stimulates the muscle cells themselves to proliferate. Thus, when part of an artery's lining is damaged, the underlying muscle cells are exposed to two abnormal influences: one stimulus to gorge themselves on cholesterol and another stimulus to increase their numbers. The result is a *plaque,* which now deforms the arterial wall and thus creates additional turbulence in the flow of blood and even further damage to the artery's lining. Eventually enough blockage occurs to limit the flow of blood to heart muscle.

Risk factors

Until atherosclerosis can be prevented at the cellular level, we must deal with a secondary level of prevention involving so-called "risk factors"—factors known to be statistically associated with an increased risk for CAD. The three major risk factors for coronary disease are:

- *Age.* The older we are, the more likely we are to have a heart attack.
- *Sex.* Until the age of menopause, women are protected by their hormones; the result is a far lower incidence of heart attacks than among men.
- *Heredity.* A history of heart attacks or strokes in family members during their thirties and forties means a marked increase in risk, unlike a family history of relatives dying of heart disease at a ripe old age.

Obviously, there is nothing we can do about the above risk factors. We therefore rightly turn our attention toward the three most important risk factors we *can* modify:

- *Smoking* (discussed extensively in Chapter 2)
- *High blood cholesterol* (discussed in Chapter 1)
- *High blood pressure* (discussed in this chapter, in the section on stroke)

In addition to these "big three" risk factors, many other items have been identified by some studies as possibly increasing the risk of coronary disease. Among the more intriguing of these:

- *Personality type.* In the 1950s, two California cardiologists published data indicating that a certain personality style (labeled Type A) was more likely to lead to heart attacks. The key ingredients of the Type A personality are competitiveness and time consciousness. This personality theory, however, has become quite controversial in recent years, and many experts question its reproducibility and therefore its reliability.
- *Obesity.* While significant obesity may indeed be associated with health hazards (*see Chapter 1*), the link between obesity and coronary disease is far from certain. No one would suggest that obesity is good for the heart, but mild forms of obesity are certainly far down on the list of coronary risk factors.
- *Coffee.* As pointed out in Chapter 2, coffee's link to heart disease is very controversial. Suffice it to say that if coffee is a risk factor, it is a very mild one—and then only when consumed in excess.

Diabetes—especially type 1 (insulin-dependent) diabetes—is associated with a clearly increased risk for coronary disease. However, there is some evidence that attention to other risk factors and reasonable control of blood sugar levels can reduce the additional risk posed by diabetes.

Coronary artery spasm

There is no question that atherosclerosis is the leading culprit in heart disease. However, during the past decade, many research and clinical findings have highlighted the fact that not all angina—the pain caused by poor blood supply to heart muscle—can be explained by fixed blockages in the coronary arteries.

Coronary arteries, as we have seen, contain a layer of smooth muscle cells that help regulate blood flow. The idea that these arteries might go into spasm—a sudden narrowing of a portion of coronary artery due to intense constriction of this muscular layer—has been around at least since 1910, when it was suggested in a lecture by Sir William Osler. In 1959 Dr. Myron Prinzmetal described an unusual type of angina (now known as "Prinzmetal's," "rest," or "variant" angina) which is characterized by chest pain occurring during rest—rather than exertion—and by electrocardiogram findings almost opposite to those associated with typical angina. In 1970 Dr. Albert Kattus actually observed a coronary artery go into spasm during heart surgery. Since then, spasm has been found many times during angiography (*see below*). Other studies have indirectly confirmed the phenomenon of spasm.

It now appears that temporary spasms of coronary arteries not only cause atypical angina but contribute to the whole clinical spectrum of coronary artery disease, ranging from typical angina (chest pain with exertion) to actual heart attacks (permanent death of heart muscle). Spasm may occur in an area of a coronary artery totally free of atherosclerosis, or the spasm may be superimposed upon an area already ravaged by a fixed blockage.

This concept provides an explanation for the wide range of cardiac problems that can occur with or without evidence of underlying permanent blockage in the coronary arteries. There is particular interest in spasm as an explanation for the statistically rare angina that occurs in younger women—a group normally free from symptoms of coronary artery disease.

Although much uncertainty exists as to the exact physiological triggers that may set off coronary artery spasm, the following areas have received considerable attention in recent years:

- *Platelets*. When platelets clump together, they release thromboxane A_2, which is a potent vasoconstrictor—a substance that causes narrowing of a blood vessel. Therefore, the role of aspirin and other anti-platelet agents that might interfere with the clotting process are of continuing interest.
- *Smoking*. Several investigators have reported dramatic decreases in the frequency of angina when cigarette smoking is stopped; it is postulated that this is due to less coronary spasm.
- *Stress*. The clinical correlation between stress and heart pain in some persons has long been noted, and current research suggests that, in some persons, spasm might be the connecting link.

Can an aspirin a day—or every other day—keep heart attacks at bay? There is some reason to think that the anti-clotting action of aspirin can have an anti-clogging effect in the coronary arteries. Currently, to test this theory about 10,000 U.S. physicians are taking an aspirin every other day and another 10,000 are taking a placebo pill as part of a controlled experiment. Until the results are announced, in another year or two, the answer to this question remains a conservative "maybe."

The final common pathway for all of the triggers that initiate spasm may be an increase in the calcium flow into the smooth muscle cells lining the coronary arteries. This calcium flow has nothing to do with dietary calcium or even the blood calcium level; it is instead a common part of the molecular machinery of all smooth muscle cells. Based on this theory, drugs that specifically interfere with calcium flow into cells are now an important mode of treatment (*see below*).

Diagnosing coronary artery disease

An important element in preventing heart attack damage is accurate diagnosis of coronary artery disease before irreversible damage to heart muscle occurs. In practical terms, this means studying the coronary circulation.

Today three methods are commonly used for studying the coronary circulation in persons with angina-like chest pain or other symptoms that might represent deficient blood flow to the heart.

EXERCISE ELECTROCARDIOGRAPHY Exercise electrocardiography (ECG) is a way of finding out whether an area of the heart begins to run out of blood during the stress of exercise. The subject walks or jogs on a treadmill while the heart's electrical activity is measured by an ECG machine (attached by wires to electrodes pasted onto the arms, legs, and chest of the subject). Changes in the ECG tracing during exercise may reveal areas of deficient circulation or indicate that further diagnostic testing is worth considering. Often today, a gentle form of this test is performed on heart attack patients before they leave the hospital. This procedure promises to identify a group of patients who need special attention in the months after discharge.

THALLIUM SCANNING Thallium scanning is sometimes used as a complement to the exercise ECG, or it may be used alone. In this test, a small amount of radioactive material is injected into a vein and, a few minutes later, a scanner to detect emitted radiation is used to measure how much of the material appears in various parts of the heart muscle. A region that does not take up the thallium can be assumed to have deficient circulation. In general, adding a thallium scan to an exercise ECG increases the probability of detecting existing coronary disease from about 70% to about 90%.

One of the most perplexing questions facing both patients and physicians is just how often a person should be tested for coronary artery disease. In the absence of any past or current symptoms—or a strong family history of heart disease—most physicians would recommend a baseline resting electrocardiogram at about age 40. However, for an individual with suggestive symptoms or a worrisome family history, an exercise ECG may be recommended even earlier—and periodically throughout life. In short, a program of testing must be tailored to each individual's family history, symptom level, and planned exercise program.

CORONARY ANGIOGRAPHY Coronary angiography (catheterization) provides the most complete and accurate diagnostic information. In this procedure, a substance that demonstrates blood flow on x-ray pictures (commonly but inaccurately termed a "dye") is injected into the coronary arteries while an x-ray movie is made of the heart. The resulting pictures give an excellent, detailed image of the coronary arteries and their larger branches. Angiography can be uncomfortable, and it occasionally leads to complications, but it is a necessary step if bypass surgery is being considered. Researchers are experimenting with less hazardous means to visualize the coronary arteries.

Treatment

For patients with clearly established coronary artery disease, three main kinds of treatment are available. The first usually considered is medication, often including calcium-channel blockers and beta-blockers. At the other extreme, bypass surgery can be performed, both to relieve severe anginal pains and possibly to prevent heart attack. There is often debate about whether surgery or medication leads to a better quality of life and longer survival in any given case. It is probable that different types of patients will benefit more from one or the other form of therapy. For many patients, however, a third type of intervention, called balloon angioplasty, has recently become widely used.

Medication

The vast majority of individuals with coronary artery disease can be successfully treated with medications. Today, three major categories of medicines are available—as described below.

NITRATES These drugs have been the mainstay of angina control for many decades. It is believed that they increase blood flow to the heart by stimulating the coronary arteries to dilate. Nitrates may also lower demand on the heart by relaxing the walls of blood vessels elsewhere in the body and thus lowering blood pressure. In their simplest chemical form, 3 nitrate groups are linked to a glycerol molecule—trinitroglycerol (TNG). Absorbed from a tiny tablet held under the tongue, TNG produces rapid, but very temporary, relief from anginal pain. After a few minutes, the effects are gone. Another nitrate preparation, isosorbide dinitrate (Isordil), can be swallowed for protection that lasts 4–6 hours. This drug will not terminate angina attacks, but it seems to help prevent them.

Because TNG can be absorbed through the skin, it can be rubbed onto the chest or arm in an ointment that also seems to provide 4–6 hours of relative protection. But this routine is a bit messy, so a new device has been introduced—a patch of material soaked with a nitrate and covered with adhesive plastic. The Band-Aid-like patch is placed in a convenient location on the skin once a day. Unfortunately, the body seems to develop tolerance to nitrate when it receives the drug in this sustained manner, and studies have shown that these nitrate patches may not provide the long-term protection against angina claimed by their manufacturers.

BETA-BLOCKERS These drugs work to lower the heart's demand for blood. The heart is largely under the control of the autonomic (involuntary) nervous system, which sends its instructions through several different kinds of nerves. One set of these nerves sends its messages to sites in the heart muscle known as beta-receptors. When beta-receptors are stimulated, they invariably respond by making the heart beat faster and harder. Beta-receptors are also found in blood vessels throughout the body. They respond to stimulation by raising blood pressure. One can think of beta-receptors as tiny telegraph receivers that sit waiting for a signal to come down the wire. When it comes, the receivers automatically activate the heart and raise blood pressure. As a result, the heart demands more blood, and if blood is in short supply because of coronary artery disease, angina results.

Beta-blockers, then, are like a little wad of paper slipped under the telegraph key to prevent it from clicking. The nerve sends its signal, but now the heart and vessels cannot "hear" it. The problem with beta-blockers is that they can also interfere with signals elsewhere in the body, and uncomfortable symptoms may result. The airways in the lung, for example, depend on beta stimulation to stay wide open; thus, beta blockade may lead to asthma-like symptoms in some people. Fortunately, it turns out that beta-receptors are not all alike. Those in the lungs are subtly different from those in the heart, and so it has been possible to design drugs which act mainly—but not exclusively—on the heart and have little effect on the lungs.

Today, a large variety of beta-blocking drugs are available—not only for the treatment of coronary disease but for such problems as high blood pressure and migraine headaches. In general, if a patient taking an older beta-blocker drug has no side effects and is willing to keep up with the dosage schedule, there is usually no point in switching to a newer, more expensive beta-blocker. However, if side effects are a problem, another beta-blocker should be considered. The most common adverse reactions to beta-blockers are depression, wheezing (usually in people predisposed to asthma), fatigue, and (in males) impotence.

CALCIUM-CHANNEL BLOCKERS As described earlier, there is growing interest in the phenomenon of coronary artery spasm, in which a segment of a coronary artery clamps down and temporarily restricts the flow of blood. What triggers spasm is not exactly known, but it is clear that a severe spasm can bring on the same kind of pain as is produced by fixed blockage from a plaque.

Enter calcium. This mineral, which is present in blood and body fluids, acts like a key that can turn on a switch leading to spasm. More precisely, the dissolved calcium moves through specific channels in the outer membrane of the cells that form the wall of the blood vessel. Once within the cells, calcium somehow stimulates them to contract, and spasm results.

By blocking the channels for calcium entry, certain drugs can prevent the spasm. Fortunately, the drugs do not gum up other essential channels in the cell membrane, so they are relatively free of side effects. Several different drugs that block calcium channels are now available. All of them have proved useful in patients suffering from angina, particularly when spasm plays a role in causing the pain. The calcium-channel blockers also have certain other effects that can be useful in some patients. Each of them, to varying degrees, can lower blood pressure and prevent, or suppress, an abnormally racing heart rate. Verapamil (available under various brand names) is most effective at slowing the heart, whereas nifedipine has little effect on heart rate and relatively more on blood pressure; diltiazem is intermediate between the others. Because each drug is somewhat different, the physician can choose an appropriate one.

Entrepreneurs promoting chelation therapy for heart disease may claim that this procedure has effects similar to calcium-channel blockers. This is simply not true. Chelation therapy temporarily lowers calcium levels in the blood; there is no evidence that it alters the rate at which calcium moves into cells.

Bypass surgery

Bypass surgery, introduced in 1967, involves attaching a short length of vein taken from the thigh—or, more commonly today, the internal mammary artery (IMA) in the chest—to a diseased coronary artery so as to convey blood around the obstructed segment (*see illustration*). Bypass surgery usually provides very effective relief of pain for people with angina that does not respond to the best available drug therapy. However, whether a bypass prolongs life expectancy is more complicated. This question is a big one, because coronary artery surgery is very costly and carries some risk of death or complications. Currently, well over 200,000 patients undergo bypass surgery each year in this country, at a cost of about $20,000 each. In major medical centers, death rates from complications of

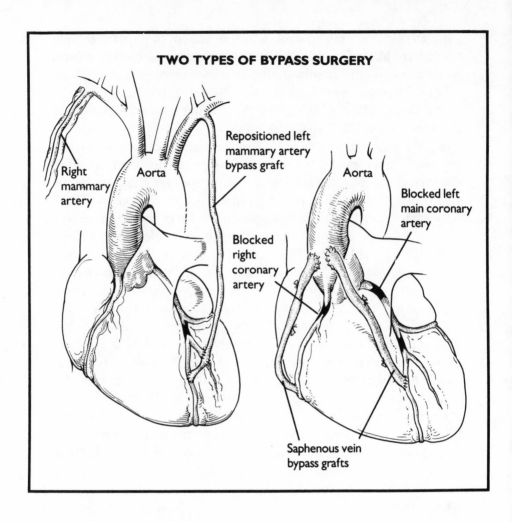

TWO TYPES OF BYPASS SURGERY

Right mammary artery

Aorta

Repositioned left mammary artery bypass graft

Blocked right coronary artery

Aorta

Blocked left main coronary artery

Saphenous vein bypass grafts

the surgery itself are in the 1–2% range. However, rates vary considerably from one hospital to another. Given these costs and risks, the decision to perform bypass surgery must be carefully weighed.

Results of a study released by the National Heart, Lung, and Blood Institute (NHLBI) in 1983 have provided information that should help to put bypass surgery in perspective.

The important conclusions from the NHLBI's study are these:

- The risks of coronary bypass surgery, though real, have been reduced to a very low level.
- About 60% of patients with moderate angina enjoy complete relief of pain during the first year after surgery, and 50% remain

pain-free 5 years later. (In the interval, of course, other people develop more pain, and some die of their basic heart disease.)

- Although surgery is effective in providing pain relief, it does not appear to "fix" the underlying problem: obstructions can continue to develop through grafts. Whether treated with surgery or medication, patients live about equally long. There is one important exception to this rule: if someone has severe obstruction near the very beginning of the left coronary artery, he or she will live longer with surgery than without. Otherwise, surgery does not make a detectable difference in survival.
- Patients report less pain with a bypass than do patients on medication, but the two groups report an equal ability to work or play.

In practical terms, these findings mean that people with mild-to-moderate angina do not risk shortening their lives if they delay surgery (except for those with obstruction of the left main coronary, who comprise a relatively small percentage of all patients regarded as eligible for bypass). That also means that people with coronary artery disease have time to try a variety of medications and see whether adequate control can be achieved without the operation. If the available drugs do not suffice, then surgery is relatively safe and is often, though not always, a highly effective treatment for the pain of angina.

Recently, heart specialists have become concerned about the high percentage of *vein-graft blockages* developing in patients approaching the 10-year anniversary of their surgery. Some studies suggest that as many as 80% of all vein bypass patients will develop potentially life-threatening narrowing. This knowledge has prompted vigorous debate as to what kind of screening should be done on asymptomatic vein bypass patients. (Obviously, patients who develop symptoms should report them immediately to their physicians.) Some have suggested that angiography should be routinely performed on all vein bypass patients as they approach the 10-year point; others have suggested waiting for symptoms to develop. Most physicians fall somewhere in between in their recommendations—using a stress ECG as a screening device and saving angiography for symptomatic patients or for those whose stress test is abnormal. Fortunately, the internal mammary artery, when used as a bypass, seems to carry far less risk of subsequent narrowing. Therefore, while the IMA bypass is often technically more difficult than grafting leg veins, heart surgeons are increasingly turning to it. Indeed, most experts advise patients to request that the IMA be used when at all possible for bypass surgery.

Balloon surgery

"Balloon surgery" on blood vessels involves inserting a thin catheter with a balloon at the end into the arterial system, pushing it to the point of blockage in the artery, and then expanding the balloon in the area of blockage for several seconds. This expansion opens up a channel for blood flow. Before it was used on the heart, balloon angioplasty (the technical name for this procedure) was tried in leg arteries constricted by atherosclerosis. When, somewhat to the surprise of physicians referring the patients, this method worked to relieve the calf pain the patients felt on walking, it was applied to the coronary arteries in the hope that it would relieve the pain of angina pectoris by increasing blood flow to the heart.

The narrowing of coronary arteries was always a target of the pioneers in this field. At first, it was felt that this treatment should be restricted to patients with disease in only one coronary artery, and then only if it was narrowed in a single place. With increasing success, patients with more than one constriction in a single coronary artery, or with narrowings in two or even all three of the principal arteries, are now undergoing angioplasty. Catheters and their operators can now reach further along the course of an artery to get to obstructions in its branches (*see illustration*). But the longer a narrowed segment is, the less amenable it is to balloon widening.

Balloon angioplasty (Greek for "shaping of blood vessels") has been performed in many thousands of patients and has become a fairly routine procedure in many cardiac catheterization laboratories throughout the country and the world. Over 100,000 coronary angioplasties are being done in the United States each year. Use of the balloon to treat constricted coronary arteries has led to the development of a whole new group of subspecialists, known as "interventional cardiac angiographers." Increased experience, along with more versatile catheters, has made it possible to correct more and more complex types of coronary narrowings (and other problems, such as valve disease). For many patients with coronary disease whose symptoms cannot be controlled by medication, balloon angioplasty is a reasonable alternative to bypass surgery.

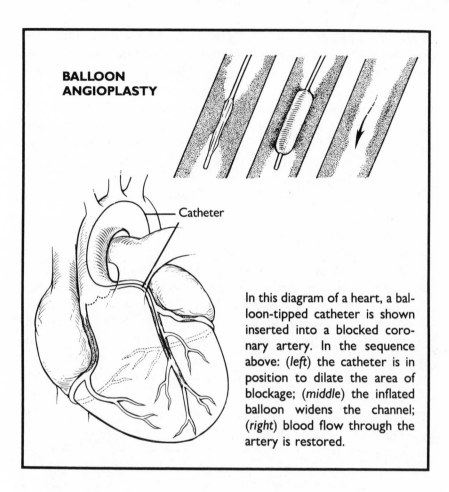

BALLOON ANGIOPLASTY

Catheter

In this diagram of a heart, a balloon-tipped catheter is shown inserted into a blocked coronary artery. In the sequence above: (*left*) the catheter is in position to dilate the area of blockage; (*middle*) the inflated balloon widens the channel; (*right*) blood flow through the artery is restored.

Balloon dilation is not risk-free. A coronary artery may be torn during the procedure, or a clot can form in the dilated area and, by blocking flow of blood, undo the treatment. These mishaps can become the *cause* of a heart attack if they are not immediately corrected. For this reason, balloon dilation is usually undertaken only when a surgical team and operating room are available on standby for rapid hands-on repair. No more than 5% of patients undergoing balloon dilation will require immediate surgical intervention. But at that point, the surgery must be done urgently, and the outcome under these circumstances won't always be as good as if the procedure had started out to be bypass surgery.

In general, success has been impressive. According to recent reports from major centers where balloon angioplasty is performed frequently by experienced personnel, the coronary vessels are significantly widened in 85% of patients. However, arteries that have been dilated will go on to narrow again within a year in almost a third of these patients. So the probability that another procedure will be required—either a repeat session with balloon angioplasty or bypass grafting—is fairly high even when successful dilation is achieved by the first balloon procedure. On the whole, patients under 65 years of age, and those with a relatively brief period of symptoms before treatment, get the most benefit from balloon angioplasty. Emerging data suggest that dilation can sometimes be used during an acute heart attack to help limit the destruction of heart muscle.

Balloon angioplasty is now a standard therapy, but it is not *the* standard therapy for narrowed coronary arteries. In many cases, it seems to be the best choice, but in many others it may be neither simpler nor safer than bypass surgery. No wide-scale, comparative trial has been completed to guide decisions as to which procedure is best for the various categories of patient. In the meantime, the availability of balloon angioplasty creates a temptation to use the procedure for a rather minimal degree of coronary narrowing, the kind that seems to do quite well on a program of diet, exercise, and drugs if needed. More information is needed to clarify when it's preferable to use the balloon and when to leave well enough alone.

Just as with bypass surgery, angioplasty is expensive and entails serious risks. As is so often the case, as much skill and judgment must go into deciding whether and under what circumstances to use the procedure as into performing it.

Limiting the damage of a heart attack

Heart attacks come in all sizes, depending on how much heart muscle dies. Blood is normally carried to the heart through the three main coronary arteries, which give off branches over the outer surface of the heart. The branches then turn toward the heart's inner surface and give off yet finer twigs that feed blood into the interior muscle tissue. Loss of blood flow affects the innermost portion of the heart wall first, because cells there work the hardest and have the greatest need for blood. They are also at the end of the supply line. If circulation through the plugged artery is not restored, the injury of a heart attack may extend toward the outer surface of the heart. Damage extending all the way through the heart wall makes the heart muscle much weaker than damage confined to a small area near the inner surface. Thus, techniques to limit the size of injury once a heart attack has begun should improve the outlook for victims.

About 85% of heart attacks are ultimately caused by the formation of a blood clot within a coronary artery, usually in an area already narrowed by cholesterol accumulation in its walls. Once the blockage occurs, the blood-deprived heart tissue dies gradually. Muscle fibers at the outskirts of the area that has been deprived may get a small amount of blood from neighboring vessels and be able to live for a number of hours. If the blocked artery can be opened before the injured heart muscle reaches its point of no return, a substantial amount of heart muscle can be salvaged.

Clot-dissolving drugs

Efforts began several years ago to treat heart attack victims with a clot-dissolving substance called *streptokinase*. At the very onset of a heart attack, a thin tube is threaded (through an arm or leg vessel) into the coronary arteries. The site of blockage is determined by squirting a small amount of contrast material through the tubing and taking x-rays. The same tubing provides the route through which streptokinase is fed to the clot.

Clot-blocked arteries have clearly been reopened by this technique—called *thrombolytic therapy*—but it does not appear to be a realistic answer for most heart attack victims. The patient must quickly be moved to a facility with specialized equipment and a highly skilled team of physicians and technicians. The procedure, which is invasive and cumbersome, must be accomplished within several hours of the heart attack.

In an attempt to simplify the procedure, streptokinase has been administered by vein to many patients, but the results have not been universally encouraging. Furthermore, streptokinase interferes with general blood clotting (thereby promoting unwanted bleeding) as well as clotting in the coronary artery. For these reasons, it's unlikely that streptokinase will have a major role to play in the treatment of heart attacks.

A newer substance, *tissue plasminogen activator* (TPA), is less apt to promote bleeding when it is injected intravenously because it becomes activated only when it encounters a clot. Thus, a very high concentration of working TPA can be delivered to just the site where it is needed, without requiring a catheterization procedure.

Until recently, TPA was too scarce to be a realistic alternative to streptokinase. But now genetic engineering has put the machinery for making this human protein into bacteria, which are now capable of producing it in quantity.

Preliminary results from the first large-scale trial comparing intravenous streptokinase with intravenous TPA showed TPA to be the clearly superior agent. Coronary arteries were unclogged within 90 minutes of the treatment period in two-thirds of TPA-treated patients and in only one-third of those receiving streptokinase by vein. These results may, however, be an underestimate of the effectiveness of TPA. Because of research requirements, treatment with TPA had to be delayed so that coronary angiography could be performed to evaluate the results. For this reason, the potential clinical benefit of very early TPA treatment could not be measured. Many authorities believe that TPA given at the beginning of a heart attack will write a happier ending to many stories.

Preventing "electrical deaths" from heart attacks

As many as half of all heart attack deaths occur before victims are able to get to a hospital. Most such deaths are believed to be due to "electrical failure" of the heart, not "pump failure." In other words, people with perfectly adequate amounts of heart muscle wind up dead because their heart's electrical signals degenerate; the muscle then twitches chaotically and can no longer pump blood. Known as *ventricular fibrillation* (VF), this rhythm disturbance is absolutely deadly if it cannot be reversed within minutes.

Lidocaine, a drug that protects against VF, is routinely given *by vein* to heart attack patients once they arrive at the hospital. Many have questioned whether this drug might be effective if given by a more accessible route at an even earlier stage of a heart attack. Evidence from one trial strongly supports the use of lidocaine given by injection into a muscle prior to transportation to the hospital. In an experiment conducted in the Netherlands, paramedics gave intramuscular lidocaine to a randomized sample of patients with acute chest pain at the start of their ambulance ride. As it turned out, only one third of all the people brought in for chest pain proved to have heart attacks; but of these, the ones who received early lidocaine were half as likely to develop VF. In fact, once 15 minutes had elapsed from the time of the injection, only two cases of VF occurred in the treated group, compared with 12 cases among the controls. Presumably, the benefit took 15 minutes to become apparent because this much time was required for the lidocaine to be absorbed from the injection site in the upper arm into the circulation and thence to reach the heart.

As a result of this study, it is likely that paramedics in many parts of the world will now be instructed to administer intramuscular lidocaine routinely whenever a patient is suspected of having a heart attack.

SELF-INJECTABLE LIDOCAINE? The provocative question raised by these findings is whether people at high risk for heart attacks—such as prior heart attack victims—should carry their own self-injectable lidocaine for use at the very onset of severe chest pain. After all, it takes a while for the paramedics to arrive. A cautionary note, expressed by Dr. Bernard Lown in an editorial accompanying the report, describes the possible dangers of overuse of lidocaine by patients who would come to regard it as an irresistible lifesaver at a time of even innocuous chest pain. Because lidocaine can, rarely, produce side effects—such as stoppage of the heartbeat and seizures—overuse of this drug could disrupt more lives than it saves. The stage appears to be set for the next study, to learn whether early self-injection with lidocaine will reduce mortality from heart attacks.

Abnormal heart valves

The pain of angina can usually be traced to narrowed coronary arteries or, in some cases, to coronary artery spasm. But chest pain and other symptoms of impaired circulation can also arise when valves that control the flow of blood through the heart are not functioning properly.

Aortic stenosis

This term refers to a narrowing (stenosis) of the valve that separates the aorta from the heart. The symptoms of aortic stenosis are most likely to appear in middle age or later. In some people, the normally supple flaps or *cusps* of the valve become thickened and infiltrated with calcium. Fibrous tissue in the body often reacts to inflammation or injury in this way, and heart valves are no exception. (Athletes who find themselves getting calcified tendons as a result of injury or overuse are experiencing another version of the same reaction.) What causes the original damage of aortic valves and triggers this process is not always clear. Sometimes, the problem begins with a congenital abnormality; the valve comes with only two flaps instead of the usual three. Males, for some reason, are more likely to have this condition. Typically, the valve works perfectly well in the first few decades of life, but as time goes on it may begin to show signs of damage. Thus aortic stenosis is not likely to draw attention to itself at ages below 40 or 50. After the age of 60, valves that began as perfectly normal ones may also show signs of thickening and calcification. Rheumatic fever sometimes affects the aortic valve, but it is not thought to be a common cause of pure aortic stenosis.

The important consequence of increasing rigidity and narrowing of the aortic valve is that the heart must pump harder to move blood through the valve. One of the first victims of this process is the heart itself, which depends for its own blood supply on arteries that originate just beyond the aortic valve. The brain, with its high demand for blood, may also suffer.

The symptoms, then, are fairly easy to predict. Most common is the chest pain of angina pectoris. Feeling light-headed or dizzy is frequently another symptom; at a somewhat more advanced stage of aortic stenosis, full-fledged fainting occurs. These symptoms are most common during exercise, when muscles, in effect, steal some of the limited supply of blood from the brain. Late in the game, shortness of breath during exertion, or even at rest, may be felt. This is a sign that the heart's ability to continue pumping blood past a narrowed opening is nearly exhausted.

The first step in diagnosing aortic stenosis is for a physician to listen with a stethoscope. A certain type of murmur suggests that blood is being forced through a narrowed valve. But relatively unimportant conditions can produce murmurs sounding like aortic stenosis, so a more specific test is an *echocardiogram,* which evaluates the tightness of the valve by using high-frequency sound. If this study indicates a very tight valve, a cardiac catheterization to examine the heart is probably warranted. This technique permits direct measurement of blood pressure on both sides of the valve, and it gives a measure of blood flow through the narrowed opening. If symptoms have begun to appear and these studies confirm that the valve is obstructed, surgical replacement is generally recommended. On the other hand, people with minor degrees of aortic stenosis can continue to lead quite active lives.

Sometimes narrowing of an aortic valve is discovered incidentally. As long as there are no symptoms and no indication that the heart muscle is becoming overdeveloped (hypertrophied) in the effort to pump blood, watchful waiting is the recommended course. But chest pain, fainting spells, or shortness of breath usually indicate that the time has come for surgery. Survival without a valve replacement is likely to be less than 2–3 years, whereas with an artificial valve, a much longer and a more active life can be anticipated.

Recent advances have made it possible to widen a narrowed aortic valve by balloon dilation, similar to the technique used to unblock coronary arteries (*see above*). However, the results are not as good as those achieved through surgery.

Mitral valve prolapse

The mitral valve is between the two chambers on the left side of the heart. Its role in life is to prevent blood from flowing back into the left upper chamber during *systole,* the moment when the heart squeezes blood out into the body. Ideally, the two flaps or *leaflets* of the valve slide together to form a taut closure. The edges of the mitral valve are stabilized at this point by a set of fine cords, like guy-wires, attached to the wall of the left ventricle. Then, as the heart relaxes to admit a new shipment of blood, the leaflets pull apart slightly, at which point they look somewhat like the item of headgear known as a bishop's mitre (hence the name).

In about 5% of people, the vast majority women, the leaflets of the mitral valve are so flexible that they tend to billow a little (prolapse) on closing. The result is an audible sound, a kind of click heard through the stethoscope, and sometimes a brief murmur, as a little bit of blood slips back through the valve. In the past 20 years or so, with the aid of such modern imaging techniques as ultrasound, this click-murmur pattern has been explained by observing the motion of the mitral valve. As a mixed blessing, the diagnosis of mitral valve prolapse (MVP) has become a very common one. The blessing is mixed because, on one hand, it may provide an explanation for disturbing symptoms that are not part of a threatening illness, but on the other hand it creates a new category of diagnosis that has more people worried than need to be.

By and large, prolapse of the mitral valve can be regarded as just one more example of human variation. It seems to be connected with a particular body type: tall, slender, with relatively long arms and "flat" rib cage. This distinctive form of the mitral valve may thus only be one aspect of a more general trait affecting the way a body's connective tissue is organized in some individuals.

In the vast majority of people with MVP, the condition is purely a laboratory finding—something that turns up when an ultrasound examination of the heart is performed. (Lots of people have click sounds that can be heard through the stethoscope, but these are not definitive evidence of MVP. When indicated, more elaborate testing is needed to clinch the diagnosis.) Particularly in thin young women, the diagnosis is often of trivial significance and it tends to go away with time. In men, MVP is more persistent, but it seems to have little clinical importance.

Once in a while, though, someone with MVP is symptomatic. Episodes of peculiar chest pain, palpitations, fatigue, dizziness, or shortness of breath may be associated with the syndrome. (But because these symptoms are so common in people generally, some experts still wonder whether MVP is actually the reason for them.) Such symptoms are often triggered by anxiety or fatigue, and appropriate modifications of lifestyle can help to prevent them. If the symptoms are disabling, they may be helped with drugs known as beta-blockers. But in the vast majority of MVP cases with no symptoms, this use of drugs is neither necessary nor desirable.

Antibiotic treatment is not needed to protect most people with MVP from developing a valve infection carried by bacteria that enter the blood stream during dental or minor surgical procedures. Frankly deformed heart valves are at risk of infection, and it appears that this is also the case if a mitral valve is loose or "floppy" enough to produce a distinct murmur (indicating back-flow of blood) during systole, in which case routine antibiotics are recommended.

So far, it is not clear whether ordinary MVP has any other potential for serious complications, but in most people the answer usually is no. The sudden popularity of this diagnosis is not due to the appearance of a new disease but rather to new technology, which allows us to recognize something that has probably existed for as long as the human race.

Arrhythmias

Heart arrhythmias—abnormalities in heart rhythm—range in severity from the incidental skipped beat in normal people to life-threatening emergencies usually associated with underlying heart disease. Arrhythmias can be an important complication of heart disease, and their consequences can be serious. If palpitations or other kinds of heart irregularity are noted, a physician should be consulted to rule out serious disease. Advances in various forms of therapy have made arrhythmias a very treatable problem in most cases.

Just as a car's engine requires a well-timed electrical system to coordinate the pistons that provide its power, so does the heart have its own system to coordinate contraction of its chambers so that blood can be pumped efficiently. Normally, electrical activity begins in the "pacemaker" area of the heart, the sino-atrial (S-A) node (*see illustration*). This area contains cells that undergo "self-excitation," triggering an electrical impulse about once a second. This impulse is

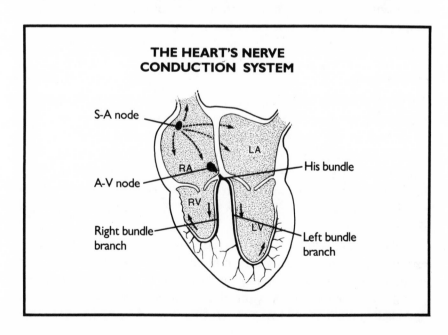

THE HEART'S NERVE
CONDUCTION SYSTEM

S-A node
LA
His bundle
RA
A-V node
RV
Right bundle branch
LV
Left bundle branch

then spread rapidly by other cells through both atria of the heart, causing them to contract and push blood into the ventricles. At the atrio-ventricular (A-V) node, the impulse is momentarily delayed before it is transmitted to the ventricles via the His bundle and its branches. Thus, the atria are signaled to contract before the ventricles, which allows blood to fill the ventricles before they pump it to the lungs and body.

Arrhythmias result from disturbances in the initiation or the spread of the electrical impulses that trigger the heart's pumping. And just as a car may lose power when its timing is off, the arrhythmic heart may lose some of its capacity to pump blood effectively if its rhythm is abnormal. When pumping becomes ineffective, vital organs that are deprived of their customary blood supply may suffer. Decreased flow to the brain, for example, can cause fainting.

Disturbances in the heart's electrical system can arise in a number of situations. A decrease in the heart's own blood supply (the ischemia that occurs with severe atherosclerosis) is a major cause of arrhythmias and is often the basis for "electrical deaths" that occur during heart attacks. Other settings for arrhythmias include stretched heart tissue (as in "heart failure"), imbalances of blood electrolytes (especially potassium), high epinephrine levels (as may occur with excitement), or the effects of certain drugs (for example, amphetamines, caffeine, or alcohol).

Diagnosis

An arrhythmia is often signaled when a person complains of a racing or pounding heart—especially when the episode begins suddenly and in the absence of exercise or emotional upheaval. The medical term for the sensation of a racing heart is *palpitation;* that word is also used to refer to the single thump of a skipped or extra heart beat. Sometimes arrhythmias are experienced mainly as fatigue, faintness, or blackouts because of reduced blood supply to the brain.

Once an arrhythmia is suspected, the initial goal is to define exactly what type of arrhythmia it might be. Checking the pulse rate (number of beats per minute) and rhythm is a big help, but the primary tool in diagnosis is the electrocardiogram (ECG) which is designed to record the heart's electrical activity. Given that many arrhythmias come and go but seem never to be present while one is visiting the doctor, the Holter monitor has taken on a major role in the diagnosis of arrhythmias. Worn on the belt for 24 hours, this lightweight electrocardiograph provides a record of the heart's activity for that full time—a record that can be quickly analyzed by computer. Finally, for very complex rhythm problems, newer electrophysiological testing (using tiny electrodes placed within the heart via the veins) is available in some specialized laboratories.

Types of arrhythmias

There are many types of arrhythmias, but the following are the more common ones:

PREMATURE CONTRACTIONS   There are two major types of premature contractions—atrial or ventricular, depending on which of the heart's chambers is contracting prematurely. The "jumping-the-gun" beats usually result from the brief appearance of an abnormally located pacemaker in one of these chambers that overrides the normal pacemaker—the S-A node. This causes the chamber to contract earlier than normal, breaking step with regular heart rhythm. A patient with premature ventricular contractions (PVCs) might feel a thump in the chest. Infrequent contractions of this sort occur in many normal individuals and do not require treatment. Too much coffee, too many cigarettes, or too much anxiety may bring on PVCs, but they also seem to occur without any type of triggering event. They usually do not represent any danger if they are not associated with underlying heart disease or other rhythm problems.

PAROXYSMAL ATRIAL TACHYCARDIA (PAT)   A person with PAT typically comes to an emergency room anxiously describing the very sudden onset of a very rapid heart rate. This fast, forceful, but regular heart beat is due to abnormal conduction pathways in the atria. Symptoms of light-headedness are frequently reported. PAT is common in young, otherwise healthy adults, and can usually be effectively treated by modifying lifestyle and using anti-arrhythmic drugs when necessary.

VENTRICULAR TACHYCARDIA (VT)   Ventricular tachycardia is also characterized by attacks of rapid heart rate, dizziness, and sometimes chest pain. But the implications are usually far more serious than those for atrial tachycardia, since ventricular tachycardias represent circuits or electrical impulses originating in the ventricles and can degenerate to fatal ventricular fibrillation. Ventricular tachycardia usually occurs when heart disease is present, and corrective treatment is almost always an urgent matter.

ATRIAL FIBRILLATION (AF)   Atrial fibrillation is due to random, chaotic electrical impulses in the atria, with consequent loss of forceful contraction by these chambers. Effective contractions by the ventricles are preserved, however, because once an atrial impulse is captured by the A-V node, it is transmitted in orderly manner to the ventricles. The resulting pulse is rapid and its rhythm is irregular. Atrial fibrillation is generally seen in association with heart disease, though occasionally episodes occur in persons who seem to be normal otherwise.

VENTRICULAR FIBRILLATION (VF)   Ventricular fibrillation occurs when ventricular electrical activity becomes chaotic. The muscle tissue does not beat in a coordinated manner. Instead, a series of localized twitching-writhing movements occur and there is no true pumping action. After a few minutes, all heart activity ceases. VF is frequently the cause of sudden death in patients with heart disease.

BRADYCARDIA   "Brady" means slow, and this label applies to a heart which beats at an abnormally slow rate. Although strictly defined as a rate below 60 beats a minute, problems generally do not occur until the rate falls below 40. Many healthy people, especially well-trained athletes, have heart rates well below 60. However, other people with a very slow rate may complain of loss of energy because the slowly pumping heart cannot deliver oxygen and other nutrients to hard-working muscle—a supply and demand problem. Bradycardia that is not related to athletic training can be caused by certain drugs, by a diseased S-A node (failure of the atrial pacemaker), or by blockage of the impulse traveling across the A-V node (so-called heart block).

Treatment

Treatment for arrhythmias can take various forms, depending on the specific situation:

DRUG THERAPY   Drug therapy is the usual method of treating bothersome arrhythmias. Commonly used medications include quinidine, digitalis, propranolol, procainamide, disopyramide, and verapamil. These work by correcting electrical imbalances so that rhythm may be restored.

CARDIOVERSION   Cardioversion is used in response to ventricular fibrillation. Metal paddles applied to the victim's chest administer a large amount of electricity to shock the heart's electrical system into regular activity. The result is known as defibrillation. Cardioversion using smaller amounts of electricity is sometimes used to treat other rhythm disorders that require prompt reversal.

ARTIFICIAL PACEMAKERS   Artificial pacemakers are used primarily for treating patients with bradycardia, including heart block. These battery-operated devices were introduced in the early 1960s, and they have become increasingly important over the years. With a wired electrode implanted into heart muscle, pacemakers can take the place of the heart's own starter system to activate contractions.

LIFESTYLE CHANGES   Coffee, alcohol, cigarettes, and very-low-calorie diets (under 500 calories a day) can contribute to the onset of some arrhythmias. Increasing evidence also points to the relationship between psychological stress and rhythm problems. (A Boston physician once described "Celtic Fever" in a patient who developed ventricular arrhythmias during the critical moments of a televised basketball playoff game.) It is obvious that when very specific lifestyle factors play a role in causing arrhythmias, efforts to eliminate them make good sense.

Heart-felt emotions

Everyone knows that the emotions can affect the heart. The question is, how often are severe rhythm disorders that can lead to sudden death preceded by intense emotional experiences? In one study, more than 200 people who had survived life-threatening rhythm disturbances, and their families, were questioned about the events of the 24 hours before the episode. In 1 case out of 5, a major and unusual emotional stress was reported. In some cases, the emotional disturbance was very unusual and seemed closely associated with the arrhythmias.

But 80% of the people in the study had gone through perfectly ordinary days. The problem with their hearts was not tied to any obvious emotional factor, and the episode of arrhythmia clearly

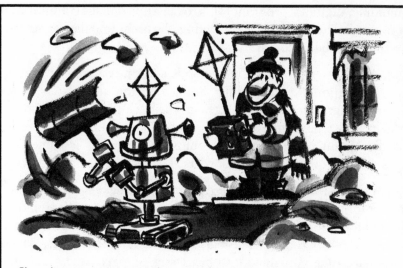

Shoveling snow is more than an odious winter chore that results in aching muscles. It can be life-threatening for anyone who is out of shape. If you're not used to strenuous exercise, help prevent a heart attack (and share the wealth): hire a neighbor kid to shovel for you. If you must do it yourself, work slowly and take frequent breaks.

required another explanation. Furthermore, the vast majority of people who go through psychological disturbances, even agonizing experiences, do not suffer a life-threatening disorder.

Isolated emotional events seldom led to severe arrhythmias in this study. Rather, a whole web of conditions usually came together to form a unique moment. Most of the people who seemed susceptible to emotional disturbances also had prior evidence of heart disease, making it likely that their hearts were especially vulnerable. Some of them gave previous evidence of rhythm disturbances or had some form of structural abnormality in their hearts. Unusual fatigue preceding the arrhythmia was a relatively common finding. After a period of exhaustion, susceptible people seem to be even more vulnerable than usual.

The kind of psychological reaction that preceded arrhythmias was typically some kind of agitation or anger, rather than despondency or simple grief. Some of the people were depressed, but they were also agitated. In one case, intensely competitive feelings seemed to produce an arrhythmia in a man who was on the verge of winning an athletic contest. None of the episodes occurred during sexual intercourse, and none of them was brought on by purely joyful feelings. Some people seemed to become conditioned to certain emotional situations and experienced arrhythmias repeatedly when the situation recurred.

Contrary to folklore, no one dropped dead the instant after experiencing a moment of terror. In all of the cases reported in this study, some time had elapsed—a few minutes to a few hours—between the emotional experience and the arrhythmia. In general, these findings suggest that emotional distress, fatigue, and possibly other factors working together make the heart more susceptible to a rhythm disturbance. But strong feelings alone do not often "trigger" the arrhythmia. Rather, they seem to make it easier for another factor, such as spasm in a coronary artery or a spontaneous abnormality in the action of the heart, to become a trigger.

Many people who have had a heart attack or other cardiac problem come to believe that they must protect themselves from the normal experiences of life—that they must give up challenging work or exciting activities. Family members, out of understandable concern, often contribute to this attitude. They feel that everybody must "walk on eggs," as it were, to protect the patient's heart. This approach can be very distressing to people who are accustomed to busy, active lives. They may be made miserable by a misdirected effort to protect them from the ups and downs of normal life.

For most people who are subject to arrhythmias, there appears to be little or no association between emotions and rhythm disturbances. The best advice to a patient who has a susceptible heart is: "Go on being yourself." A person who is "hyper" by nature cannot reasonably be expected to change. Those who are used to responsibility might do just as well to continue in responsible positions. But they may be able to modify their life in ways that can help with this problem.

Obviously, if some specific situation predictably sets off an arrhythmia, patients and their families should work on changing that situation. Avoiding extremes of fatigue or emotional tension may reduce risk. One patient in the study described above became angry, left his house to go jogging, pushed himself harder than usual, and passed out from an arrhythmia. Such a man should not stop all jogging, but he should pay more attention to how he is feeling and avoid adding physical stress to any emotional stress he is experiencing at the moment.

The mainstay of prevention is proper medication. People who are subject to life-threatening arrhythmias should be protected by adequate doses of the right drugs. And finally, patients seem to benefit from having a doctor who understands their lives as well as their hearts. A doctor who can also be a confidant may indeed provide preventive care for the emotions.

Stroke

Strokes are the third leading cause of death in this country after heart disease and cancer. Even though the stroke rate has been reduced rather dramatically in the United States during the past decade, approximately 750,000 people will have a stroke in the next year, and 1 out of 3 of them (250,000 people) will die. Of those who survive, about 1 in 6 will require permanent care in an institution; almost 3 out of 4 will have a reduced working capacity. Despite these gruesome statistics, most people have little understanding of what causes a stroke and, more significantly, what can be done to try to prevent one.

Definition

A stroke may be simply defined as a change in body function caused by interference with the blood supply to the brain. Since the major part of the brain is called the cerebrum, strokes are often referred to as CVAs—*cerebral vascular accidents*. Usually, the "accident" is rather sudden, and the resulting loss of function may range from a minor change in speech to severe paralysis or coma. While the possible causes of decreased blood flow to the brain are many, the vast majority of strokes are caused by one of three events:

THROMBOSIS   Thrombosis means a "clot"—in this case, a clot or plug somewhere in the vessels of the neck or brain (cerebral thrombosis). Atherosclerosis—the villain that causes plugging of arteries supplying blood to the heart and thereby leads to heart attacks—also causes the narrowing that leads to "brain attacks" or strokes.

HEMORRHAGE   Rupture of a blood vessel in the brain (cerebral hemorrhage) will interrupt blood flow to the part of the brain supplied by that vessel. Extensive bleeding can also cause direct damage to brain tissue. Hypertension (high blood pressure) may cause damage to blood vessels, thus setting the stage for rupture to occur.

EMBOLISM   Embolism refers to the dislodgement of a piece of material—such as a blood clot or cholesterol plaque—from the coronary arteries or arteries leading to the head. The material is carried into the smaller arteries of the brain, where it blocks the flow of blood (cerebral embolism).

Transient ischemic attacks

Many strokes can be prevented through early intervention. The people at highest risk for stroke are those who have experienced warning signals in the form of a *transient ischemic attack* (TIA). A TIA is a temporary (transient) episode (attack) of abnormal function caused by decreased blood flow (ischemia) to the brain. Obviously, the distinguishing feature of a TIA is that the loss of function is *temporary*—versus the longer-lasting and often permanent damage of a stroke. Many TIAs are caused by a narrowing of the blood vessels in the neck (carotid arteries), where surgical correction is possible if the abnormality is discovered before a stroke occurs (*see illustration*). When surgical correction of narrowed vessels is not possible (as in the vertebro-basilar arteries in the posterior part of the neck), anti-coagulant medicine may be useful.

Stroke specialists often describe two major types of transient ischemic attacks:

TRANSIENT MONOCULAR BLINDNESS   A disturbance in vision in one eye occurs that may take many different forms—visual blurring, a "blackout" or "whiteout" of vision, or a "shade coming down" over the eye. The anatomical basis for this kind of attack is that the back of the eye (retina) is supplied with blood by the first branch of the internal carotid artery. Narrowing in the carotid artery can mean decreased blood flow to the eye.

TRANSIENT HEMISPHERAL ATTACKS   Blood flow to the affected side (hemisphere) of the brain is diminished, causing more "typical" stroke symptoms—numbness or weakness (or both) of the face, arm, or leg on one side of the body or difficulty in speaking or thinking. These symptoms are also typically caused by dimin-

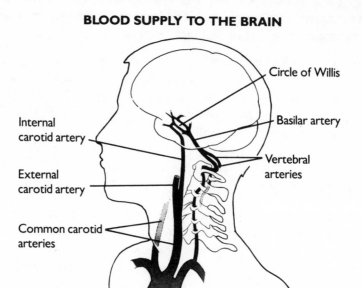

BLOOD SUPPLY TO THE BRAIN

Circle of Willis

Internal
carotid artery

Basilar artery

External
carotid artery

Vertebral
arteries

Common carotid
arteries

One pair of blood vessels toward the front of the neck (the carotid system) and another in the back of the neck (the vertebrobasilar system) supply blood to the brain. These systems join at the base of the brain via the so-called circle of Willis.

ished blood flow through the carotid vessels. Other symptoms (double vision, vertigo, nausea), however, may be caused by diminished blood flow through the vertebro-basilar vessels. Dizziness is a particularly difficult symptom to evaluate since the vast majority of dizzy spells are not significant. However, when dizziness is combined with other symptoms—or when in doubt—a physician should be consulted.

In most people, the internal carotid arteries on each side of the neck are the major suppliers of blood to the brain. A build-up of fatty plaques in these arteries leaves many people at risk for stroke. Of those whose disease has progressed to the point where they are having transient ischemic attacks, 1 in 3 will have a stroke during the subsequent 5 years, if no treatment is given. Put another way: a TIA increases the risk of a stroke during the following year about

17 times. Therefore, the response to a possible TIA should be, first and foremost, to recognize that something is wrong and to head for a competent physician—possibly a neurologist, the medical specialist in diseases of the nervous system.

Testing for a narrowed artery

Tests are available—if a physician finds them necessary—to determine if narrowing of a blood vessel in the neck is responsible for the reported symptoms. Methods of assessing blood flow through the carotid arteries can be grouped roughly as follows:

FEELING AND LISTENING   A trained examiner can often pick up signals of diminished blood flow by simply feeling the pulse of the carotid arteries (palpation) or listening for sounds of abnormal flow (bruits) by using a stethoscope placed over these arteries. Comparing the two sides of the neck is often useful, and should be an expected part of a routine physical examination in anyone over age 50. If dramatic evidence is discovered—such as the marked reduction of a pulse—further studies are obviously indicated. However, other changes can be difficult to interpret. These simple examination measures, while often useful, are not enough to make a final judgment of the status of the blood flow through the carotid arteries, so further studies may be done.

ARTERIAL ANGIOGRAPHY   The ultimate diagnostic test for blood vessel disease in the neck or head is the injection of contrast material into the arteries (via a tube inserted into the arterial system) as x-ray pictures are taken. The x-rays are done in rapid succession so that the movement of contrast material through the vessels can be examined for evidence of narrowing.

While it is a widely used procedure, arterial angiography is expensive, requires hospitalization, and carries a small but real danger of causing serious side effects, including a stroke or death. (In medical centers experienced with this procedure, the rate of such serious complications is less than 1%.) Angiography therefore is largely reserved for those people in whom there is a high likelihood of finding a narrowing that requires surgery. A newer version of the technique (digital subtraction angiography or DSA) involves injecting contrast material into a vein—making the procedure much easier and safer. For many, DSA can be substituted for arterial angiography.

NONINVASIVE STUDIES Within the past decade, several tests have attempted to combine the safety of "feeling and listening" with the accuracy of angiography. These studies are usually described as noninvasive because they do not involve the risk of inserting a tube (catheter) into the arterial system.

New tests and new versions of old ones are constantly being developed, but the following are examples of tests currently in use:

- *Doppler ultrasonography.* This test uses ultrasound to detect changes in the circulation in vessels around the eyes or in the carotid artery.
- *Ultrasound imaging.* This method provides direct images of the carotid arteries in the neck and can depict even mild narrowing.
- *Oculoplethysmography (OPG).* This tongue-twisting word refers to a technique of measuring pressure or the rate of circulation in vessels that arise from the carotid arteries to supply the eyes. If pressure or circulation is abnormal, there can be a narrowing in the carotid artery.

The fact remains that arterial angiography is still the most accurate diagnostic test. But even with this kind of final evidence of narrowing or plaques, the decision whether to clean out the plaques in the carotid artery using a surgical procedure (carotid endarterectomy) is difficult and often controversial.

To operate or not?

One highly regarded textbook of medicine states that there is as yet "no evidence that surgically treated patients fare better than medically treated patients with respect to ultimate stroke or survival rates." However, the textbook also points out that apart from the question of long-term survival, there is little doubt that properly selected patients with TIAs who have successful carotid artery surgery usually improve in terms of symptoms and quality of life.

Indeed, given the dismaying outlook for an individual with evident transient ischemic attacks, most well-informed physicians today will opt for carotid artery surgery when the following circumstances are met:

- *If arterial angiography confirms a significant narrowing.* There is considerable debate as to what is significant; but all would agree that *at least* 50% narrowing must be present to consider surgery; many insist on 80% or more narrowing.

- *If the individual is under age 60.* Since the risk for stroke is actually higher in younger persons with a TIA, since they usually tolerate surgery better than older people, and since the risks of alternative medical therapy increases with duration of use, the decision may often tip toward surgery in younger patients. Obviously, one's general medical condition must be considered at any age.
- *If adequate surgical experience is available.* There can be an enormous difference in complication rates between hospitals where carotid surgery is done only occasionally, versus major centers with a typical mortality rate in the 1% or below range.

The question of surgery for individuals without symptoms (that is, who have not experienced a TIA) but with evidence of carotid narrowing is even more controversial. However, there is a trend toward *at least considering* surgery in such cases when firm evidence of major narrowing is demonstrated on angiography.

In short, the question of whether or not to place your neck in a surgeon's hand remains controversial. Most experts would argue for consideration of such surgery under the conditions described above, and for medical treatment (blood-thinning, anti-platelet drugs, and so on) when surgery is not the treatment of choice.

Anti-platelet drugs

It has long been known that certain drugs—including ordinary aspirin—interfere with the role of blood platelets in forming clots. Intensive interest in the use of these anti-platelet drugs to prevent clots associated with heart attacks and strokes has led to several important treatment trials. In 1978 the Canadian Cooperative Study reported striking results concerning the use of aspirin to prevent strokes in those at risk. The Canadian study involved the use of aspirin (4 regular tablets per day) in people who had experienced a "threatened stroke" (their phrase for a TIA). The effect of aspirin in the absence of warning symptoms was not studied. People with ulcers were excluded from the study, and coated aspirin was not tried.

Five hundred eighty-three subjects who had experienced at least one threatened stroke during the previous 3 months were given either a placebo, aspirin, sulfinpyrazone (another anti-platelet drug), or sulfinpyrazone and aspirin together. No reduced risk for subsequent stroke could be attributed to sulfinpyrazone, but males taking 4 aspirin tablets per day—during an average follow-up period of 26 months—demonstrated a reduced risk for stroke or death of 48%, as compared with males not receiving aspirin. There was no substantial protection for females in this study, but subsequent ones have suggested that women can also benefit.

So who should take aspirin? The answer is not an altogether straightforward one. Persons who experience warning symptoms should not simply start popping aspirin but should see a specialist (usually a neurologist) to learn what treatment is most appropriate. When diagnostic studies show a significant blockage and surgery can be done without complications, the results, in terms of symptom relief and stroke prevention, may be better than with any medication—including aspirin. Aspirin is an effective treatment in some cases, and the Food and Drug Administration has now approved it for use as a measure to protect against recurrent TIAs.

What about the person without symptoms who thinks about taking a daily dose of aspirin "just to be safe"? Obviously, it will not be safe for everyone to take aspirin—though most people without known ulcer disease or bleeding tendencies can take aspirin without side effects. Most experts are reluctant to recommend daily aspirin for a person who has not had warning symptoms of a stroke.

Who is at risk?

Those who have experienced a TIA are at highest risk for stroke. But other risk factors have been identified which, if eliminated, may reduce one's chances of having a stroke.

HIGH BLOOD PRESSURE   Detection and control of high blood pressure is the single most important stroke-prevention measure. High blood pressure contributes to both the process of atherosclerosis and the increased likelihood that weakened arteries will rupture. Hypertension is appropriately described as a "silent killer" because the initial damage to blood vessels occurs without warning symptoms (*see below.*)

BIRTH CONTROL PILLS   Studies clearly show that women using the pill are at a slightly higher risk for the development of strokes. While this increased risk is quite small, especially for women under age 35, women with a family history of strokes or a history of other risk factors for stroke should seek another form of contraception.

Especially worrisome is the combination of migraine headaches and pill use; such headaches should eliminate the pill from consideration as a form of contraception at any age. Also, some women taking the pill develop hypertension while on it.

HEART RHYTHM ABNORMALITIES   Persons with certain arrhythmias of the heart have an increased chance of blood clots traveling to the brain, especially if they have heart murmurs or congestive heart failure. Such persons often require anti-platelet drugs to minimize clot formation. Minor rhythm disturbances (such as occasional skipped beats) are not worrisome as risk factors for stroke.

OTHER RISK FACTORS FOR HEART ATTACK   Most experts feel that the same risk factors that have been identified with an increased chance of heart attack also contribute to strokes, since the same process of atherosclerosis is often involved. Besides hypertension, these include smoking and elevated cholesterol.

Although stroke has usually not been mentioned as one of the prominent risks of smoking, more and more evidence is adding this indictment to the already long list. A study recently reported by the Honolulu Heart Program has demonstrated that among men of Japanese ancestry, smokers are 2–3 times as likely to suffer a stroke as nonsmokers. This risk is *in addition to* any other underlying risk factors for stroke, such as coronary disease or hypertension. Those smokers who were able to break the cigarette habit reduced their risk of having a stroke.

There's no reason to believe that Japanese are more vulnerable to cigarette-induced strokes than others. The Honolulu results probably apply to all smokers.

The hypertension story

It is now well known that hypertension is a common problem and that people with untreated high blood pressure have an increased risk for strokes, heart disease, and kidney failure. At present, almost all physicians recognize the importance of treating an otherwise healthy person whose diastolic blood pressure (the second number) consistently exceeds 100. But what about that gray area of milder elevations below 100? That is often a difficult question for both patient and doctor.

Terminology

High blood pressure means that at a given moment, one's blood pressure is "up" compared with the normal range. As is now widely appreciated, temporary elevations can frequently occur during moments of tension or even quiet concern—as is often the case when blood pressure is being checked. The diagnosis of hypertension—meaning a disease of persistent elevation—should be made only after at least 2 separate blood-pressure measurements by a competent examiner using reliable equipment. There is good reason for being cautious in labeling anyone with the diagnosis of hypertension because this usually leads to a recommendation for extended, if not lifelong, treatment.

Blood pressure is recorded in numbers equivalent to the pressure exerted by a mercury column of varying height—expressed in millimeters of mercury. Two numbers make up a blood pressure reading; they refer to the pressure within the arteries during the two phases of the heart cycle. The first number (*systolic pressure*) designates the pressure during the brief period when the heart is actually contracting and forcing blood into the arteries under a temporarily increased pressure. The second number (*diastolic pressure*) designates the lower pressure which is present during the longer resting phase between the heart's contractions. By the way, the prefix "hyper" has nothing to do with personality type; many passive and placid people have hypertension and many "hyper" individuals have perfectly normal pressures. That's why the only way to find out your blood pressure is to have it taken.

Screening and diagnosis

As indicated, the key question is this: What level of systolic or diastolic pressure is high enough to be labeled hypertension—and to warrant treatment designed to prevent long-term complications?

The extremes are no problem; it's the territory in between that provokes disagreement. For example, the World Health Organization has placed the upper limits of normal at 160/95 (spoken as "160 over 95" and meaning a systolic pressure of 160 and a diastolic pressure of 95). However, the latest guidelines issued by the Joint National Committee on Detection, Evaluation, and Treatment of High Blood Pressure use 160/90 as the upper limit of normal; using these guidelines, nearly 58 million Americans over age 6 are estimated to be hypertensive. And data from the National Heart, Lung and Blood Institute suggest that treating individuals with diastolic pressures in the 90–104 range can reduce deaths from all causes (primarily heart disease and strokes) by about 20%.

Insurance companies have long been rigorous in setting upper limits of normal; their actuarial projections clearly show that even apparently mild elevations of blood pressure predict a reduced life span. (One actuarial example: a 35-year-old man with a blood pressure of 150/100 will have a shorter lifespan by 16.5 years if his hypertension remains untreated.) Not surprisingly, premiums are usually higher for persons with hypertension, but successful control of hypertension can qualify one for a waiver of the higher premium.

Factors other than just the numbers must often be considered in dealing with the gray area of mild hypertension. These include:

SYSTOLIC VERSUS DIASTOLIC ELEVATION While both pressures are considered to be important, many experts make a distinction between them. For example, the systolic pressure is often elevated by itself when arteries "harden" as a part of the aging process. Some clinicians still allow for this factor (100 plus your age) before deciding that true systolic hypertension exists. And elevation of the systolic pressure alone can also be caused by other diseases, such as an overactive thyroid gland. Diastolic elevations, however, virtually always mean hypertension.

AGE, SEX, AND RACE Mild pressure elevations have more serious meaning when they occur at a younger age. Also, there is general agreement that men are more likely to suffer from the complications of high blood pressure than women. And the complication rate (as well as the prevalence) of hypertension is higher in blacks than in whites. However, the general trend in recent years has been to initiate treatment for consistent pressure elevations, regardless of race or sex.

OTHER RISK FACTORS   In ultimately deciding whether a given level of pressure deserves treatment, many physicians will also consider the presence of other factors that tend to increase the risk of complications—such as smoking, diabetes, elevated cholesterol levels, and a family history of atherosclerosis.

PHYSICIAN BIAS   Some doctors who are strongly prevention-minded are persuaded that the evidence at hand is sufficient to urge treatment for patients with very mild hypertension; they argue that even patients with borderline hypertension will, in time, develop more strokes than those in lower ranges. Other doctors are less convinced of the need to recommend lifelong therapy (with its attendant expense and inconvenience) to combat what they perceive to be a slight risk.

In short, the diagnosis and treatment of mild hypertension is a tricky business that requires thoughtful consideration of many factors other than just the numbers. The very uncertainty about criteria for diagnosis and treatment carries implications for screening policy. Persons should not conclude that they have hypertension on the basis of a single blood-pressure reading taken on a drug-store machine or at a street-corner booth. While such screening programs may be valuable in alerting someone to the possibility of hypertension, the diagnosis must be confirmed under the conditions described earlier.

Causes—primary and secondary

The overwhelming majority of cases of hypertension turn out to have no easily identifiable cause; indeed, because high blood pressure of this type is so common it was, in the past, often referred to as "essential"—a terrible misnomer in light of present understanding. Today this type is referred to as *primary,* and while the exact basis for this kind of hypertension is unknown, the following factors are of interest in terms of their prevention and treatment potential:

SALT INTAKE   Evidence for the role of salt in the development of hypertension comes from both animal investigations and studies of human populations. For example, researchers can produce hypertension in certain animals simply by feeding them high-salt diets. And human societies in which individual salt intake averages less than 4 grams (about 2 teaspoons)—versus the average American consumption of 12 grams—have much less hypertension.

Few experts claim that salt is the sole cause of hypertension; rather, they describe salt as an important contributing factor in the 10–20% of Americans who are genetically susceptible to high blood pressure. And for such persons, the hidden salt in the processed food of the typical American diet is a real hazard. For example, one ounce of corn flakes contains twice as much sodium (the component of salt related to high blood pressure) as an equivalent serving of salted peanuts, and a Big Mac comes loaded with 5 times as much sodium as the 1-ounce serving of corn flakes. Salt is everywhere in the American diet, but it is a learned taste which our children can be trained to live without.

CALCIUM In recent years, several research centers have reported that increased calcium intake might reduce blood pressure in some individuals. However, other experts are much less certain about a role for calcium in preventing or treating high blood pressure.

EXCESSIVE WEIGHT Many studies have now documented the fact that obesity heightens the risk for hypertension. Similarly, there is evidence to show that substantial weight loss (20 pounds or more) can be effective treatment for mild high blood pressure in someone who is overweight.

EXERCISE Regular exercise may cause a mild reduction in blood pressure but its effect is considerably less predictable than that of weight loss. And some forms of exercise—such as weight lifting—can produce temporary elevations in blood pressure that might be dangerous for some individuals.

The above factors are less relevant for individuals with *secondary hypertension,* who are rare among the many with high blood pressure. Secondary hypertension results from a potentially treatable underlying cause—such as an adrenal gland tumor or a narrowed artery leading to a kidney. In these instances, surgical correction can replace the lifelong drug therapy required in most cases of primary hypertension. The dilemma arises in deciding which persons with accurately diagnosed high blood pressure should be subjected to further diagnostic tests to detect secondary hypertension. The initial evaluation of *all* persons with newly diagnosed hypertension should include a complete blood count, urinalysis, blood levels for urea nitrogen and/or creatinine (tests of kidney function), and an electrocardiogram. Additional studies looking for causes of secondary hypertension are usually reserved for those with any of the following conditions:

- Hypertension before age 35
- A rapid onset of hypertension and no family history of the disease
- An unsuccessful response to initial medical treatment
- Unusually severe hypertension
- Symptoms or appearance suggesting an adrenal tumor

However, the vast majority of patients with moderate and uncomplicated hypertension can be treated without costly and potentially risky testing.

Treatment

The good news is that death rates from hypertension have been dramatically reduced in the last 10 years. With today's effective drugs, it is rare for a person to die of heart or kidney failure due to uncontrollable hypertension. Beyond this, many experts think that the recent decline in the death rate from heart attack and strokes is largely attributable to the greatly improved treatment for hypertension developed during the past quarter century. Such treatment includes:

LIFESTYLE CHANGES As mentioned earlier, salt restriction, weight loss, and exercise may be all that is needed to control very mild elevations of blood pressure. In these cases, some would even quibble about using the term "hypertension."

BEHAVIORAL THERAPIES Several studies have reported mild lowering of blood pressure using techniques of relaxation, meditation, and biofeedback. These approaches (particularly those that involve no expensive equipment or investment) may be worthy of trial by themselves in cases of very mild hypertension and in combination with drug therapy for more severe cases.

DRUG THERAPY Given the new guidelines described above, most persons with diastolic blood pressure levels remaining over 90 will be encouraged to take one or more drugs to bring it into a lower range. Understandably, the idea of having to take drugs, often for the remainder of one's life, is not appealing. Yet it is not an optimistic overstatement to suggest that the great majority of persons requiring drug therapy will find a program of treatment that produces very little interference with normal living. Honesty also requires mentioning that some persons now taking anti-hypertensive drugs must learn to live with unpleasant side effects—including fatigue and impotence.

The drugs used today to treat high blood pressure can be categorized as follows:

- *Diuretics* ("fluid" pills). The exact reasons for the effectiveness of these drugs, which promote increased urinary excretion of sodium, are not known. However, many patients require no other medication. The long-term effectiveness and safety of diuretics is well established for most people, with abnormally low potassium levels (easily corrected by diet or supplement) being the most common problem. The many different diuretics available today are roughly similar in effectiveness.
- *Beta-blockers*. These drugs—Inderal being the oldest example— are now often used as the first-line treatment for mild hypertension. There are a number of beta-blockers now available, differing primarily in terms of dose and side effects.
- *Calcium-channel blockers*. More recently, the use of calcium-channel blockers has been found to be useful in the treatment of some cases of high blood pressure. The exact reasons for their effectiveness are not clear, but many physicians are now using them as initial treatment.
- *Sympatholytics*. These drugs (such as Aldomet) modify nervous-system control of blood vessels in a manner that allows the vessels to dilate and thus decrease pressure. More side effects typically occur with these drugs than with diuretics or beta-blockers.
- *Vasodilators*. These drugs (such as Minipress) widen blood vessels by acting on them directly. Like sympatholytics, they are usually combined with other drugs, and side effects may occur.
- *ACE inhibitors*. These newest anti-hypertensive drugs act to interfere with so-called angiotensin converting enzyme, thought to be important in the development of many cases of high blood pressure. ACE inhibitors are being reported to typically cause fewer side effects than those mentioned above—and therefore to have a higher rate of patient acceptance.

The skilled use of anti-hypertensive medications requires thorough familiarity with the many kinds of drugs now available. In difficult cases, specialist care may be necessary. For most patients, however, internists or family physicians should be able to provide adequate supervision.

Cancer

Cancer is a condition in which previously normal cells undergo a change that makes them proliferate in an uncontrolled fashion. The clump of diseased cells may form a swelling (*tumor*) at the point of origin. Sooner or later, some cells may cut loose from their anchorage and spread to other sites in the body (*metastases*).

Cancer cells cause damage both by distorting the normal structure of tissues and by interfering with normal metabolic processes. Exactly what happens depends on the kind of cell that is affected. Each type of cell in the body produces a distinctive type of cancer; but even within a single tumor the cells may behave in different ways, so that treatment effective against one cell type has little or no effect on another. Moreover, two cancers of the same type may act differently. For example, two different patients may have cancers that appear in all respects to be identical (arising from the same kind of cell, similar in size and growth rate). Yet one patient will respond to treatment and the other will not. To add to the complexity of cancer, some people appear to resist cancers more effectively than others, even people exposed to the same potentially damaging influences.

We now understand something of why all cancers are not alike. Most, if not all, cancers result from damage to the hereditary material (DNA) of a cell. In the normal course of events, many of the cells in our bodies must repeatedly divide throughout life to allow for growth or replacement of tissue. At each division, the hereditary instructions are duplicated so that a complete copy of the genes can be passed on to the daughter cells. Each of these divisions provides an opportunity for a genetic error to occur. (We are talking about a mistake that occurs in cells of the body, not in the egg or sperm. Therefore, the genetic error in question is *not* passed to the patient's children, but rather disrupts the normal growth of cells in the patient's own body.)

Much current work is aimed at untangling the genetic process leading to cancer. Some evidence suggests that large disruptions of the DNA threads called chromosomes are responsible for cancer. But there are strong indications that certain genes, known as *oncogenes,* which normally are switched off, cause cancer when they are switched on by mistake. It appears that at least two such errors must accumulate for a cancer to develop. This process usually takes many years.

Environmental factors

If indeed oncogenes are implicated in the uncontrolled growth of cancer, what causes them to be switched on? It has been known for well over a hundred years that exposure to certain chemicals could cause cancer in humans and in laboratory animals. Still, as recently as 10 years ago, many authorities thought that hereditary factors and perhaps viruses were the major causes of cancer. Viruses have proved to be extremely useful in producing cancers in laboratory animals. Although they are clearly involved in some human cancers, they seem unlikely to be primarily responsible for causing the majority of them. As for heredity, it is important in establishing a person's susceptibility to cancer, but other factors are undoubtedly involved in causing the disease. Certainly, the common cancers are not "inherited" in any straightforward fashion.

Thus, the focus of attention is shifting to environmental chemicals as the primary causes of cancer. But contrary to the popular belief, most chemicals responsible for most of the cancers occurring today probably do not come from chemical factories. Even though the number of man-made chemicals in the environment has markedly increased in the last 50 years, the overall frequency of cancer has not changed very much in that period (after lung cancer, which is usually caused by smoking, is subtracted and a statistical correction is made for the increasing proportion of older people in our population). Other chemical culprits may be natural substances, contaminants such as molds in our food, or even chemicals that are produced from food by bacteria present in our large intestine. The way food is cooked may also make a difference; charcoal broiling, for example, has been implicated in creating carcinogens.

Epidemiologic studies

Most of the evidence for the important role played by environmental factors (much of it accumulated only in the last 20 years) comes from studies of the frequency of various cancers in different human groups.

The prevalence of the various kinds of cancer differs from one part of the world to another, but when people migrate from their home culture to a foreign one (for example, Japanese moving to the United States or European Jews to Israel), they tend to acquire the cancer pattern of their adopted country within a couple of generations, even without intermarrying.

By now there are perhaps two dozen known settings in which cancer has arisen from occupational exposure to chemicals such as dyes, asbestos, certain solvents, and plastic components.

And there is the most powerful evidence of all: the death rate from lung cancer. Between 1900 and 1950, American men increased their consumption of cigarettes by about 10-fold, and their death rate from lung cancer went up nearly 100-fold. (Women, who began smoking in earnest around World War II, are now making history repeat itself.) As John Cairns, a prominent cancer researcher, has said, "It is almost as if Western societies had set out to conduct a vast and fairly well-controlled experiment in carcinogenesis bringing about several million deaths and using their own people as the experimental animals."

Next to lung cancer, cancers of the colon (large intestine) and breast account for the greatest mortality in the United States, and these two diseases have hardly changed in frequency for decades, despite changes in our environment and lifestyle. Changes in other types of cancer have occurred, however. Stomach cancer has been diminishing for several decades—nobody knows why. The death rate from cancer of the cervix has also fallen in the past 30 years. On the other hand, more deaths are being caused by cancers of the pancreas and nervous system. The leukemias increased in frequency from 1930 to 1950 but have not changed much since then. These facts suggest that changing environmental influences are at work, but they do not support the notion that our increasingly industrialized environment has, so far, produced an epidemic of new cancers in the general population.

But just because epidemiologists do not yet see evidence of a big risk in cancer deaths does not mean that it cannot happen. Experience has taught us that there is a delay period. As a rule, cancer usually appears 10–30 years after exposure begins. A potent carcinogen brought into our chemical environment today would probably not begin to show up as cancer deaths until the year 2000; a carcinogen introduced in the 1960s could start to reveal itself any time now. The only way to be truly certain that a new chemical is carcinogenic for humans is to find out over a period of time that it causes cancer. However, if the chemical were to produce cancer at fairly low rates, its effect on people might be undetected because so many other causes can contribute to the development of cancer.

Testing for carcinogens

In the early years of coal mining, it is said, the miners brought canaries with them into the tunnels. The birds, being more sensitive than the men to deterioration of the atmosphere, would collapse in time to warn the miners to seek safer air. Obviously, we would all be a great deal more comfortable in making decisions about the chemicals that we swallow, inhale, or rub on our skins if we had a warning system of this kind. This is the principle that underlies present-day testing for carcinogens. Instead of canaries, modern researchers use mice, rats, hamsters, guinea pigs, or, sometimes, larger animals.

Animal testing

For each chemical to be tested, about 500 animals are needed, of which half are not exposed while the other half receive the suspected agent in various doses. In a test of this sort, which costs about $250,000 when properly conducted, between 200 and 250 animals are put at risk. In other words, each animal is "standing in" for a million Americans.

If animals and people were equally sensitive to the chemical, the test could easily miss carcinogens capable of causing many deaths, unless some method was used to increase the frequency of cancers in the animals. To compensate for this statistical disadvantage, the animals are usually given the highest daily dose of the chemical that they can tolerate without immediate ill effects. The alternative would be to expose more animals to lower doses. But the cost of such an approach would rapidly become prohibitive, especially in light of the fact that there are as many as 63,000 chemicals in common use in the United States, of which more than 5,000 have been identified as prime candidates for testing. The National Cancer Institute has funds to test about 100 substances a year using present methods.

There is a misconception that high doses of virtually anything will produce cancer sooner or later and, thus, that the high-dose approach is bound to "invent" carcinogens which really are not injurious at common levels of exposure. In fact, many chemicals appear incapable of producing cancer at any dose compatible with life. As scientists become more knowledgeable about carcinogens in general, they are able to predict more reliably the chemicals that should be tested.

When the announcement is made that a substance has been shown to produce cancer in rats or mice, a natural question is whether the same will hold true for people. The best answer to date appears to be, "Yes, maybe." Certainly, the reverse appears to be true; chemicals known to cause cancer in people also produce the disease in animals. It seems likely that people will almost always be susceptible to carcinogens that work in animals. But, and this is a big "but," people may be either more or less sensitive than the test animals. For example, the chemical 2-naphthylamine, formerly used in dye and rubber manufacture, is a potent carcinogen in people and dogs, but not in rats, mice, guinea pigs, or rabbits.

The government's position, expressed in a provision known as the Delaney clause, has been that if a substance has been shown to cause cancer in a well-conducted animal test, it may not be added to foods. The official rule is based on the assumption that thresholds do not exist, that is, lowering the dose of a carcinogen may result in fewer cancers, but some people are still going to get cancer from even a low level of exposure. The policy implicit in the Delaney clause is that no exposure in food additives is worth the risk.

The Ames test

In addition to being inexact, animal tests are expensive and time-consuming; they present a formidable barrier to anyone hoping to test the thousand-odd chemicals introduced each year, not to mention those already in use. But new systems for evaluating carcinogens may help us out of this bind. They are based on the fact that chemical carcinogens produce their effects by damaging DNA in cells of the body. In other words, they produce mutations. If a mutation occurs in a sperm or egg cell, one's offspring may be affected by the genetic damage. If the mutation occurs elsewhere, that cell may begin to behave abnormally within the body and go on to the kind of unregulated growth that we call cancer.

Capitalizing on the fact that carcinogens act by producing mutations, researchers have developed several tests that use bacteria or cultured animal cells to display such mutations. The best known of these is the Ames test, named after its developer, Bruce Ames, of the University of California, Berkeley. In this system, slightly abnormal bacteria are placed under conditions in which a mutation is required for them to thrive and grow within their carefully controlled environment. When they are exposed to a chemical that causes mutations (a carcinogen), the bacteria begin to multiply, which would mean a positive test. If no growth of bacteria occurs, the test is regarded as negative.

The Ames test is much less expensive and much more rapid than animal testing, yet its results appear to correspond rather closely to the results obtained in animal tests. It may become possible, by using the Ames test, to identify prime suspects in the world of chemicals and then, if need be, subject them to further testing with animals. There is even some hope that the relative potency of various carcinogens can be determined in this system.

Improved techniques will not, in the end, make decisions about carcinogens for us. To be sure, poor or insufficient testing may lead to either excessively restrictive or inappropriately lax policies. Because animal testing is cumbersome and subject to human error, there have been frequent disputes about results obtained with relatively weak carcinogens, such as saccharin. Even with good testing, however, certain questions may always remain unanswered: How comparable are animals and people? How much of a threat are low doses of a "proved" carcinogen? Is it possible that one low-risk chemical will interact with others in the environment to increase the threat it poses to people?

And there are other questions that cannot be scientifically answered because they are matters of economic and moral choice. Is the benefit from, say, an artificial sweetener worth the potential risk that it poses? What reason is sufficiently compelling to allow a potential carcinogen into the human environment? Should a policy of absolute prohibition in food and drugs be modified, and whose interest is served by doing so? Unfortunately, there are no easy answers when scientific uncertainty coexists with disagreements on values.

Early detection and treatment

Of the approximately 965,000 people in the United States with newly diagnosed cancer each year, about 40% will survive for at least five years. Some cases of cancer are cured completely. Nevertheless, the American Cancer Society estimates that about 170,000 people will die of cancer in this country this year because of late diagnosis or inadequate treatment. It is true that certain cancers (pancreas and lung cancers, for example) are very difficult to diagnose early and treat effectively. Cancers of the bowel, breast, cervix, and skin, however, often can be detected early enough for effective treatment and a permanent cure.

The warning signs

It is easy to ignore or forget the warning signs of cancer. However, we can and should remember that any persistent (more than 2-week) change in body appearance or function is cause for concern and should prompt a visit to a doctor. Usually the problem is not cancer; but studies indicate that most people unwisely wait too long before checking on changes that are obviously abnormal. An immediate investigation of symptoms has a much greater pay-off than a postponed routine check-up.

The following are some common and important warning signs worth having checked by an experienced physician:

SKIN CHANGES Any significant new growth or change in previous skin growth or marking should be investigated by a dermatologist (skin specialist) if a satisfactory explanation is not given by your usual source of medical care. Remember, too, the "skin" inside your mouth; it should be examined carefully for unusual white or red areas, especially if you smoke heavily (including pipes and cigars), drink heavily, or chew tobacco.

CHANGE IN BOWEL HABITS Most people experience occasional upsets in bowel habits, the vast majority of which are not due to cancer. However, any persistent change (of more than 2 weeks) should be reported to a physician.

ABNORMAL BLEEDING OR DISCHARGE Any bloody material that is coughed up or vomited is clearly abnormal, as is any vaginal bleeding in a post-menopausal woman or any discharge (bloody or otherwise) from the breast. More confusing is minimal bleeding from the rectum (often due to hemorrhoids) or in the urine (often due to infection). Also confusing is unusual bleeding in a woman still menstruating. The safest course is to report such changes to a physician.

LUMPS AND BUMPS Most important is a lump found in the breast. Other lumps, however, should not be ignored even though most turn out not to be cancer—including 80% of all breast lumps. Men should examine their testicles for lumps every 3 months.

COUGHING AND HOARSENESS Coughing and hoarseness are common complaints, usually secondary to inflammation of the vocal cords. However, hoarseness of more than 2 weeks' duration may be an important warning sign of cancer of the larynx. Coughing is *not* helpful in detecting lung cancer at an early stage.

Remember: This list is only partial. Any persistent changes in appearance or function should be reported.

Treatment concerns

If cancer has been diagnosed, many patients and their families ask where the very best treatment can be obtained. When people ask about the "best" place for cancer treatment, it is often with the idea that treatment by a local specialist working in a community hospital will be inadequate. Instead, the thought is, they would do better by going to a cancer research center, probably a long distance away, and preferably one that has recently reported encouraging experience with a new (that is, experimental) form of therapy. Such research centers, it is imagined, have three potential advantages. They are likely to offer advanced—but proven—treatments that are not in use outside a few big-city centers. They can use therapies still in a research stage that others may not have access to. Or they have so much skill, technology, and experience that standard therapies work better in their hands than at smaller centers. In reality, each of these supposed advantages is often illusory.

Information about cancer therapy is widely available to physicians. Regional cancer centers give advice and consultation to doctors who ask for it. There is also a computerized data base called "PDQ" (Physician Data Query) that all doctors have access to. From it they can rapidly retrieve the latest information on treatment results for virtually any type of cancer. Thus, no doctor in the United States is cut off from the most up-to-date published information just because of his or her remoteness or lack of connection to a research center. The information that is typically available from these sources tells what methods were used on what types of patients, and it reports their response rates and survival results. Patients themselves may obtain similar guidelines tailored for the general public through the "hotline" operated by the Cancer Information Service for the National Cancer Institute (1-800-4-CANCER).

When patients learn about a new treatment program touted as a "breakthrough," it stands to reason that they would be eager to seek this new treatment. Most such breakthroughs, however, represent the early results of an innovative form of treatment that has been offered to only a handful of people, has been associated with partial—but usually not total—shrinkage of tumors, has not resulted in cure, and may have caused relatively severe side effects. Such research treatments, which are often only being used in specialized centers, are not necessarily right for everyone, may not offer any advantage over existing therapy, and in some cases may even lead to less favorable results.

Many cancers, including the most common ones of later life, may be managed as well in a community hospital as in a research center. These include breast, bowel, stomach, and pancreatic cancers, as well as most forms of lung cancer, to name a few. But with certain diseases—including the acute leukemias, Hodgkin's disease and some other forms of lymphoma, and testicular cancer—it *is* often advisable to go beyond a community hospital, at least to have a consultation at the nearest center that is organized to provide comprehensive care for cancer patients. The same advice seems appropriate for women who are contemplating a lumpectomy and radiation therapy (as opposed to mastectomy) as the first-line treatment for breast cancer. It's also a step that should be considered by anyone who has been advised to undergo radical surgery or intensive, intricate radiation therapy, as may be recommended to someone with cancer of the prostate. There are several reasons for going outside a community hospital in these cases: (1) if correctly treated, some malignancies, even in advanced stages, have cure rates in excess of 80%; (2) many of the highly treatable cancers are relatively rare, so most doctors are not very familiar with their management; (3) giving optimal therapy in these diseases, or performing technically difficult procedures, requires an unusual level of experience, judgment, and skill.

As a general rule in medicine, if a treatment is complicated and has the potential for injury, and implementing it requires the efforts of a skilled team, then the treatment is likely to work better when given in a referral center where many cases are seen every year, rather than in a setting where the therapy is given only occasionally. This is as true of some kinds of surgery, radiotherapy, or chemotherapy for cancer as it is of open-heart operations. The common cancers of adults, on the other hand, are seen so frequently that specialty centers need not be involved in the care of each patient. Even in this situation, though, the specialty center may be able to offer useful advice without requiring that a patient be transferred.

In most situations what is needed is not some sort of exotic, high-tech treatment but the guidance of an intelligent, sensitive, caring primary physician. Rather than searching for the most overworked specialist they can find, many patients and their families would do far better to seek a doctor who relates well to patients, who will act as an advocate, and who can undertake the responsibility of coordinating all treatment efforts, including consultation with specialists.

The following survey describes the most important points of prevention and early detection for the most common cancers in the United States.

Skin cancer

Over 400,000 new cases; 7,800 deaths*

The vast majority of skin cancers are basal cell or squamous cell cancers—easily curable if detected early. However, over 25,000

* The numbers after each cancer represent 1987 estimates of the American Cancer Society as to numbers of new cases and numbers of deaths per year.

new cases of melanoma occur each year, and they will account for the majority of skin cancer deaths because they are much more likely to spread before detection occurs. Thus, a regular survey of the skin, with special attention to moles, should be one of the routine self-examinations. This rule applies mainly to white people; melanoma is quite rare in blacks, and the risk is intermediate in other races. However, areas of unusual pigmentation, especially mottled light areas on the hands and feet of a black person, should be evaluated for possible melanoma.

White adults normally have 10 to 40 moles on the body, which increase in number up to middle age and then gradually disappear. During their career on the skin, these moles tend to grow imperceptibly, become darker, and develop a slightly raised surface, even as they keep a sharp border and a relatively even color. Eventually they lose their color and/or slough off. Such moles are thought to be normal and to have little potential for harm.

But one type of mole (technically a *dysplastic nevus*) carries an increased risk of melanoma. This type often runs in families. People with dysplastic nevi usually acquire lots of them, mostly between the ages of 5 and 8. The moles typically have an irregular margin and a mixture of colors (*see illustration*). The surface may be

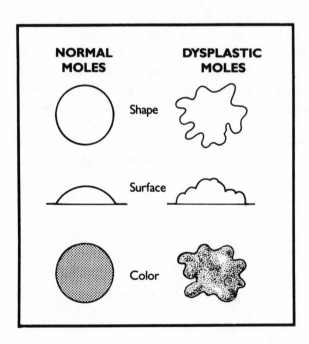

smooth, but more commonly is somewhat "pebbled." Sometimes these moles look a little like fried eggs, with a raised center on a pigmented base. People with dysplastic nevi would do well to be regularly monitored by a dermatologist or family physician. Other family members should probably be evaluated as well.

Any mole is suspicious if it is changing noticeably and especially if it has one of the following features: a highly irregular border, a very uneven surface, or a mixture of colors (especially black, gray, or blue). A dermatologist should examine such an area and make a decision about whether to do a biopsy. Unfortunately, it is not possible to be absolutely certain about the nature of a mole simply by inspecting it. But these guidelines should help to catch many cases of melanoma at a point when they are eminently treatable.

Finally, a reminder that the risk for all skin cancers—including melanoma—is greatly increased by exposure to the sun, and particularly by intensive exposures that cause tanning or burns. When such sun exposure cannot be avoided—or when it is chosen—the use of a sunscreen should be mandatory.

Lung cancer

150,000 new cases; 136,000 deaths

As the figures above indicate, this cancer is still very lethal; only 10–15% of all lung cancer patients will be alive 5 years after diagnosis. This dismal situation reflects both the difficulty of detecting lung cancer at an early stage and the inadequate treatment methods available for most forms of lung cancer. The tragedy of lung cancer is compounded by the fact that we know the cause in most cases— and it is preventable. Cigarette smoking accounts for nearly 90% of all lung cancer—quite apart from its contribution to many other major diseases. Even though it takes 20 years or more for the link between smoking and lung cancer to show itself, current trends illustrate the connection. As smoking has increased among American women since World War II, the lung cancer rate among women has increased to the point where it now causes more cancer deaths than breast cancer. However, the lung cancer rate among *men* has begun to drop, reflecting the decreased smoking in American men since World War II. In thinking about whether or not to smoke—or to continue smoking—you should keep in mind the following facts about lung cancer:

- There are no reliable early warning symptoms; by the time such symptoms as blood in sputum, chest pain, or recurring pneumonias appear, it is usually too late to effect a cure.
- There are no reliable screening tests that can pick up a lung cancer at an early, curable stage; by the time a lung cancer is seen on chest x-ray, it is beyond the stage of surgical cure in the majority of cases. This is not to say that smokers should not have regular chest x-rays—they might get lucky; it is to say that they should take no comfort from a "normal" chest x-ray because such an x-ray may easily miss the early stages of a lung cancer. In short, the only important statement to make in relation to lung cancer is this: do whatever it takes to *stop smoking*!

Sputum cytology (checking a sputum sample for cancer cells) is advocated by some experts as a regular screening test for heavy smokers. The test is far more expensive and complicated than a chest x-ray but may slightly increase the odds of early detection when combined with a chest x-ray (cytology tends to pick up different lung cancers than a chest x-ray). However, like chest x-rays, cytology detection usually comes too late.

Colon cancer

145,000 new cases; 60,000 deaths

Colon cancer is almost as common as lung cancer, but far less deadly. That is because colon cancer—unlike lung cancer—does offer the opportunity of early detection, from both warning symptoms and screening tests.

Far and away, the most important warning sign of cancer in the colon (large intestine, including the rectum) is blood from the rectum or in the stool. Such bleeding should be brought to the immediate attention of a physician. The truth is that most rectal bleeding is caused by hemorrhoids or fissures (tears) around the anus. But it might be fatal to assume this is the case without checking with a physician.

The other warning symptom often cited is a "persistent change in bowel habits." This description is often difficult to translate into practical advice about detection, since bowel habits are notoriously variable from day to day—and from one individual to another. However, when someone notices a marked change from the usual pattern that does persist—we will arbitrarily say for more than 2 weeks—such change should be called to the attention of a physician, who must then decide if further diagnostic tests (barium x-ray, sigmoidoscopy) are in order.

The basic idea of a *screening* test, on the other hand, is to find a cancer before it would otherwise be noticed—to find it in the absence of any warning symptoms. In the case of colon cancer, there are three such tests currently recommended.

Rectal exam

Anytime a physical exam is done on a person past age 40, a rectal exam (gloved finger inserted by the examining physician into the rectum) should be done. Such an exam is actually a "triple-threat" maneuver—it detects cancers within reach of the finger, removes a stool specimen for testing for hidden blood (*see below*) and, in a male, checks the posterior surface of the prostate gland (*see "prostate cancer" below*).

Sigmoidoscope (procto) exam

Such exams involve the insertion of a lighted tube into the last part of the large intestine—the rectum and sigmoid portions. For many years, this exam was done with a rigid tube that would reach approximately 10 inches into the lower colon; today, a flexible tube that can reach 20 inches is often used instead.

Testing for occult (invisible) blood in the stool

By one estimate, more than half of all bowel cancers shed blood in quantities large enough to be detected by a test performed on the stool. These tumors may otherwise be silent for long periods of time. But they don't remain so. Thus, checking stool specimens for occult (hidden) blood has become the first-line approach to screening for colon cancer in adults over 40. The test is painless, inexpensive, and easy to perform—which makes it far more suitable as a screening method than other diagnostic techniques.

THE THREE-CARD APPROACH As an increasingly standard practice, cards designed for rapid stool checks are being issued by physicians at periodic examinations. And do-it-yourself test kits can now be purchased at most drugstores. Many different test kits are commercially available; they almost all rely on the same set of chemical reactions. The most popular is known as Hemoccult; others have been marketed with such descriptive names as Fecatest, ColoScreen, Col-Rect, and Haemoscreen. But these devices only accomplish the easy part: determining whether a stool specimen contains hidden blood. The difficult problem, for which there is no easy solution, is deciding how vigorously to search for bowel cancer once a positive stool test has been obtained from someone with no symptoms and no family tendency to develop bowel cancer.

Two simple steps are required to test a stool for hidden blood. First, a small amount of feces is transferred with an applicator stick to a test card. Each card has 2 chemically impregnated test areas, one for a sample of the stool surface and the other for a sample of the stool interior. As a rule, 3 cards are prepared in this way from 3 different bowel movements. Second, several drops of peroxide solution are added to each specimen on the card. If blood is present in a sample, the hemoglobin reacts with the peroxide to turn the test paper from white to blue within 30 seconds or so. Just one "positive" result from among the 6 samples is currently regarded as sufficient reason to pursue the diagnosis of bowel cancer with more elaborate techniques.

The 3-card approach to early detection of bowel cancer sounds straightforward. For a variety of reasons, though, it isn't. Most patients who receive the cards don't complete the test and return them as instructed. Often, fewer than a third of them follow through. Even when a positive result is obtained, many physicians fail to take appropriate measures to search for the source of bleeding and determine whether it is cancerous. Until these problems can be solved, stool screening will not be as effective in practice as it could be in theory.

RELIABILITY The advantage of using test cards for stool screening is the ease of the procedure. The trade-off is that the method is not totally reliable. Under different conditions these tests may produce very different results. Among the variables that can affect the test are stool texture, storage time of the loaded cards before testing, moisture content of the samples at the time of testing, the site of blood loss in the bowel, content of the person's diet, and drug use.

Normally less than 2 milliliters of blood (about half a teaspoonful) is lost each day into the bowel. The test cards are set to register positive only at considerably greater blood loss (10–20 ml daily) to avoid the distress and expense that would arise if an excessive number of tests were to be falsely positive. But again there's a flip side: as false-positive tests are reduced by lowering the sensitivity of the test, false negatives are increased. Some cases of cancerous bleeding thus become undetectable. At the degree of sensitivity currently employed, it is estimated that 33–50% of bowel cancers will be missed in a population screened by stool exams. So, a set of negative stool tests does not provide absolute assurance that the person tested is free of bowel cancer.

In order to maximize accuracy, several recommendations on diet and drugs are generally handed out along with the cards. Because meat intake is apt to produce false-positive tests, a meat-free diet is recommended for several days before and during the stool sampling period. A high-fiber diet is sometimes advised in the belief that the increased fiber will roughen up a bleeding point and provoke added blood loss during the testing period. However, there's much skepticism about this "roughage" recommendation. Some high-fiber foods contain peroxidases, chemicals that will act on the test cards in the same way that the hemoglobin of blood does and thus produce a false-positive result. On the other hand, a high fiber diet could conceivably produce a stool that was bulky enough to dilute the hemoglobin and make it undetectable on the test cards (a false-negative result).

Certain drugs should be avoided at the time of stool collections. Iron can cause a false-positive reading. Aspirin and other anti-inflammatory drugs can produce gastrointestinal bleeding in some people, so these drugs should also be discontinued. So should vitamin C pills, because ascorbic acid suppresses a positive result even when blood is present in the stool.

Studies to date show that when large numbers of symptom-free people are screened by the 3-card method, about 5% of them will test positive. But this does not mean that they all have cancer. In fact, when further studies are performed, only about 5% of those with a positive test prove to have a bowel malignancy. The remainder either have polyps (nonmalignant growths), other minor disorders such as hemorrhoids or diverticula, or no evident source of blood loss. Thus, for a symptom-free person entering a screening program, the likelihood of having a positive test is 1 in 20, and then there is only 1 chance in 20 that the positive test will be due to

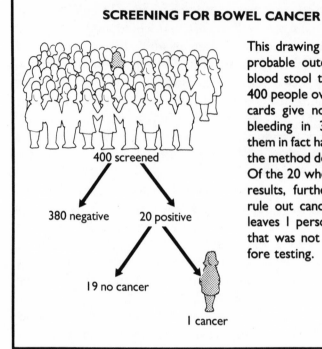

SCREENING FOR BOWEL CANCER

400 screened

380 negative   20 positive

19 no cancer

1 cancer

This drawing illustrates the probable outcome of using blood stool tests to screen 400 people over age 40. The cards give no indication of bleeding in 380, but 1 of them in fact has a cancer that the method does not detect. Of the 20 who have positive results, further testing will rule out cancer in 19. This leaves 1 person with cancer that was not suspected before testing.

bowel cancer (*see illustration*). With advancing age, the odds increase that bleeding due to a cancer will be found.

IS IT CANCER? Determining whether cancer is the cause of a positive stool test can take a bit of doing. A thorough evaluation may require any or all of three tests to learn the answer: a barium enema (colon x-ray), sigmoidoscopy (inspection of the rectum and lowermost colon through a tube), and colonoscopy (examination of the entire colon using a flexible fiberoptic instrument). These tests are expensive and uncomfortable. In the case of colonoscopy, there is a slight risk of bowel perforation. For the person in whom a small, localized cancer is ultimately detected as a result of a positive stool test, the cost and discomfort of the subsequent procedures are easily acceptable. But for every such beneficiary of stool testing, 19 others may have to undergo these tests to be assured that they do not have a cancer.

Apart from the worry level and physical discomfort brought on by tracking down each positive test, the economics of doing so bear consideration. On average, the cost for a barium enema is $125, sigmoidoscopy $50, and colonoscopy $750. If all three procedures were performed to follow up each positive test, any widely implemented screening program would have a staggering cost.

Alternative strategies might be adopted, however. For example, the threshold for undertaking further studies could be set at 2 positive samples of the 6 submitted, rather than just 1. (A "single-positive" subject might first be followed up with an additional round of stool testing.) Another strategy would be to employ only 1 or 2 of the follow-up procedures for people with sporadically positive stool tests. The choice of procedure would not be particularly easy, however. Colonoscopy, the most reliable technique, is also slightly risky, and it is by far the most costly. Barium enemas are intermediate in expense and will inevitably miss some small cancers—perhaps 15% of them. Sigmoidoscopy is a very accurate method of examining the rectum and lowermost colon, where nearly half of all bowel cancers occur, but others are out of range of the rigid instrument often used in this procedure. (The flexible sigmoidoscope gets about twice as far up the colon as the rigid one, costs about twice as much to use, and will still miss about 35% of bowel cancers.)

To date there is no way of knowing the best approach for dealing with a positive stool test in an asymptomatic person who is at no particular risk for bowel malignancy. Until several large clinical trials are completed, we can't even be certain that stool screening indeed reduces mortality from bowel cancer. In the meantime, most physicians feel that the difficulties posed by the current screening tests are outweighed by the potential benefit of finding a bowel cancer at an early stage. The reason for all of the emphasis on early detection in colon cancer is that the 5-year survival rate is 80–90% when the cancer is detected at an early, localized stage and removed surgically. After spread has occurred, the 5-year survival rate falls below 50%.

Breast cancer

130,900 new cases; 41,300 deaths

One in 11 American women will develop breast cancer during their lifetime; that means, of course, that 10 of 11 will not. That also means that most breast lumps turn out not to be cancer. And even if cancer is discovered, more than two-thirds of the American women who develop breast cancer live over 10 years and about one-third of them survive at least 20 years after the diagnosis is made. Detecting the cancer in its earliest stage offers the best hope of cure, and treatment of small, localized tumors is much less taxing for the patient than treatment of later-stage cancers.

Early detection

Monthly self-examination of the breast is one very effective means of early detection. Most lumps are discovered this way. But by the time a tumor has grown large enough to be felt, it has already been present for a while and, thus, has had an opportunity to spread. Sometimes, also, the size or texture of a breast makes a tumor hard to feel. Consequently, a lot of effort has gone into developing methods to detect breast cancers by various imaging techniques even before they can be felt.

Screening refers to the search for disease in apparently healthy individuals. To be useful for screening, an imaging technique should be able to detect cancers smaller than those which can be felt—generally those less than half an inch in diameter. It should be inexpensive, harmless, and readily accessible to the people who need it.

Some methods are not useful for screening, but they can help the physician decide whether a lump, once found, is cancerous or not. By far the majority of lumps are not cancer, but often there is no way to tell for sure unless the tissue in question is surgically removed for examination under a microscope (a process known as *biopsy*). In the future, better imaging techniques might make some biopsies avoidable.

X-RAY MAMMOGRAPHY This is currently the most effective screening method for routinely demonstrating cancers smaller than half an inch in diameter. One reason the technique is so sensitive is that it can find tiny calcium deposits in breast tissue. These "microcalcifications" frequently indicate that a tumor is present.

The x-ray mammogram is basically an x-ray snapshot of the breast, done in such a special way as to reveal the soft-tissue components. The image can be obtained in either of two ways—xeroradiography or film-screen radiography. At their best, these two

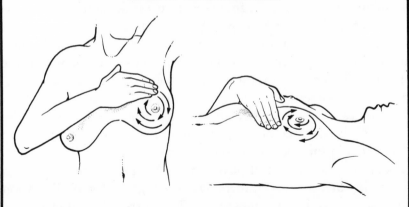

BREAST EXAMINATION

Breasts should be examined 2 or 3 days after the end of a menstrual period. (When your period begins, mark the likely day so that you'll remember.) Women who do not have periods, or have them infrequently, should set a regular day, such as the first of each month. In brief, this is the procedure: Feel each breast while standing up (say in a shower) and while lying down. Pass your fingers in a circular motion around the breast, repeating this motion in smaller circles until you have felt every part. The object is to become familiar with the usual feeling so that you can recognize any changes, specifically a lump or thickening. Also press each nipple between thumb and forefinger to check for any discharge. Before or after feeling your breasts, look at them in the mirror to check for a change in contour, dimpling of the skin, or a change in one of the nipples. Discuss any abnormal finding or change with your doctor. As you get used to self-examination, the chance of a false alarm will diminish.

techniques are about equally informative. Which one is used depends mostly on the type of x-ray equipment available and the experience of those who are doing the tests and reading the results. Currently, xeroradiography is the more common procedure.

With xeroradiography the x-rays are beamed onto a specially coated metal plate, which is processed by a variant of the familiar Xerox machine. The blue-on-white picture that comes out (a "xerogram") is easy to look at and has the advantage that detail in the thicker portion of the breast is as sharp as it is in the thinner part.

In film-screen mammography, the x-rays strike a kind of fluorescent screen, which in turn exposes a piece of film in contact with it. This device has two advantages: it uses a very low dose of radiation, and it can be adjusted to emphasize the kinds of tissue within the breast. It also has two disadvantages. One of them affects the physician: the film-screen image is slightly more difficult to interpret than the xerogram. The other one affects the patient: the breast must be fairly tightly squeezed between two plastic plates so as to minimize differences in thickness from back to front.

Because of a theoretical possibility that x-rays themselves could be causing breast cancers, there has been a great deal of discussion about the risks of mammography. The current situation can be summarized as follows:

- There is no evidence that the incidence of breast cancer in women who have undergone mammography is higher than in those who have not.
- Modern equipment uses such a low dose of x-rays that the theoretical risk of dying from a mammogram appears to be no greater than the risk of traveling in a car for 300 miles or riding a bicycle for 10 miles.

Many studies now support the benefits of mammography. For example, reports from the Netherlands suggest a 50–70% reduction in breast cancer deaths in women who are screened by this technique. But recommending routine screening for all women has several drawbacks. One is the problem of false positives—seeing a possible breast cancer when none exists. Such a false-positive diagnosis, or even a question raised, will inevitably result in biopsy studies that ultimately prove to be unnecessary.

The other major problem with mammography today is its excessive cost. In a physician's office or clinic the cost of mammography is usually $80–160. And because it is a screening technique, mammography is often excluded from health insurance coverage. Specialized clinics are beginning to offer lower prices, however, and health insurance will sometimes cover mammography if a physician certifies that there is a need for it.

For women with no prior personal or family history of breast cancer, the American Cancer Society recommends an initial mammogram between the ages of 35 and 40, a repeat every 1–2 years from ages 40 to 49, and yearly mammograms after age 50. The challenge is to develop inexpensive screening programs that can approach this frequency without snapping the nation's medical purse string, and with an acceptable accuracy rate to avoid the problems of a false-positive diagnosis.

ULTRASOUND Ultrasound produces images using a device that first emits a pulse of high-frequency sound and then records the echo. Sometimes the device (a "transducer") is placed directly on the breast, or the breast is immersed in a water bath through which the sound waves are transmitted. Sound waves pose no apparent risk to the tissue, but on the other hand they do not have the sensitivity or reliability of x-rays in detecting either the tiny calcium deposits of a tumor or a lump too small to be felt. Consequently, ultrasound cannot be used in screening for breast cancer, but it can be used to determine whether a lump is only a cyst (a noncancerous pocket of fluid), or to differentiate between infection and malignancy. As an aid to diagnosis, rather than a screening technique, ultrasound has a useful role to play.

Treatment options

During most of this century, an extensive operation called a *radical mastectomy* was regarded as the standard and proper treatment for breast cancer. This surgery removed not only the breast itself but also the muscles under it and as many as possible of the lymph nodes forming a network in the adjacent underarm tissue. The radical mastectomy was always disfiguring and often somewhat disabling. Use of this operation was justified by prevailing beliefs about the nature and behavior of breast cancer—namely, that breast cancer originated in a single, small part of the breast and then spread in an orderly fashion first to surrounding tissue and then to the lymph nodes located in the armpit. Only from these lymph nodes, it was thought, would tumor cells jump to the blood stream and then to remote parts of the body, where they would form secondary deposits known as metastases. Based on this concept of the disease, the best hope for cure was believed to be removal of not only the original malignancy but also much of the neighboring tissue and as many lymph nodes as possible in the hope of catching invasive cells before they escaped the area of origin.

This scenario was called into question by studies conducted in Europe and Canada, beginning 15 or 20 years ago. As the rationale for extensive surgery was challenged, a more limited form of mastectomy came into use and by now has virtually replaced the radical operation. Called a *modified radical mastectomy,* this procedure still requires removal of the entire breast and a small muscle from under the breast, but the contours of the chest wall are not altered by it, and strength of the arm is not significantly affected. As with any surgical procedure currently in use for breast cancer, the lymph nodes are removed from the adjacent armpit, but for diagnostic rather than treatment purposes.

Results of several major clinical trials have indicated that less extensive procedures can accomplish the same result as the modified radical mastectomy. In one of these studies, women were randomly assigned to undergo either a *simple mastectomy*—removal of the breast only—or the more traditional modified radical surgery. Survival rates in the two treatment groups have proved to be virtually identical. Modified radical mastectomy was not better than the simpler procedure at preventing recurrence of tumor in the chest wall. However, as a group, patients whose tumors had not yet spread to the nearby lymph glands by the time of diagnosis fared better than those who did show evidence of metastases—no matter which treatment group they were in.

These results strongly suggest that if a breast malignancy has already spread beyond the original area of growth, surgery cannot rid the body of cancer. Thus, removing a large amount of tissue from the area around the primary tumor does not serve any protective purpose. Rather, the main obstacle to cure is the fact that cancer has already found its way in minute amounts to sites remote from its point of origin. The underarm lymph glands are no longer thought to be a funnel through which all errant tumor cells must emigrate. Instead, when they contain cancer cells, they are an indication that the malignancy may be present in other parts of the body.

In more recent studies, patients were randomly assigned to receive either a simple mastectomy or an even less extensive operation in which only the cancerous lump and surrounding tissue were removed. This procedure, technically called a partial or segmental mastectomy, is colloquially known as *lumpectomy*. It was deemed appropriate only if the primary cancerous lump was less than 1.5 inches in diameter and had not involved the skin or chest wall. Survival of the women in these two groups has also remained similar. But it was also demonstrated that radiation therapy after a lumpectomy reduces the likelihood that cancer will reappear in the breast or chest wall.

All patients in these trials had lymph nodes removed from the armpit and examined microscopically for the presence of cancer. When tumor cells were found in these nodes, the women were begun on a course of chemotherapy in an attempt to eradicate the cancer presumed to be elsewhere in the body.

These important studies, which could not have been conducted without the courageous consent of the women who participated, have led to a major re-evaluation of ideas about the biological behavior of breast cancer. It now seems clear that many women with small breast tumors may be given a choice by their physicians as to whether they prefer to have the entire breast surgically removed or to undergo an operation restricted to the segment of breast that contains the tumor, with radiation therapy (and possibly chemotherapy) to follow.

The new knowledge has not simplified matters, however. A number of issues remain unresolved. Patients with certain types of breast cancer (as identified by microscopic study of samples removed at biopsy) may have a better chance of achieving control of disease in the area of the breast if they undergo a modified radical mastectomy, rather than one of the less extensive procedures. Precise identification of these individuals has not yet been achieved, how-

---

▪ Keep checking ▪

New findings about breast surgery have not altered the role of regular breast examination as the first line of defense against breast cancer. Most breast cancers do not form metastases until they reach a certain size. Monthly self-examination, periodic checks by a professional, and mammography improve the chance of catching breast tumors in the early stages.

ever. And radiation therapy appears to be an important component of treatment when a lumpectomy is chosen. However, radiation may be accompanied by discomfort, and it has the potential for long-term side effects. While no reports of serious problems have yet appeared, many years of follow-up will be needed to establish any level of risk. Radiation therapy to the breast is a relatively new technique, requiring technical experience that is not yet available in every radiation therapy department.

In seeking a surgeon to treat breast cancer, women should bear in mind that radical mastectomy is no longer standard therapy. Decisions concerning which surgical approach to use—mastectomy or lumpectomy plus radiation—should take account of an individual patient's physical and emotional needs. At least three major considerations must be weighed in choosing a treatment: (1) evidence that the cancer has spread, thus reducing the likelihood of long-term survival; (2) the size and character of the tumor itself, which must be effectively removed to prevent discomfort and disfigurement; and (3) the patient's preferences with respect to appearance and intensity of treatment. It is obvious that in such a situation, the patient can, and should, be encouraged to take an active part in making the necessary decisions. Unfortunately, although the range of choices has expanded, there are as yet no certain answers about true long-term results.

Prostate cancer

96,000 new cases; 27,000 deaths

Although it is less common than benign prostate enlargement, cancer of the prostate gland is one of the major causes of cancer deaths in men. Most cancers of the prostate—especially in older men—grow at a slow pace and are not likely to spread excessively or cause death. Indeed, the majority of males over age 80 probably have small amounts of this slow-growing type of cancer. When prostate cancer is established by microscopic study to be of this indolent type, most experts advise no treatment other than annual check-ups and transurethral (through the penis) removal of the obstructing tissue (*see illustration, p. 312*).

When the prostate cancer is a more aggressively spreading kind, various initial treatment measures can be employed. For example, radical prostate surgery—more extensive than simple tissue removal for enlargement—has often been used. However, recent studies indicate that the results of radiation treatment may be comparable to those of surgery in some of these cases. In short, the exact form of treatment that should be used in any given case will depend on the stage of the disease, the age of the patient, the latest information from studies comparing treatment methods, and, most important, the skill and judgment of an experienced urologist.

The most critical theme concerning prostate cancer is the importance of annual rectal exams in males over age 40. If a prostate cancer can be detected in early stages before spread has occurred, chances for cure are considerably improved. Most prostate cancers occur in the rear part of the gland, which can be easily felt during a rectal exam. Therefore, any male over 40 who does not receive a rectal exam as part of a routine physical exam is getting shortchanged.

Unfortunately, by the time a cancer can be felt, it may have spread beyond the gland, making a cure much less likely. Thus, there is enormous interest in current research to develop a simple blood test to detect chemicals from the prostate gland that indicate early cancer. Such tests are in advanced stages of refinement, but there is still considerable uncertainty as to how they should be used—given that results showing elevations may signify an indolent cancer that should not be treated. As with all screening tests, results become important only if there is a clear strategy for responding effectively to positive findings.

More recently, there has been growing excitement about newer forms of ultrasound screening exams of the prostate—"pictures" of the prostate resulting from an ultrasound probe inserted through the rectum. Many urologists believe this will become the most important screening tool of the future for early prostate cancer.

Cervical cancer

12,800 new cases of invasive cancer; 6,800 deaths

If cervical cancer is detected early enough, the cure rate approaches 100%. The traditional method of early detection has been the yearly Pap smear. But questions regarding its necessity have been circulating within medical circles for years, and have recently gone "public." The basis for this somewhat startling attack on one of the sacred cows of preventive medicine is two-fold.

First, there is increasing evidence that a woman who has had several negative Pap smears in consecutive years is highly unlikely to develop cervical cancer in immediately succeeding years. Some experts are now saying that women who have had 2 normal Pap smears a year apart need only have a Pap smear at 3-year intervals and even less during late life.

Second, some surveys have suggested that the Pap smear is not as reliable in detecting early changes as is assumed. However, most experts insist that if the test is well done, it is indeed very effective in detecting early changes. Recent evidence suggests that if 2 smears are taken, the sensitivity of the test (ability to detect changes) is significantly increased.

It is important to recognize that the value of an annual Pap smear goes beyond the possible detection of early cervical cancer. Visiting a physician to obtain a Pap smear may provide the opportunity for a blood pressure check, breast examination, and complete pelvic examination, all of which are relatively low-cost but effective screening procedures. If indeed the Pap smear provides an opportunity for other checks, it may be worth preserving as an annual health practice.

It is also important to stress that the Pap smear does not reliably detect the other major cancer of the uterus—namely, endometrial cancer, which arises from the inner lining of the uterus. Therefore, a negative or normal Pap smear means that cervical cancer is highly unlikely, but does not rule out endometrial cancer. (Sometimes a Pap smear will discover, coincidentally, cancer cells from the endometrium, but the test is not designed to do so predictably.) Indeed, there is no *simple and reliable* screening test for endometrial cancer comparable to the Pap smear for cervical cancer. However, when symptoms suggest endometrial cancer—unexplained vaginal bleeding at any age or *any* bleeding in a post-menopausal woman—then procedures which can sample endometrial tissue are available.

8 | Dealing with the Medical Establishment

Medical discovery and change are occurring at an unprecedented rate. Powerful new diagnostic techniques such as CT scanning, colonoscopy, and mammography have become standard within just a few years. Dazzling treatment breakthroughs quietly settle into routine use in a similar pattern: coronary artery surgery, organ transplantation, joint prostheses, and any number of drugs that are unique in the way they combat disease. New entries are constantly being evaluated to learn every possible way that they may be used to relieve suffering in the future. Laser beams, interferon, interleukin, stone-smashers, and internal drug delivery pumps promise to be counted among the darlings of tomorrow.

The organization of medical care delivery is also evolving at a dramatic pace. Some indication of what is to come can be gained by listening to the new language of planners and analysts: *corporate medicine, managed health care, health maintenance organizations,* and *gate keeper.* This last term refers to a physician, believe it or not, who is expected to play the pivotal role in controlling the expense of medical care by limiting the access of patients to consultants, procedures, appliances, and hospital beds. His difficult role will be to decide who really needs top-of-the-line attention among the many who are potential candidates for it.

Keeping Things in Perspective

For reasons that are hardly obscure, people confronting this brave new medical world are likely to harbor a mixture of confusion, optimism, anxiety, and loneliness. There is no easy way to respond to all of the questions each of us may have, but a few general themes may help in developing a sensible personal approach to the so-called medical establishment.

More can be too much

Not every person with a headache needs a CT scan to exclude a brain tumor, and most instances of belly pain are nothing more than that. Yet, surrounded as we are by the miracles of modern medicine, we tend to feel that every measure should be used to check out every bodily complaint. Until a few years ago, almost everyone believed that for the privileged few who had the opportunity to get so-called executive health check-ups on an annual basis, a vast panoply of expensive diagnostic tests were desirable even in the absence of any symptoms. But experts who have analyzed the real benefits of indiscriminately applied medical attention express genuine concern about the overuse of resources at hand. A well-known graph of diminishing, and then negative, return for the cost incurred helps highlight the argument.

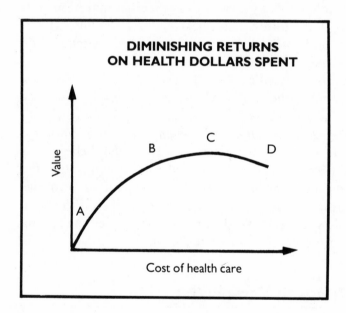

At the steep upslope of the curve (A) is the investment of money in vaccines to prevent polio and tetanus or in screening newborn infants for an underactive thyroid gland which, if left untreated, would result in cretinism. Here, a relatively small outlay of money reaps tremendous benefit by thwarting debility or death at the start of life's span.

At the gradual portion of the curve's ascent (B), more money is being spent with less incremental gain, but few would argue against the purchases: organ transplantation, coronary artery bypass grafting, intensive care units. The flat part of the curve (C), on the other hand, is where doctors and patients often scratch their heads as diseases enter advanced stages. Is there enough benefit to justify the expense and discomfort of chemotherapy when a cancer has spread widely through the body? How extensive should the effort be to discern a reversible cause of dementia in an elderly person who has gradually lost the ability to recognize family and surroundings?

The downward slope of the curve (D) describes circumstances where spending more could actually have a negative value. Examples would be decisions to embark on screening for coronary artery disease by coronary angiography, or to treat minimally narrowed vessels (by balloon dilation or bypass grafting) in advance of symptoms. The complications from the procedures, when coupled with the discomfort involved, would quite likely outweigh any advantage that might be achieved in respect to prolonging life.

On a personal level, it's wise to think of this curve as it might apply to the risks of "going for more" within the medical establishment. Fancy tests often carry perils as well as high price tags. Even routine tests used to screen for disease in healthy persons carry the hidden danger of giving false-positive results, which then prompt wild-goose chases to search for diseases that were never there in the first place. Being hospitalized is often an opportunity to obtain the best that modern medicine can offer, but it also exposes one to additional risks in the form of infections, invasive procedures, and drug reactions. In the final phase of a chronic, fatal disease, heroic interventions almost always cause more suffering than relief. Yet, even at the extreme, many will opt for a shot at a miracle.

> It seems a necessary move
> In an unnecessary action,
> Not for the good that it will do
> But that nothing be left undone
> On the margin of the impossible.
>
> *T. S. Eliot*

It ain't necessarily so

Most thoughtful doctors feel far more comfortable with probabilities than absolutes. This causes dismay in those patients who want unqualified answers. But the world of biology, disease, and human variability is filled with exceptions to just about any rule. Even the best medicines don't work for every person taking them. Differences among individuals with respect to drug metabolism, vulnerability to side effects, and allergic reactions to foreign chemicals will always result in some disappointments.

Many diagnostic tests are notoriously subject to mistakes for a variety of reasons. Equipment malfunction and human error are frequently the source of faulty results, but even if these could be eliminated, virtually no test can ever separate out all of the sick people from the healthy ones. The biological variability of individuals, again, makes this impossible. Some normal, healthy people will turn out to have an abnormal laboratory result (a false positive), which leads to unnecessary worry and follow-up testing. Conversely, test results sometimes come out normal even when the person being checked harbors the illness in question (a false negative). This test result can lead to a false sense of security.

Although medicine is inherently probabilistic, this does not mean that reasonable expectations and decisions cannot occur. The key is to attempt to identify the *degree of probability* that obtains in a given situation. We know, for example, that the chance of getting into trouble from silent gallstones (ones that give absolutely no symptoms) is about 18% over a 20-year period. Moreover, surgery performed only after symptoms arise will usually be just as effective as if it had been done at an earlier time and will carry a very small risk (less than 1% fatality rate for an otherwise healthy person). Therefore, it makes sense, all other things being equal, to adopt a stance of watchful waiting rather than early surgery for silent gallstones. More is not necessarily better in this situation.

Experienced physicians can explain the odds in most circumstances with reasonable accuracy. Obviously, these odds vary with the patient. The chance that a shadow on a chest x-ray is a cancer is much greater in a smoker than in a nonsmoker. A racing heart is more worrisome in a person with known heart disease than in an otherwise healthy young adult. Spells of wooziness are much more often due to hyperventilation than to heart disease or vascular

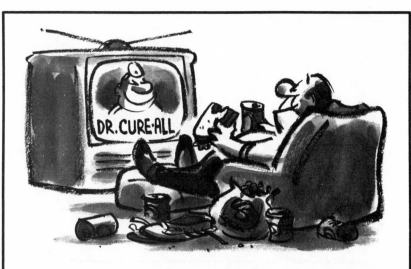

Television may be hazardous to your health. According to one study, frequent viewers have more confidence in members of the medical profession and are more complacent about eating, drinking, and exercise than are infrequent viewers. Fictionalized medicine on TV seems to decrease interest in prevention by fostering the unrealistic notion that physicians can cure any problem that might arise.

insufficiency of the brain; in low-risk persons, vigorous testing for cerebral vascular or cardiac abnormalities is usually wasteful. Assurance can be provided by simpler measures, such as having the patient reproduce the symptoms by deliberately hyperventilating.

The downside of probabilism is that every once in a while there are surprises. The "one-in-a-thousand" likelihood will turn out to be true for one person in a thousand. This fact, coupled with a more litigious attitude in our society, has prompted many doctors to abandon sound medical judgment when they embark on a diagnostic evaluation. Expensive and sometimes uncomfortable testing for improbable diseases is being performed increasingly to guard against malpractice suits for "being wrong" on rare occasion. In an age when so much is expected of the medical establishment, it is hard for many patients to recognize that a good decision will be the wrong one for that one victim of chance in a thousand.

An ounce of prevention

Some of the least glamorous practices have the most dramatic impact on health. Examples include wearing seatbelts, taking needed medications on schedule, keeping immunizations up-to-date, and avoiding native water and raw vegetables in areas of poor sanitation. To call the results of these practices dramatic is paradoxical, because *nothing happens*. That is the goal. The drama comes only from the contrast with what *could* have happened if these basic measures of prevention were not employed. Success means not having to deal with the medical establishment at all.

Any doctor who has worked a Saturday-night shift in a busy

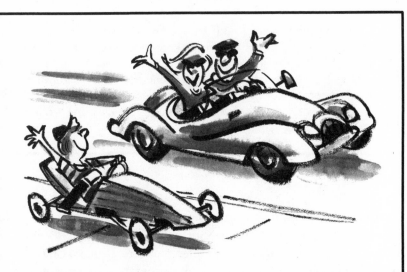

Children can crash, and be injured, even when the car doesn't, and isn't. In fact, about 15% of serious traffic injuries to children under the age of 14 occur without a crash. For example, the child crawls out the window of a moving car, or bangs against something inside the car when the driver suddenly swerves, stops, or accelerates. All the more reason to protect your child with a restraint system.

And despite the popular fear, being "trapped" in the car is safer than going without a seat belt. So buckle up yourself as well as your children: You'll not only serve as a role model but also remain around and intact for the years ahead.

emergency ward has witnessed the graphic consequences of not wearing a seatbelt. Death and disfigurement are especially gruesome when one considers that they could have been so easily avoided by a simple tug and a snap. Thus, it was no surprise to learn in our survey of Harvard Medical School faculty physicians that 73% routinely wear seatbelts (see p. 484 for the complete survey).

Other preventive measures widely employed by this faculty include limiting alcohol to no more than two drinks per day (93%); abstaining from cigarette smoking (92%); restricting red meat intake to 3 times a week (44%); eating no more than 3 eggs a week (79%); substituting margarine for butter (69%); and performing aerobic exercise at least 3 times a week (49%).

Not all of these practices are as simple or effective in preventing tragedy as snapping on a seatbelt. And no matter how careful we are, so long as we are mortal the chances are high that we're in for a stretch of serious illness at some time in our lives. The goal is to delay that period of intensive interaction with the medical establishment as long as possible. To this end, the cost of an ounce of prevention—usually counted in units of inconvenience rather than dollars and cents—is a superb investment.

Selecting a Health Plan

For most of us, a sense of security includes the expectation that any health problems we may have will be handled competently and at an affordable price. Since World War II, health insurance has become one of the great equalizers in American society. Although many people, even now, are not covered by insurance, the large majority have some form of financial protection from the cost of unexpected illness. However, it's widely believed that health insurance in this country has also helped to increase the total cost of health care and thus to create an economic crisis. To cope with this rising expense, various cost-cutting alternatives have been developed. Just in the past few years, the number and type of insurance plans offered by most employers have proliferated—and so has the confusion of people who must choose among them. We offer here a brief guide for the perplexed, with some principles that should be applied in making choices between competing health plans.

Fee-for-service payment

The simplest financial transaction with a doctor (or hospital) resembles any other purchase of services. You go in with your problem, you get taken care of, and then you get a bill for the amount judged to be appropriate. This is called *fee-for-service-care*. It was standard practice when health insurance was introduced, and at the time it was vigorously defended by practicing physicians as the only acceptable method of payment. So insurance programs were designed simply to pay the bills. In this system, which is still the most common, you pay an annual premium, in return for which the insurance company pays at least a portion of your health-care bills.

The case against this form of insurance is that it removes barriers to overspending. The provider benefits from offering care, whether it is essential or of only uncertain worth to the patient. Professional judgment guides the choices that are made, but financial incentives to offer more rather than less care are undeniably present. The patient, especially when coverage is good, likewise has no reason to be cost-conscious about care. Thus, in a doubtful situation, there's little barrier to spending extra money.

Over the years, insurance coverage has become more complete, and its cost has often become buried in the "benefits package" offered by employers. Employees have thus tended to lose sight of the fact that the care they receive is costing them money. Both doctor and patient can make choices without directly considering what the cost will be. The result, according to most students of this subject, has been an inclination to take the medical high road, to buy excessive amounts of medical care, regardless of expense.

Neither doctors nor patients have objected, and as long as insurers have been able to balance premiums against payments, they have been able to stay in business. The insurer's profit is not the major issue here. The organizations insuring fee-for-service care are not necessarily, or even usually, profit-making companies. The bulk of fee-for-service coverage is provided by Medicare (the federal program for retired people), Medicaid (state programs for low-income people), and Blue Cross/Blue Shield (nonprofit organizations that offer coverage for hospitalization and doctors' fees, respectively). In the past, it has been feasible for insurers to make the adjustments needed to balance their books, but recently premiums (or tax payments) have threatened to go so high that nobody would be prepared to pay them.

Cost-conscious alternatives

There needs to be some way to have the protection of insurance coverage, while holding on to the sort of restraint that comes from balancing the value of a treatment against the expense. The burden of making this kind of decision can be assigned to the patient, to the provider, or to both.

A *prepaid plan,* currently the major alternative to fee-for-service insurance, puts the main burden on the doctor. In this type of plan, the provider (a doctor or group of doctors, hospital, or other organization) essentially offers a binding estimate of what a given amount of health care will cost the average patient for a year. Patients enroll in the plan and pay that amount. (This system is often referred to as *capitation,* because the plan is paid "by the head.") If total costs go higher than the sum of these prepayments, the provider loses money; if they stay below the estimate, the provider gets to keep the difference. In many ways, this arrangement reverses the incentives of the fee-for-service style of practice. The provider benefits financially from delivering less care rather than more, so long as patients remain in good health.

Prepaid plans are usually called *health maintenance organizations* (HMOs) and they come in several forms. A *closed-panel* HMO hires a staff of physicians and pays each one a salary, usually with the understanding that any money saved by the end of each year (for all intents and purposes, the profit) will be distributed among the medical staff. The HMO charges each patient a predetermined amount (usually negotiated in a group contract with the patient's employer) and in addition may charge a few dollars each visit.

An alternative is the *open-panel* HMO, also known as an *independent practice association* (IPA). Instead of maintaining its own staff and clinic buildings, the IPA contracts with a group of physicians to provide its members with care. IPAs are structured in a variety of ways, but commonly each doctor is paid, in advance, a set amount per patient. The doctor, in return, must cover the costs for all services to that patient. The same doctor may have fee-for-service as well as prepaid patients.

Critics of prepaid plans argue that they can put too much pressure on doctors to limit care for the sake of protecting their income. A desirable feature of fee-for-service care, as they see it, is the doctor's sense that it is financially worthwhile to care for difficult cases. One strategy that seeks to preserve this aspect of the fee-for-service philosophy is the *preferred-provider organization* (PPO). The insurer, representing its clients, does some comparative shopping in the medical marketplace. It contracts with a group of providers who agree on a predetermined list of charges for all services, including complex and unusual procedures. Then it pays that rate. The patient is covered for care offered by the list of "preferred providers," though with this type of plan, as with any other, one may choose to go elsewhere and pay for treatment.

Coverage and price tags

The real price tag for any health coverage includes not only the amount of the premium or prepayment but additional costs that occur at the time of treatment. These take three forms. Any treatment that is not covered at all (for example, routine dental care or eye examinations in many plans) is an additional cost to be considered. And insured care may be only partially covered, with *deductibles* and *copayments* required to make up the rest.

Insurance plans vary widely in the number and type of services they will cover. In some cases, however, the list of services is regulated by law. Groups calling themselves HMOs, for example, must provide a certain menu of services. In evaluating a plan, one should learn whether dental work, appliances (canes, eyeglasses, wheelchairs, and the like), and medications are included. It is also worth looking at how much mental health care is covered.

In some instances, extra services may not be a particularly good buy. Routine dental care, for example, is a fairly predictable expense, which one must pay for either directly or through an insurance premium. Insurance, because of the costs of administering and marketing it, may wind up costing more for routine care than just paying the bills. On the other hand, because an employer's contribution to insurance premiums is untaxed income, extra coverage may prove to be economical even when theory indicates that it would not be. Preventive health services (Pap smears, screening for bowel cancer, mammography, immunizations) tend to be covered by prepaid plans but are rarely covered by fee-for-service insurers.

A *deductible* is a portion of the bill that the subscriber must pay before insurance coverage begins. The idea behind this provision is to remove the incentive to get all kinds of minor care simply because it is covered by insurance, and to reduce the administrative costs that come from handling small claims. Much as with automobile insurance, the higher the deductible, the lower the premium.

A *copayment* is a contribution the patient must make to cover some portion of each bill. With fee-for-service coverage the copayment may be a percentage, say 20%, of the total. The copayment is usually higher for outpatient visits than for hospitalization, which is likely to be almost completely covered, once the deductible is paid. A fee-for-service provider may charge more than the insurance company is willing to pay; the remainder is then billed directly to the patient—a practice known as *balance billing*, which may be restricted by law in some states. With prepaid plans, there is typically a fixed amount of copayment—say a few dollars—charged at every visit.

Taking all this into account, the price tag for a prepaid plan is now generally less than with fee-for-service insurance. The major reason appears to be that patients cared for by HMOs spend, on the average, fewer days in hospitals than do patients who pay fee-for-service. Since inpatient care is very expensive, a lot of money can be saved by limiting the amount of hospital time that is "convenient" rather than strictly necessary. In a prepaid plan, the amount of money spent for laboratory and other diagnostic tests is also reduced, because the plan has an incentive to perform these tests as efficiently as possible.

Choice

A clear advantage of fee-for-service coverage, in principle, is that the patient can choose any desired provider. Any qualified doctor offering a recognized health-care service can submit a bill to the insurer; for all intents and purposes, one can choose any primary physician or specialist. In the event of an emergency, care can be sought at any site with the expectation of at least partial reimbursement.

In a prepaid system, on the other hand, a member must obtain virtually all care from doctors and hospitals participating in the plan. It is unusual for consultation or care to be covered if it comes from outside the plan without prior approval. As a rule, treatment for a true emergency is covered, no matter where it is given, but the administrators of the prepaid plan define what a "true" emergency is. These rules do limit the member's freedom to choose providers.

No matter what the type of insurance, an individual or family must often meet certain qualifications before being accepted for coverage. Prepaid plans are usually somewhat more restrictive, and may be available only to those who are eligible through an employer, union, or other group. Virtually anyone can buy individual insurance to cover fee-for-service care, but the cost for an individual policy may be exceedingly high. Prepaid plans typically have limited periods of time when new members may enroll. Regular insurance plans often require that applicants wait for a period of months before coverage begins. Both of these restrictions are intended to prevent people from trying to save premium payments when they are well and then sign up when they become sick.

In general, those who are self-employed, unemployed, working part-time, or retired may have the most difficulty finding suitable and affordable coverage. Retired people are usually, of course, eligible for Medicare, but Medicare coverage is often quite incomplete. It is wise to plan for supplementary coverage a few years in advance of retirement.

Quality

At present, health care in a prepaid plan costs about 15% less than fee-for-service insurance for corresponding coverage. Most of this saving, as we have noted, comes from reduced amounts of hospitalization. Other economies may also be noticeable, although they play a somewhat smaller role in cost-containment. For example, HMOs are more likely than private physicians to employ nurse practitioners or physician's assistants. There is no clear evidence that the less expensive care in prepaid plans results in poorer health for their members—nor, for that matter, that it is measurably better. Measuring quality of health care is, however, notoriously difficult. If it were easy, there would be no problem in choosing the best of all possible systems.

Theoretical arguments can be made on both sides. Full insurance coverage for fee-for-service care is expensive, but it puts neither physician nor patient at risk if large numbers of tests or procedures are thought to be needed. This may mean that disease can be detected earlier and thus prevented, and it means that when serious illness occurs, there is no financial reason to hold back on the maximum course of treatment. The counter-argument is that excessive medical care can create problems of its own (complications, discomfort, and so forth).

The financial interests of a prepaid plan dictate that tests and procedures not be prescribed in a wasteful manner. On the other hand, the prepaid plan is also more "profitable" if its patients are healthy. In theory, this is an incentive for judicious use of preventive care, including diagnostic tests to ensure that patients stay well. In reality, many preventive measures—such as screening programs— seem not to lower net cost. So, if HMOs are offering more preventive services than fee-for-service practitioners, the reason may be more a matter of philosophy and federal regulation than purely financial incentive. Some critics have also argued that HMOs maintain a healthier membership by admitting mainly younger, healthier people. This situation can be expected to change as people enrolled in HMOs continue to age.

The bottom line

To summarize, in looking at health-care options, the purchaser should keep the following points in mind:

COST Currently, a prepaid plan will almost aways cost less, whether only the size of the premium is considered or the benefits per dollar are calculated.

FREEDOM OF CHOICE This issue is probably most important to people who are already happy with a fee-for-service practitioner, and to those who are comfortable and knowledgeable in making choices among doctors. The prepaid plan never eliminates freedom of choice, but it does narrow the options to a panel of participating doctors or a few hospitals.

QUALITY This is the most difficult aspect of care for anyone to evaluate. So far, prepaid plans have not been shown to save money at the cost of their members' health. But this statement must still be made with caution, because research in this area is difficult and the results of available studies cannot be regarded as conclusive. By law, HMOs must have built-in quality-control systems and grievance procedures. On the other hand, the patient in a fee-for-service relationship may simply "fire" his or her physician and start over. In either case, the patient does not have to continue with care that he or she regards as unacceptable.

Although the wide range of options for health-care coverage is currently bewildering, this development is probably a good sign. We can regard the present period as one of experimentation in which we, as a society, are looking for ways to provide the highest quality of medical care at the most reasonable price.

Choosing and Using Your Doctor

Like most important questions, "Who should I have for my doctor?" is not easily answered. Preference for a man or woman doctor, for one who is older or younger, or for a particular personality type will naturally affect your choice. A particular medical need, such as bowel problems, allergies, or arthritis, may lead you to a doctor with special interest and experience in that area. What we would like to offer here are some suggestions on selecting a "primary" physician—the one you turn to first for medical help and the one you rely on to help prevent illness.

Whether your choices are limited by membership in a health maintenance organization or whether you have the freedom offered by fee-for-service insurance to range widely when it comes to choosing a physician, it pays to ask around. A single person's experience may not be representative, but a consensus of several patients and colleagues can be a useful guide to a physician's strengths, weaknesses, and idiosyncrasies. You can tap into the general opinion in the medical community by asking other doctors or nurses, pharmacists, hospital workers, or other members of your HMO.

You cannot be sure that a doctor is the right one for you until you have had a chance to work together, but a little homework can tell you a surprising amount about how your partnership is likely to develop. When personal "chemistry" prevents a relationship from working, however, nobody is obliged to stick it out. It is possible and even desirable to part company, with all due respect, and try again. This should be as true in a health maintenance organization or group practice as it is with a solo practitioner.

Training

It is important to know about a physician's training. Fortunately, this information is easy to find. The American Medical Association publishes *The Directory of Medical Specialists* and other directories, which are available in most local libraries. Find out whether your doctor has graduated from a fully accredited medical school (as is now true of the overwhelming majority). Going beyond that information to find out whether the physician has graduated from a so-called prestige school may be of some interest, but post-graduate training (residency) probably has more influence on the quality of a doctor's work than basic schooling.

For several decades it has been standard to expect doctors entering primary care (usually internists or family practitioners) to acquire 3 full years of training after medical school. Following training, the doctor must pass an examination to become "board certified." Someone who finishes the training but has not taken or passed the examination is sometimes described as "board eligible," and such a designation should at least raise questions as to why certification was not achieved. Physicians over age 60 or so may not have gone through the formal process of certification at the end of their training, but younger physicians in practice normally have done so.

A doctor's hospital appointments—the places where he or she is authorized to admit patients—also tell you something about qualifications and professional standing. Most hospitals carefully screen the physicians appointed to their staffs; the better a hospital, the better qualified its physicians are likely to be.

The superstar young physician of 1960 would be worse than mediocre today without a continuing effort to keep abreast of medical progress. There are many ways to do this. Reading is important. If books are around a doctor's office, look to see whether they are of relatively recent vintage, instead of dusty with disuse and yellowed with age. Attending courses at a medical school, meetings of a specialty society, or weekly "rounds" at a hospital is an important means of staying up on recent advances. Teaching in a nearby hospital or medical school is both an excellent means of keeping the teacher informed and an indication that his or her ability is recognized by these institutions. Many specialty boards have realized that "certification" early in a career cannot guarantee competence for a lifetime. A number of them now offer or require recertification at intervals.

Practice patterns

To be any good at all, primary medical care has to be available in time of need. A good primary physician responds to truly urgent problems by fitting the patient into his or her schedule, returns calls, and sees to it that there is ample coverage when he or she is away or off duty.

An orderly office, defined office hours, equipment in good working condition, a secretary who knows where to find the doctor, overall cleanliness, and correspondence that is punctual are all indications of a well-run medical practice. When you sit down with the doctor, he or she should give you a chance to describe the problem initially in your own words without a barrage of yes-or-no questions before you get two sentences out of your mouth. (Yes-or-no questions, later on, can be important in clarifying things.) The physical examination should be performed carefully and with due consideration for your modesty (but not at the expense of neglecting breast, rectal, and genital examinations). If you come in with what seems to be a minor complaint and many expensive tests are ordered, find out why.

Your primary physician should be prepared to refer you to competent specialists when serious or complicated problems come up. When difficult decisions must be made, the best physicians will welcome a second opinion. If yours doesn't, you should find out why not. On the other hand, the doctor who refers routine, minor complaints (trivial rashes, mild headaches of long standing, brief digestive disturbance) to specialists is either exercising poor judgment or evidencing deficient skills.

Communicating

Your doctor may be harassed and distracted by the problems of others, but that's small solace when you need attention. Ask yourself if your physician is really concentrating on your specific complaints. On the other hand, remember that medical care is a partnership of the patient and the physician. Each member of the partnership has responsibilities. Prepare for your visit to the doctor's office.

Begin by saying clearly why you have come. Have a list of questions in mind. (There is no harm in writing them down so you'll remember them.) Evidence from doctors' practices indicates that nearly half the time, the patient's main reason for seeking help is not acknowledged. This occurs partly because doctor and patient often have different priorities and partly because patients often are not explicit in making their concerns known. One of the physician's jobs is to help allay your anxieties. Some patients avoid the question that worries them most by talking about less threatening topics. Perhaps they hope that the matter will come up by itself. If it does not, they may bring up their real reason for seeking help at the end of the visit with an, "Oh, by the way." And then there is not time for the physician to deal with the problem effectively.

Many people go to the doctor because they want relief from a troublesome symptom. The doctor, on the other hand, is sometimes more focused on the underlying condition than the particular symptom. Because of this difference in perspective, many patients misinterpret the purpose of treatment or fail to recognize when the treatment is effective. They quit taking medication too soon because they feel better or they discontinue because of unpleasant side effects. To counteract this danger, always ask the doctor how to evaluate your progress, since symptoms may be an unreliable clue.

When you get instructions from a physician, be sure you understand them. Doctors sometimes speak their own language. Make sure your doctor speaks yours. Once you understand what the doctor wants you to do, be explicit about your reactions to the recommendation. Many patients leave the doctor's office with reservations about the prescribed treatment; but the doctor knows nothing about their reservations because the patient has smiled graciously and said "thank you" without expressing any reluctance or asking questions about what he or she is expected to do. If scheduling problems will get in the way of complying with the doctor's recommendations, or if time conflicts will make it difficult to keep follow-up appointments, the patient needs to take the initiative to make these problems known.

The impaired physician

An impaired physician is a doctor whose ability to work is compromised by one of the following problems: abuse of alcohol or other drugs (about 80% of all cases), senility (perhaps 10%), mental illness, or aberrant behaviors that appear to be part of a stress reaction (uncommon).

"Impairment" should not be confused with "malpractice." A doctor may be impaired before he or she commits any obvious act of malpractice—and most malpractice seems to originate with doctors who don't have any of the problems listed above. Malpractice implies a harmful interaction with a patient due to ignorance, poor judgment, or deficient technical skill. The danger here is that, by confusing impairment with malpractice, colleagues or other observers will think that nothing can, or should, be done about a doctor's impairment until a patient is injured. (The cases that make headlines are just these: an addicted or alcoholic doctor who is tolerated on a hospital staff until something dreadful happens.)

When a physician appears to be impaired, some important, but admittedly difficult, distinctions must be made. The focus of concern is professional conduct—not the person's private life. For example, a physician who sometimes goes on weekend binges but is always sober and appropriate during working hours certainly has a drinking problem. But it is not so clear that he or she is professionally impaired. At the other extreme, someone who lies to, cheats, steals from, or sexually exploits patients may have serious emotional problems. But the real problem is a breach of ethics, and the general assumption must be that the person's character is incompatible with the practice of medicine.

Although it's hard to collect reliable data, a plausible estimate is that 3–5% of physicians, at some time in their careers, are impaired as a result of drug or alcohol abuse. Careless interpretation can make the situation look worse than it is. If you counted anyone who self-prescribed a sleeping pill in the past year as a drug abuser, you would come up with much higher numbers—implying an "epidemic" of abuse that doesn't exist.

In general, doctors don't appear to be much different from the general population with respect to drug and alcohol abuse. Drugs are most used when they are most available, however. So doctors who work in hospital or clinic settings (where a supply of drugs is kept on the premises) are more likely to use drugs than others.

Anesthesiologists, who must constantly handle narcotics, among other substances, are at high risk.

Some doctors are at especially high risk because of their personality characteristics or personal history. Those with a background of abusing drugs, especially in their teens, may continue or resume that pattern in adulthood. It also seems that doctors in high-stress settings—perhaps especially those who feel that they must carry the ball on their own—are pretty vulnerable. They may come to see stimulants and sedatives as a way of holding themselves together—and not be able to conceive of the alternative of getting human help either with their work or with their problems.

Identifying and treating impaired physicians

Impaired physicians have to be reported by someone. Occasionally, a doctor is self-referred, but questionable behavior is more likely to be reported by a patient, colleague, or relative—and very often in a compassionate spirit.

In most states, people who report a suspicion of impairment are protected from lawsuits—provided the report is made in good faith without malicious intent. Patients who have reported a probable impairment almost inevitably have to change doctors, though, simply because the situation would be too tense otherwise.

A real problem is with getting physicians to report the impairment of their colleagues. Taking this first step seems to be most difficult. Many states have laws requiring physicians to report themselves if they have an impairment. Once an impairment has been identified and acknowledged, state medical societies usually have a formal way of responding, and many doctors are ready and willing to commit their time and effort to helping with the remedy.

Most impaired physicians are highly treatable. They can usually continue to work, or return to work fairly quickly. The real difficulty is identifying them at an early phase and getting them into a program. Once they have been identified, the stakes are so high, and methods of control so effective, that relapse is uncommon.

The medical societies in all 50 states have some kind of program for monitoring and treating impaired physicians. To take one example, in Massachusetts when a report comes in that a doctor is impaired, two members of the Committee on Impaired Physicians are assigned as a team to evaluate the situation and, if need be, confront the physician. In fairly short order, as a rule, the impaired physician agrees to a plan. The cost of not cooperating is simply too high.

The first order of business is to establish whether the doctor's patients are safe. This may entail a period in which he or she does not practice and receives intensive treatment.

In any event, there will be a follow-up plan. Virtually always, this means setting up a contract through which the doctor's behavior is monitored for a matter of years. The team of two doctors follows the impaired physician on a personal basis, takes responsibility for monitoring compliance, and, as appropriate, confers with the physician's superior or a responsible colleague. The full committee of 25 meets regularly to review problem cases and decide whether the program is working. If it is not, referral to the state's licensing board may be recommended.

In the case of drug addiction, there is a very high rate of successful treatment and control—at least 85% is the usual experience. The rehabilitation plan includes therapy, participation in a group such as Narcotics Anonymous, and regular urine drug monitoring.

Alcoholism is more prevalent than drug addiction and is harder to treat. There tends to be a lot of denial of the problem. "A few drinks" are socially acceptable—often even encouraged when they should not be. The first step—confrontation—can help the person begin to regain control. There are physician and professional AA groups, which alcoholic doctors are encouraged to attend. Alcohol can be monitored by smell, behavior, breath analysis, and blood detection. Alcoholic doctors are one group for which the drug disulfiram (Antabuse) can be very effective. This drug makes people sick if they take a drink, but it only works when the person is highly motivated to take it regularly.

Rather uncommonly, compulsive behaviors may emerge as part of a physician's reaction to stress. These may range from inappropriate friendliness during a consultation (described as "creepy" by patients), to bizarre gestures during examination, to bizarre behavior outside a practice setting. In these cases, there is usually "sexual" content to the behavior, but patients are not violated. The behavior is isolated, not part of an overall pattern, and in each case appears to be part of a reaction to unusual stress in the doctor's private life. When physicians are confronted, therapy is almost always effective in ending the behavior. Where there is a potential for inappropriate behavior during an an examination, the presence of a female chaperone is usually required (good practice in any case).

Other kinds of mental illness less commonly require intervention. The main form that affects practicing physicians is depression, and a severely depressed doctor most often withdraws from practice until recovery is adequate.

Senility—the loss of mental, emotional, and physical capacity to practice as a result of age—must be handled in a different way. Here, the essential task is to get the physician to recognize the need to retire. A team may have to visit several times and confront the aging practitioner to bring this about.

Taking Your Medicine

When you are given a prescription, you need to know, at a minimum, the name of the drug being prescribed. Many drugs have names that sound alike, and many of them look alike. There is no substitute for knowing exactly what you are taking. The dose and schedule should also be clearly understood. If the drug must be applied, as is the case with skin preparations, you will need to know the procedures and place for application.

Many very effective treatments, such as drugs to reduce high blood pressure, have a rather disappointing overall record because at least one-third of the people receiving prescriptions fail to take the drugs regularly. Some drugs, such as antibiotics, are usually given for limited periods, usually 10 days, whereas pills for high blood pressure are generally prescribed for much longer duration. If you discontinue a course of treatment prematurely for any reason, this should be reported to your doctor.

If bothersome side effects are the reason for stopping a drug, sometimes the physician can prescribe a different drug that will serve the same purpose but without causing discomfort. Your doctor should always mention common side effects of any drug being prescribed. The mild stomach upset caused by some medications is easier to tolerate if it is expected. You should also be warned about possible incompatibilities of drugs taken at the same time. Any drugs that have sedation as their side effect can have serious consequences. It is a good idea to compile a list of all the pills that you take, prescribed or over-the-counter, and ask questions about side effects and possible adverse reactions to drugs taken together.

Whether a specific drug is taken with food or on an empty stomach may or may not be important. Some drugs are absorbed better when there is no food in the stomach to interfere. Others require food (or the intestinal juices it stimulates) for maximum absorption. Food may also be recommended as a way to prevent the stomach upset that some drugs can cause. Whenever you begin a new medication, it's worthwhile to ask your doctor or pharmacist whether the drug should be taken at a specific time with respect to meals.

If you have trouble remembering to take medication, certain tricks may help—say, putting a pill bottle in the shoes you plan to wear the next morning, next to your toothbrush, or in some other conspicuous place. If daily activities prevent you from keeping up with the dosage schedule, your physician may be able to prescribe a newer drug that does not need to be taken so frequently. But beware of an overemphasis on using the latest drugs. A few important drugs become available each year. Many, however, are just more expensive versions of the older ones, but with the disadvantage that their side effects are not as well known.

Generic drugs

In order to encourage pharmaceutical companies to develop drugs, companies are given an exclusive right to market a new product for 14 years. After that time, any company can make and sell that same drug as long as it is proven, to the satisfaction of the Food and Drug Administration (FDA), to be equal in potency and purity to the brand-name drug that is being copied. These "copies" are usually sold under their chemical name and are called *generics*.

Price

A generic equivalent will often be less expensive than a brand-name drug, but not always. In an extensive study of nearly 900,000 prescriptions filled in 1,363 pharmacies across the country, 6 times out of 10, conjugated estrogen (the generic hormone) was *more* expensive than Premarin (the brand). This was also the case with the diuretic furosemide (generic) and Lasix (the brand). However, for the other 19 pharmaceuticals studied, the generic most often cost *less* than the brand.

In that same study, the price-per-pill at different pharmacies showed rather astounding fluctuations. Four- or five-fold price differences were commonly observed with both brand and generic products. And even though generics tended to be priced lower than brand names, the difference was often trivial. In part, this is because drugstores often mark up the generic version more than the brand. In other words, the full wholesale saving is often not passed along to the retail purchaser.

On average, pill costs were lower in chain pharmacies than in independent ones, but this is only a very rough guide. The basic message of the study is that the price of a given drug varies widely, and that the distinction between generic and brand products may not be the ultimate key to savings. Although shopping around may save an appreciable amount of money when a drug must be taken regularly or is very expensive, the time spent may not be worthwhile for many prescriptions.

Quality

Some people have had the concern that a generic may not meet the same standards of quality as its brand-name counterpart. Yet the FDA has strict criteria that must be met before a generic can be marketed as "equivalent" to its brand-name counterpart. In past years, there have been problems with two products: phenytoin, a seizure medication, and digoxin, a drug used in the treatment of heart disease. The generic form of these drugs turned out to be less well absorbed than the original brands. The problems with digoxin but not phenytoin have been solved. Unfortunately, these isolated differences have given generics as a whole an undeservedly bad name.

In some states, the routine substitution of generic drugs by the pharmacist is allowed. In others, however, the physician has to specify on the prescription that a substitution can be made. If you are unsure of the regulations in your state, ask your pharmacist.

Drugs and the elderly

One of this country's major drug problems gets very little publicity: it is the "invisible overdosing" that occurs among older people who are taking prescription or over-the-counter medications. This can happen even when the dose range appears not to be excessive. The usual drug dosages recommended for adults are based on expectations concerning the speed with which the medication will be inactivated or removed from the body. The liver and kidneys play the major role in disposing of most drugs. With age, these organs become less efficient, even in otherwise healthy individuals. Thus, a "standard" dosage schedule for the "average" adult liver or kidney often leads to accumulation of the drug in an older person.

Even when the blood level of a drug seems to be in the proper range for an adult, it may be too high for the elderly person. This is because certain organs, particularly the brain and heart, become more responsive to drugs as they age. Thus, ill effects may be observed even when blood levels of a drug are in a range that is quite safe for a younger adult. Body size, the amount of fat, and the proportion of muscle also influence the way drugs are processed, stored, and removed. In general, the changes that occur with aging conspire to intensify the effect of many drugs given at the usual doses.

As people get older, the number of diseases they have is likely to increase, and so is the number of drugs they are given. The more medications a person takes, the more possible interactions and side effects he or she will be exposed to. Indeed, the risk increases dramatically with each additional drug or disease. Furthermore, as dosage schedules become more complicated, the chance of making a mistake, such as taking the same dose twice, also goes up. This tendency is greatest in the small fraction of older people who suffer from confusion or have impaired memories. When the drugs themselves interfere with thinking, otherwise normal individuals also run the risk of making dangerous, even life-threatening, mistakes.

Most physicians in practice have no formal training in the use of drugs with elderly patients, although they may be generally aware of the factors just mentioned. Unfortunately, some physicians

▪ Stuck pills ▪

A pill can stick in the esophagus or "foodpipe," and remain lodged there for many minutes or even hours. Even though the swallower is usually not aware of it, the stuck pill can injure the esophagus, producing inflammation, ulceration, and eventually scar tissue. To avoid this problem, drink lots of liquid whenever you take a tablet or capsule, and remain standing or seated for a few minutes after swallowing.

choose incorrect medications, prescribe too much of them, or combine drugs that are not compatible with each other. Then, if the elderly patient suffers fatigue, confusion, or depression, the symptoms may be written off as evidence that he or she is merely "growing old." To make matters worse, the symptoms may then be inappropriately treated with a tranquilizer or antidepressant. Such a misguided attempt to "cure" a drug-induced condition with another drug just compounds the difficulty.

The scope of this problem should not be underestimated. Older people take a lot of pills. Although only 11% of the U.S. population is over 65, this group takes fully 25% of all prescription drugs. Elderly people receiving care in nursing homes are the most heavily medicated members of our society. They typically receive anywhere from 4 to a dozen or more drugs every day. Half of them are on tranquilizers, although there is little evidence that these agents need to be so extensively used.

What to do

There are several measures that can be initiated by any patient, health-care professional, family member, or concerned friend. Here are some steps to consider:

THE "BROWN-BAG" TECHNIQUE   Encourage a regular review of all medications taken by the patient. For example, put everything from the medicine cabinet into a bag and take it into the doctor's office. Patients often keep drugs that were prescribed years ago, "in case I have that problem again." This is a dangerous practice. Patients receiving prescriptions from two or more physicians are especially likely to benefit from a brown-bag review, as one doctor may not know what the other is prescribing.

REMINDERS   If the individual is affected by confusion or poor memory, a special strategy to manage pill-taking can help. One method is to enter the list of drugs on a calendar and check off each dose as it is taken. Or a set of small envelopes, marked with time of day, can be used. Sometimes it is necessary for a visiting nurse or a family member to allocate pills dose-by-dose to the envelopes to make sure that the patient is taking the right amount of a prescribed drug. The latest wrinkle in this approach is an inexpensive "high-tech" medication container that beeps at pre-programmed intervals to remind the patient that it is time to take a pill.

KEEPING IT SIMPLE   Working with the physician to keep a drug schedule as simple and straightforward as possible is very important. This may mean eliminating drugs that are not strictly necessary and choosing drugs that can be taken once or twice a day instead of more frequently. Selecting pills that look different from one another can help the patient to keep track as long as this strategy does not compromise the quality or nature of treatment.

OVER-THE-COUNTER CULPRITS   Sleeping aids, cold remedies, diet pills, or laxatives are among the preparations that an elderly patient can buy without a prescription and without the doctor's knowledge. Yet these agents can also produce adverse effects or interact badly with other drugs the person is taking. Be sure to include them in any brown-bag review.

A HIGH INDEX OF SUSPICION   Any new symptoms, especially nonspecific complaints such as fatigue, weight loss, abdominal distress, or confusion, could be the adverse effect of a drug rather than a dread disease or simple aging. Raising this possibility is always worthwhile.

Because drugs are not covered by Medicare or most other insurance systems, they are one of the highest out-of-pocket expenses for the elderly. When possible, lower-priced generic drugs, or the less expensive of two equivalent drugs, should be prescribed.

Used appropriately and carefully, drugs can improve the quality of life for an older person. But they have the potential to make a big difference in the opposite direction. Asking the right questions at the right time can tilt the balance in the patient's favor.

Immunizations

No other medical practices are more justified by low cost, preventive impact, and relative safety than the routine immunizations of childhood—or those which are sensible in adult years, such as tetanus boosters and, for senior citizens or people with chronic illnesses, the pneumonia vaccine and the flu vaccine. This section provides guidelines for purchasing what is probably the best set of bargains available from the medical establishment.

Childhood immunizations

The following schedule is currently recommended for children. Although it may be modified because of illness or allergy, an interruption does not necessitate starting all over again.

DTP

The DTP shot combines protection against 3 diseases that were at one time childhood killers: diphtheria (D), tetanus or lockjaw (T), and pertussis or whooping cough (P). These vaccines can be given separately in special circumstances; but for the vast majority of children, the simplest plan is a combined DTP shot given 3 times during the first 6 months of life, again during the second year of life, and just before entering school. In other words, the DTP shot should be given 5 times before school to afford optimal protection.

THE PERTUSSIS CONCERN   The pertussis component of the DTP shot has come under intense scrutiny in recent years because of safety issues. Relatively minor reactions from pertussis vaccine are common. About one-half of all children receiving the vaccine will experience temporary local pain and modest fever. More serious reactions are rare. According to commonly accepted estimates, high fever or convulsions occur in approximately 1 in 7,000 children inoculated with the vaccine; permanent brain damage occurs in about 1 in 310,000 inoculations. Children who have had truly serious reactions to previous pertussis shots should not receive the further doses of the vaccine except under careful medical supervision.

However, the routine use of pertussis vaccine as part of childhood inoculations is recommended. Since its introduction, the annual death rate from whooping cough in the United States has dropped from about 7,000 deaths per year to less than 20. As expressed by the American Academy of Pediatrics, "The risk of death and suffering caused by this highly infectious disease of infancy is far greater than the possible side effects of the vaccine."

Newer and presumably safer versions of pertussis vaccine are being tested.

TOPV

TOPV stands for "trivalent oral polio vaccine." There are two forms of polio vaccine, the so-called inactivated form (also known as the *killed* or *Salk* or *injectable* vaccine) and the attenuated form (also known as the *live* or *Sabin* or *oral* vaccine). Since there are three types of polio viruses, protection must be achieved against all three. The most common method of giving protection against polio is the attenuated (oral) form, which contains all three in one swig. The oral polio vaccine should be given 4 times during childhood, and it is usually given at the same time as the DTP shot.

THE POLIO CONCERN There has been some worry about the danger of contracting polio from the oral (live, but weakened) virus versus the injected (killed virus) vaccine. Many European countries use only the injected vaccine. But since 1962, the official policy in the United States has been to use the oral vaccine. Recently the Institute of Medicine confirmed that the safety of both vaccines is outstanding. No cases of polio have been attributed to the injected vaccine. The risk for the oral vaccine is estimated to be about 1 case of polio for every 11.5 million persons vaccinated, with a further risk of 1 household contact case for every 3.9 million vaccinated. Only 1 death since 1969 has been attributed to the use of the oral vaccine, as compared with the hundreds or even thousands of deaths annually from polio before the vaccine was available.

Given the minimal risk from oral vaccine versus no risk from injected vaccine, some ask why the injected form is not recommended for widespread immunization. The answer is that the oral vaccine provides better immunity in the general population because the live virus spreads to and immunizes some contacts of the vaccinated person.

The Committee for the Study of Poliomyelitis Vaccines of the Institute of Medicine has therefore unanimously recommended that the oral vaccine continue to be the vaccine of choice for routine immunizations in children. In addition, it recommends that children receive an oral polio booster before entering the seventh grade (age 11–12) to provide continued protection into the adult years. Injected vaccine should be available for persons with immunological disorders that make them unusually susceptible to infections, for adults undergoing first-time polio vaccination or traveling to areas where polio is a problem, and for persons who wish to receive this vaccine after understanding the relative merits of the injected and oral vaccine.

Measles-mumps-rubella (MMR)

Measles, mumps, and rubella are three other recommended immunizations of childhood. They have often been given separately, but increasing use is now made of a single shot which combines all three. It is usually given in the second year of life.

MEASLES   Until recently, the measles (rubeola) shot was usually given as a single vaccination at 1 year of age. That recommendation has now been changed to 15 months following studies which demonstrated more protection if the vaccine is given then. Children who were previously vaccinated before 12 months of age should be revaccinated.

Measles vaccine was introduced in 1957, but until 1963 the only available form of vaccine was made from killed virus. Unfortunately, it was not apparent until 1968 that this type of vaccine gave inadequate protection. In that year, reports began to appear that people given the killed-virus vaccine were developing so-called atypical measles. As a result, the killed-virus vaccine was withdrawn and only the highly effective live-virus preparation, which had been introduced in 1963, remained on the market.

Both the live and killed vaccines for measles were licensed for use in 1963, and the majority of people immunized between 1963 and 1967 received the more effective live vaccine. Nevertheless, a significant number of people now in their twenties received an ineffective killed-virus preparation and remain vulnerable to measles infection, which may take an unusual, and sometimes very severe, form in adults.

People born between 1957 and 1967 should be revaccinated unless: (1) they had a case of measles confirmed by a physician's diagnosis, (2) they are immune, as demonstrated by a blood test, or (3) they have a record of receiving live vaccine no earlier than their first birthday. Severe allergy to eggs is a reason not to vaccinate, but people with a mild allergy to eggs (in which the vaccine is grown) can safely receive current preparations. Patients with cancer can be vaccinated unless their immune systems are judged to be impaired by disease or medication. Pregnant, or possibly pregnant, women should not be vaccinated.

People in the vulnerable age group who are exposed to measles have 3 days in which to be vaccinated in order to have a reasonable likelihood of being protected.

RUBELLA So-called German measles is a mild disease in children but can cause severe damage to the developing fetus of a pregnant woman who contracts the disease. Therefore, the reason for immunization is not to protect children but to protect pregnant women from exposure. Some believe that the best way to do this is to achieve widespread immunity (so-called "herd immunity") among children—hence the official recommendations described above. Others argue that this approach will not work, and we should instead concentrate on immunizing those at risk, namely girls, just before they enter child-bearing age.

Despite the controversy, the key point is that each female who reaches child-bearing age ought to be protected against rubella. About 15% of adult women in the U.S. are not. It is important to urge women of child-bearing age—preferably in early adolescence—to find out if they are protected against rubella by means of a simple blood test. For anyone who is susceptible, a vaccination should be given. An adult woman who is vaccinated against rubella must not become pregnant for 3 months, as the vaccine itself carries a small risk of harming a fetus.

Hemophilus influenzae

"H-flu," in doctors' slang, is a bacterium that causes a variety of infections in infants and toddlers. Sometimes it affects only the skin, but it can infect the airways to produce croup or pneumonia. H-flu is the leading cause of meningitis in children, especially babies in their first year of life. This disease is fatal about 5% of the time and leads to learning disabilities or other forms of brain injury in as many as a third of the children who survive it.

Current estimates are that 1 in every 200 children will come down with a serious infection caused by H-flu before the age of 5. Children who attend day care centers are thought to be at somewhat higher risk.

That's the bad news. The good news is that a vaccine has been developed. Studies here and in Finland have shown the vaccine to be safe and also effective, at least in children past age 24 months. And although mild reactions, such as fever and discomfort at the injection site, are relatively common, major side effects are extremely rare. The H-flu immunization belongs to a class of vaccines that is relatively free of problems.

The current recommendation is that every child be immunized against H-flu at the age of 2 years. Those children with problems that put them at special risk (for example, sickle-cell disease or absence of a spleen) and those in day care centers should probably get the shot at 18 months of age (even though evidence of effectiveness is less at this age) and again at 2 years. Because the risk of H-flu infection falls as children approach the age of 5, it is unclear what the cut-off age for vaccination should be. Decisions will probably have to be individualized. For example, unvaccinated children in day care may be good candidates for immunization, even when they are as old as 4 or 5 years. Newer versions of the vaccine are expected to be effective even before age 2, when the majority of H-flu infections occur.

Adult immunizations

Immunizations for adults are a less central feature of comprehensive health care than are childhood immunizations. Indeed, a certain degree of nonchalance on the part of both physicians and their patients may account for the fact that the great majority of adults are inadequately immunized against the infectious diseases for which protection is both recommended and widely available. Because these diseases can have disastrous outcomes, achieving a full complement of appropriate immunizations should be a high priority in the health care of every adult.

The basic strategies of immunization in adult life can be divided into three groups: looking back, keeping up, and raising guard. "Looking back" refers to the simple measure of reviewing one's medical history to determine whether the significant risks of young adulthood have been nullified during childhood—either by being immunized or by having acquired the natural disease. In practical terms, this means checking the nature of protection against measles for any person born after 1956, against German measles for women of childbearing age, and against mumps, a potential cause of male sterility. "Keeping up" highlights the importance of maintaining protection against tetanus and diphtheria by obtaining a single shot of the combined toxoids once every 10 years. "Raising guard" addresses the need to immunize persons who are especially vulnerable to serious complications from certain common infections (influenza, pneumococcal pneumonia) or who are at higher than normal risk to contract certain others (hepatitis B, rabies).

Influenza

Because the risk of death from influenza increases with age, all adults over age 65 are strongly advised to have an influenza shot once yearly. The same recommendation extends to persons of any age who may be unable to fight off influenza because of chronic illness. Conditions that impair resistance include heart and respiratory diseases, chronic kidney failure, diabetes mellitus, chronic anemia, and certain malignant diseases.

The influenza shot must be repeated every fall because the vaccine is prepared anew each year to combat the strains of influenza that are most likely to cause outbreaks of the disease during the upcoming winter. The protection afforded is not complete, as the vaccine is only 70–80% effective in establishing a high level of defense against the virus. Even when immunized persons come down with influenza, however, they appear to have a relatively mild version of the illness by virtue of having a "partial" defense system.

Soreness at the injection site occurs occasionally, but generalized symptoms such as fever and diffuse body aches are rare. Even though the modern vaccine is quite pure and safe, the viruses used in preparing it are grown on chicken eggs, so persons known to have severe allergic reactions to egg protein should not receive the vaccine. Influenza vaccination has not been associated with development of the Guillain-Barré syndrome, a neurological disorder linked only to swine-flu vaccine shots given in 1976.

Pneumococcal pneumonia

The same group of people at high risk for complications of influenza are apt to have problems dealing with pneumococcal pneumonia, caused by the bacterium *Streptococcus pneumoniae*. The most recent vaccine against this streptococcus is designed to stimulate antibody production against 23 of its strains, the ones which account for the vast majority of virulent infections in humans.

Overall, the pneumonia vaccine is about 70% effective in protecting against serious pneumococcal infections, defined as those in which the bacterium can be grown out of the blood.

The pneumococcal vaccine is quite safe. Most reactions are limited to a few days of soreness at the injection site. Only a single shot is recommended, in part because revaccination causes a significant risk of more severe reactions.

Hepatitis B

Although only about 1 in 20 Americans will be infected by the hepatitis B virus over the course of a lifetime, some groups are at extremely high risk. Once acquired, hepatitis B infection can have a variety of outcomes. Most people will fight the virus off successfully, but about 10% are unable to rid themselves of it. When the virus persists, about a quarter of those infected will develop chronic hepatitis, which may lead to cirrhosis or even liver cancer.

Hepatitis B immunization is recommended for health workers who handle blood frequently, homosexually active men, users of illicit injectable drugs, hemodialysis patients, recipients of blood products to control bleeding disorders, prison occupants, workers at institutions for the mentally retarded, and household and sexual contacts of hepatitis B carriers. Immunization requires 3 injections (the first two 4 weeks apart and the third 5 months after the second) and costs around $100. For many potential vaccine recipients, prior blood testing makes sense to be certain that hepatitis B infection has not already occurred.

Only occasional local or mild systemic side effects have been reported from hepatitis B vaccine. The theoretical possibility of its transmitting AIDS has been raised because it is prepared from human plasma, but many careful studies (on both the vaccine and subjects who have received it) have shown this fear to be groundless. Nevertheless, the concern has deterred people from receiving the vaccine. For this reason, a new hepatitis B vaccine, not derived from human plasma, has been produced by genetic engineering.

Periodic Check-Ups

With the new emphasis on personal responsibility for health has come an increased questioning of such practices as the complete head-to-toe check-up—an annual ritual still enacted by many physicians and patients despite the criticism of too much, too soon. The concern is that the cost—and even the risk—of many traditional procedures far outweighs the rare benefit derived when they are done routinely on healthy persons. These costs and risks arise in great part because no test is foolproof. Inevitably some healthy people will show false-positive test results that will lead to further testing, sometimes with invasive procedures that require hospitalization.

The favored alternative to the complete check-up is a selective health examination. Just as in automobile maintenance inspections, only specific high-risk parts are checked to ascertain whether a breakdown is likely in the months ahead. Many of the choices about *which* tests and *how often* are matters of judgment because the definitive research has not been done.

Both science and common sense argue that physical examinations should be individualized according to the special needs posed by the person's age, family history, lifestyle, and work exposures. For example, frequent checks on height and weight are critical during the first year of life, but not in adulthood; mammography examinations should be more frequent for the woman with a strong family history of breast cancer; a patient with an addiction to alcohol requires more intense scrutiny for liver disease than someone who does not drink; and regular hearing tests make sense for the person who works on a very noisy production line.

Individual differences aside, what follows is a list of the tests chosen by the Advisory Board of the *Harvard Medical School Health Letter* for their value as compared with their expense, inconvenience, and risk. Tests at the top of the list are a better value than those at the bottom. The Advisory Board members agreed on the relative importance accorded to the different tests and the stage of life when each becomes relevant. How *often* a specific test should be given remains a debatable issue. Remember, we're considering the healthy person: any test may assume greater priority if it provides information about specific symptoms or lifestyle patterns the patient brings to the doctor's attention.

Screening tests for the healthy person

BLOOD PRESSURE MEASUREMENT   The evidence is so clear as to the value of lowering high blood pressure—which is usually symptom-free until its catastrophic complications occur—that the simple act of checking blood pressure yearly should be high on anybody's list of important tests.

CHOLESTEROL MEASUREMENT As indicated in Chapter 1, the blood cholesterol level is an important risk factor for coronary artery disease. An ideal goal for most persons is a value below 200 mg/dl. If blood cholesterol is elevated, other tests may be ordered (triglycerides, HDL-cholesterol) prior to initiating a cholesterol-lowering program. It's probably wise to check blood cholesterol level at age 25 and every 3–5 years thereafter.

MAMMOGRAPHY (FOR BREAST CANCER) Mammographic screening for early breast cancer has been shown to reduce breast cancer mortality. Improved equipment has lowered the radiation exposure to an acceptable level. The current guidelines of the American Cancer Society call for an initial mammogram between the ages of 35 and 40, a repeat every 1 or 2 years for the next decade, and annual mammography after age 50. Considerations of expense make this schedule unrealistic for many at this time, but fortunately costs are starting to come down.

PAP SMEAR While scientific evidence supports the recent American Cancer Society recommendation of a Pap smear every 3 years in women between 20 and 40 who have had 2 previous negative Pap tests a year apart, there is concern that the extended time intervals may result in their dropping the periodic Pap habit altogether. Obviously, a yearly Pap smear is a better investment than none at all.

STOOL CHECKS FOR HIDDEN BLOOD Screening kits, available to check for hidden blood in stools, allow samples to be checked in a doctor's office or even at home. Although the test is not perfect, it is a simple, useful, and inexpensive way to screen for cancer and other bowel problems (see Chapter 7). The test should be performed at age 40 and repeated every 1–2 years thereafter.

TONOMETRY Glaucoma—increased pressure within the eye which can lead to permanent visual loss—has no early warning signals in most cases. Tonometry is a painless procedure to check for elevated pressure that should be employed every 2–3 years past age 40 or annually if there is a family history of glaucoma. Reducing the pressure with medicine prevents the loss of vision that might otherwise occur.

MULTIPLE BLOOD-SCREENING TESTS   The large number of tests that can be done inexpensively on a small sample of blood by modern technology can lead to undue concern about "abnormalities" that later prove to be unimportant or erroneous (*see below*). But there are reasons to obtain particular blood tests to screen for specific health problems. For example, an elevated blood sugar often means early diabetes. A blood urea nitrogen is a good check of kidney function. A calcium level tests for overactivity of the parathyroid glands. Once every 3–5 years is reasonable.

TESTS FOR SEXUALLY TRANSMITTED DISEASE   Tests for these diseases are important for those who engage in sex with a number of partners, especially casual acquaintances. The blood test for syphilis and swab tests (vagina, urethra, rectum) for gonorrhea are simple and inexpensive. They should be done every year or two in all sexually active persons who are not part of a monogamous relationship—including teenagers.

SKIN TEST FOR TUBERCULOSIS   The value of periodic skin testing (every 5 years until age 35) for tuberculosis is that when "conversion" from prior negative tests to a positive one occurs, it means that tuberculosis bacteria have invaded the body in the interim. Treatment of recent conversions is not necessarily a matter of routine, but there should be a search for evidence of clinical tuberculosis (for example, a chest x-ray) as a minimum response.

SIGMOIDOSCOPY   An examination of the lower segment of the large bowel with an instrument called a sigmoidoscope is extremely important in a patient with bowel symptoms or one whose stool contains blood, as well as a person with a strong family history of bowel cancer. But the discomfort and expense of this test have raised debate about whether it should be used as a primary technique to screen for bowel cancer in the general population. Practical considerations would argue against the likelihood that sigmoidoscopy could ever become widely adopted for this purpose. But in many physicians' offices, the examination is routinely given every 2 years or so in adults past 50.

ELECTROCARDIOGRAM (ECG)   The resting ECG is overused to screen for coronary artery disease. While a single ECG at age 35 will give a "baseline" pattern with which to compare subsequent deviations, frequent cardiograms in the absence of chest pain or other symptoms suggesting heart disease are probably a waste. Exercise stress testing is too expensive and too apt to yield misleading results to recommend for routine screening purposes.

CHEST X-RAY   Many will be surprised to find this common test at the very bottom of the list, and a few medically sophisticated persons may wonder why it is mentioned at all. While the chest x-ray is an outstanding tool for evaluating patients with chest symptoms, the simple fact is that it has rather little pay-off when used in the absence of symptoms. Lung cancer is rarely detected by chest x-ray early enough to affect the eventual outcome; smokers can take no comfort in relying on chest x-rays to pick up cancer at a stage that is early enough.

Adding it up

Visiting one's physician periodically, perhaps every 2 or 3 years in mid-adult life, remains reasonable. Such visits sustain a useful doctor–patient relationship. A review of personal habits and health practices can occur, a physical exam can be performed, and the technique of self-examination—for example, of the breasts or testicles—can be taught. But extensive testing (x-rays, electrocardiograms, lung function studies, and so forth) should not automatically occur as part of each visit for the well person.

What lab tests can reveal

Did you ever wonder what might happen to the specimens of blood and urine you often leave behind after a visit to a doctor? The actual number of tests that can be done on even a single tube of blood is vast. The urine sample alone yields 5 or 6 separate measurements.

Here is a look at some tests your physician is likely to order—and others that may be reported anyway, courtesy of microprocessing techniques employed when the specimen is handled in an automated laboratory. Often, a whole series of tests is reported out, even when only a few are of real interest. As medical testing goes, each of these items is relatively low-cost—but which ones are really needed by otherwise healthy people is still a matter of hot debate.

In medical jargon, tests are commonly assigned to one of 3 categories—more or less corresponding to the laboratory that does the analysis.

"Hematology"

Several studies are routinely performed on cells from circulating blood. Taken together, these procedures give a reasonably detailed picture of the number and quality of the red and white cells.

COMPLETE BLOOD COUNT (CBC)   This test has several components. The *hematocrit, hemoglobin,* and *red blood cell count* are checks for anemia. The *white cell count* tells how many of these cells (which are part of our defense system) are present in the blood. Along with the white cell "differential" (*see below*), this information is used primarily to evaluate bone marrow function. If obtained because of a fever, the white cell count may help distinguish between a bacterial and viral infection.

Microscopic examination of a blood smear (a drop of blood spread thinly on a glass slide) makes it possible to provide a count of each white cell type—the so-called *white cell differential.* This exam can also give a rough idea of how many platelets are present to help blood clot, whether the body's iron stores are adequate, and whether other nutritional factors—such as folic acid and vitamin B12—might be deficient.

In addition to the CBC, two other tests of the blood are common, though not routine.

ESR (ERYTHROCYTE SEDIMENTATION RATE)   This test measures the rate at which red cells settle out after a sample of blood is placed in a thin, vertical glass tube. A high "sed rate" may mean any one of a number of things—infection, malignancy, active arthritis, inflammatory bowel disease—or nothing.

STS (SEROLOGIC TEST FOR SYPHILIS)   This test is sometimes called a "VDRL" or "Wasserman," the names of particular techniques used to screen for unrecognized syphilis. Screening tests for syphilis are intentionally oversensitive, so a positive result needs to be confirmed by another test that is more specific.

The "chemistries"

A vast amount of information can be revealed by the chemical composition of the fluid carrying blood cells. After the cells are separated, the remaining liquid is called either *plasma* or *serum*, depending on how it was prepared. The following tests may be performed.

ELECTROLYTES   This term is commonly used to describe four important substances dissolved in body fluids: sodium, potassium, chloride, and bicarbonate. These "ions," their correct designation, are intimately related to the metabolic health of the body. Their concentration in the blood gives information about the distribution of water in blood and tissues, about kidney function, about the acidity or alkalinity of body fluids, and so forth. Electrolyte values almost always turn out to be normal in people who feel healthy, so they are rarely helpful for screening purposes. But periodically checking blood electrolytes is important in managing patients taking diuretic medications as well as those with liver, kidney, or heart disease.

BUN (BLOOD UREA NITROGEN) AND CREATININE   The two substances urea and creatinine are both products of protein breakdown in the body and are efficiently excreted by normal kidneys. Thus, unless a person is dehydrated, an elevation in these two chemicals usually signals diminished kidney function.

CALCIUM   Elevated serum calcium can reveal any of several disorders: an overactive parathyroid gland, a malignancy, excessive vitamin D intake (or sensitivity to this vitamin), or other, more exotic possibilities. If an elevated calcium level is found, further testing to uncover the cause should follow, even though no other signs or symptoms of disease are present.

CHOLESTEROL   A high serum cholesterol level is an important sign that one is at elevated risk of atherosclerosis. Measuring the so-called "good cholesterol" (meaning high-density lipoprotein, or HDL) fraction can provide even more information (*see Chapter 1*).

TRIGLYCERIDE   Another kind of blood fat, triglyceride, is often measured after an overnight fast. This test is less popular nowadays than it was a decade ago, mainly because we have come to rely on the cholesterol value as a better indicator of coronary risk.

GLUCOSE   Levels of blood sugar must be interpreted in relation to when food was last eaten. A very high test result is evidence of diabetes mellitus. A modest elevation may be difficult to interpret and thus is often followed up with an "oral glucose tolerance test." Beware of undue attention paid to glucose levels in the low range, especially if the person had no symptoms at the time blood was drawn. Even if the term "hypoglycemia" is used, there is usually no basis for worry, and no reason to start a special diet if the person felt normal when the sample was taken.

URIC ACID   This normal breakdown product of tissue DNA and RNA is usually harmless in its own right, even though high values tend to keep company with such risk factors as high cholesterol and high blood pressure, as well as obesity. A minority of people with high uric acid will develop gout, a form of arthritis caused by tiny sodium urate crystals forming in joint tissues. But there is usually no need to treat increases of serum uric acid unless gout (or kidney stones made up of uric acid) are a problem.

THYROXINE (OR T$_4$)   This is one of several hormones released by the thyroid gland and it is the most abundant. The serum concentration of thyroxine is a good measure of whether the thyroid gland is underactive, overactive, or on target in its production of hormones.

ALBUMIN AND GLOBULIN   Often mentioned in the same breath, these two kinds of blood protein tell us very different things. A normal serum albumin means that one's liver is healthy enough to produce needed amounts of this protein and that the kidneys and intestines are free of certain disorders that could permit excessive loss of body protein. Serum globulin, if elevated, may reflect inflammation anywhere in the body. But as with the sedimentation rate, a high value may not mean very much at all.

BILIRUBIN   This yellow pigment is mainly derived from the hemoglobin released by aged red blood cells as they are dismantled in the spleen. An elevated bilirubin may mean liver disease, an obstruction to bile flow, or excessive destruction of red cells within the body. But in some individuals it reflects the presence of a hereditary abnormality that is entirely harmless. The yellow color of the eyes and skin (jaundice) in patients with hepatitis is due to bilirubin accumulating in these tissues.

ALKALINE PHOSPHATASE   An elevation of this enzyme can mean that there is a problem in the liver, bile ducts, or bone. Additional blood tests can help distinguish liver from bone alkaline phosphatase.

TRANSAMINASES Several somewhat similar enzymes with the general name "transaminase" enter the blood when their parent tissues undergo damage. An elevated transaminase level generally means liver disease; less often it reflects inflammation in muscle tissue.

AMYLASE This starch-dissolving enzyme is usually produced by the salivary glands or pancreas—so if it is elevated in the blood, one of these organs may be inflamed.

LDH (LACTIC ACID DEHYDROGENASE) There are 5 sub-species of the enzyme—and numerous potential sites for disease if an abnormality is observed. In a healthy-seeming person, an elevated LDH is often a puzzle without an easy solution.

The urinalysis

Here are the routine tests performed on a urine sample:

The *specific gravity* tells whether the kidneys are able to effectively conserve body fluid. The *urinary pH* provides a rough guide as to whether the kidneys are able to excrete acids from the body. The test for *protein* in the urine is a way of checking for inflammation or other forms of damage within the kidneys. If *glucose* is present in the urine, it may mean the person has diabetes mellitus, but such is not always the case. *Bilirubin* in the urine indicates a problem in the liver or bile ducts. Finally, *microscopic examination* of a drop of urine can reveal pus cells and bacteria (evidence of an infection) or too many red blood cells (which could mean, among other things, kidney stones or a tumor in the bladder or kidneys).

Having it all

"Routine blood work" and a urinalysis can provide a lot of information at relatively low cost. Given the number of possible diagnoses one can make from performing these studies, why not do them frequently—say once a year—on everybody? Although some have argued for just such a practice, it's important to repeat that two kinds of cost would inevitably emerge from frequent testing on people who are not complaining of ill health. One is the cost of the tests themselves, if done often and on large populations. The second is the cost of the abnormal test result—whether a minimal departure from "normal," with no clinical meaning, or an alarming "false-positive" result that stems from a mistake, such as an incorrectly processed sample, or an error, human or computer, in transcribing a piece of data. The needless worry generated by an abnormal result, as well as the more expensive tests that are apt to follow, raises legitimate doubt about ordering too many tests on healthy people. Nobody has yet devised a solution to the problem of having too many answers.

Biopsies

The word *biopsy* is often more frightening than the procedure itself. The Greek roots mean "life look"—in other words, "removing a piece of tissue from a living patient in order to have a look." But the person in question almost always takes it to mean: "there's a very high likelihood that cancer is lurking here, so let's get at it and prove the suspicion is correct." The reality, though, is often quite different. Cancer may or may not be in the picture.

Obtaining the tissue can be quite simple, and the amount required is usually minute. Skin biopsies are probably the most common type; they are quick, easy, and often cure the problem (when an abnormal area is small enough to be entirely removed by the biopsy procedure). When another tissue must be examined, the sample can often be maneuvered out of its surroundings through a needle. This is, unsurprisingly, called a *needle biopsy*. When the location doesn't permit insertion of a needle, when more control is needed, or when a larger sample is needed for accurate diagnosis, tissue may be removed with a scalpel. Currently, needle biopsies, which minimize the disruption and discomfort a patient may experience, can be used to obtain samples even from relatively deep sites. In these procedures, newer imaging techniques, such as ultrasound or CT scans, make it possible to place the tip of a needle very precisely. Topical anesthetics akin to those employed by dentists make the procedure fairly easy to take.

Once removed, the tissue can be studied in a variety of ways. Almost always, a portion is sliced into extremely thin sections, which are chemically preserved and stained so that they may be examined in detail under a microscope. The size and shape of individual cells and their arrangement with respect to one another are among the clues used to make a diagnosis. Sometimes special dyes, or other markers attached to antibodies, can be used to detect chemical alteration of the cells. These methods may be useful when an abnormality of the immune system is suspected. Microbes, such as bacteria, viruses, or fungi, can often be spotted. When infection is one of the possibilities, a portion of the sample can be put into a fluid or gel that will nourish the invading organism so that it can be grown and identified. Test-tube growth may take a while, but the ability to identify a germ precisely can lead to more effective use of antibiotics.

Even with this background information, a person may still be terrified by the prospect of having a biopsy. One way to get a notion of how frightened to be is simply to ask the doctor for more information. Sometimes you may be reassured that the thought of cancer hadn't entered your physician's head until you mentioned it. For example, a liver biopsy is often recommended during care for chronic hepatitis. Or a small artery from the scalp may be biopsied as part of a work-up for headache, jaw pain, fatigue, and muscle aches. If inflammation is found in the artery the provisional diagnosis of temporal arteritis is confirmed, and this condition, which has nothing to do with cancer, is highly treatable.

Many times, of course, the reason for a biopsy is to ascertain whether a newly discovered lump or a mole is cancerous. But even in this situation, the chance of bad news may, in the physician's mind, be low. Cancer is not found in 4 out of 5 breast biopsies. The odds are even better with moles. In any case, a cancer detected at biopsy may well be curable because it has been discovered at an early stage.

A doctor may request a biopsy even if his or her instinct is that a particular lump, spot, or suspicious x-ray finding is really nothing to worry about. The most capable physician cannot always be *entirely* sure. Usually, a doctor will reassure the patient when recommending a biopsy to check on a diagnostic possibility that seems quite unlikely. But sometimes that doesn't happen. When a biopsy is suggested, it's always fair to ask, "How worried should I be?"

Predonating Blood

The gift of blood is often life-saving. But increased awareness that blood can transmit serious illness has led to a new apprehension about receiving transfusions. A misplaced fear of contracting AIDS looms large, even though current blood screening methods have lowered the risk to near zero. Hepatitis is a much more prevalent complication, mainly because there are no good techniques to screen blood for the so-called "non-A, non-B" hepatitis virus (or viruses). About 5% of people who receive 2 or more units of blood acquire this type of hepatitis. And about half of these infections become chronic with the potential, ultimately, to cause cirrhosis and liver failure.

For many people who may require transfusion, the key to complete safety is very straightforward, very practical—and very underused. It goes by the name of *predonation,* which simply means banking one's own blood prior to planned surgery.

Modern technology permits blood to be stored in liquid form for as long as 6 weeks. If there is time enough before an elective operation, say a hip replacement or coronary bypass surgery, a unit of blood can be deposited every week or 10 days in a blood-bank account and then reinfused as needed during surgery. Usually, the only added expense is the couple of dollars or so needed for iron pills to support the bone marrow as it meets increased demand for red cell production.

At surgery, when lost blood must be replaced, what goes into the body is what came out in prior weeks. Nobody else's blood, nobody else's viruses. The procedure is simple in concept—yet somehow difficult in practice. At least that was the conclusion of a recent survey conducted at 18 medical centers. Among patients who underwent elective surgery in these hospitals, only 5% of those considered eligible to predeposit blood actually did so.

A Guide for Human "Guinea Pigs"

Medical experiments are important because properly conducted research, not patient testimonials or an individual doctor's clinical impression, is the foundation of sound medical care. Although preliminary experiments are usually conducted on animals in the laboratory, eventually human "guinea pigs" are needed in clinical trials if we are to find treatments that are safe, effective, and economical. Everyone benefits from the willingness of some people to be subjects in properly designed experiments. But what about the subjects themselves? Are they benefiting or losing?

At the start of a trial, nobody really knows whether the experimental treatment is truly better than the older one. That is why the trial is being done. Obviously, experimenters usually would not undertake such a project unless they had some reason to believe the new therapy might be better than the alternative. But they could be wrong, and a clinical trial is usually not undertaken unless the predicted outcome is uncertain or too close to call. From the subject's point of view, then, entering a clinical trial makes no appreciable difference to his or her chances of getting a more effective treatment. Later on, however, if the condition were to require further treatment, the subject would certainly benefit from the knowledge gained during the experiment.

Risks and safeguards

No study has been done comparing the risk to experimental subjects with the risk to a comparable group in standard treatment. At least one survey has indicated that subjects in medical research do not suffer higher rates of death, disability, or injury than they would in daily life. But it is crucial to have safeguards, and there are many built into medical research.

First, any trial supported by federal funds must be approved by an institutional review board (IRB) to decide whether the possible risks of an experiment are worth taking. The IRB must determine whether the projected benefits clearly outweigh the potential hazards. Large trials often must receive the approval of several IRBs. The IRB's judgment must be tailored to the situation. Obviously, any trial in a healthy population—such as the testing of a new vaccine—should come with a very low risk. On the other hand, a new treatment for a life-threatening cancer could justifiably carry a relatively higher risk. Preliminary tests provide information on which these decisions are based.

Second, during any trial, monitoring for safety is built into the system. The subject of an experiment is watched much more closely than the average patient. If something seems to be going wrong, an individual is removed from the trial and given appropriate treatment. Third, many trials are designed in a way that the results can be continuously analyzed. As soon as firm evidence shows that one treatment is working better than the other, or has a higher rate of complications, the trial is stopped and all remaining subjects are offered the better approach.

An informed decision

Nobody should feel a blanket obligation to become a subject in medical research. Certainly, before participating, a potential subject should receive a full and understandable explanation of the possible benefits and risks of entering the trial. And then he or she should feel completely free to say yes or no. This is called giving *informed consent* and it means just what it says. A hasty recital of facts about the experiment, or an obscurely written description, does not suffice. If you do not understand, you cannot give informed consent and you should not agree to go ahead. Likewise, if you feel any pressure to say yes or fear that your treatment will suffer if you say no, your consent cannot be freely given and is not valid.

The signs of a well-designed trial are also worth keeping in mind. If a study is not designed according to the following principles, you may want to question the value of participating.

There should be at least 2 groups of subjects in the trial (or treatments alternated on 1 group), because the experimental treatment has to be compared with something else (usually a standard treatment or a placebo). For the study to be statistically valid, subjects should have no choice as to which group they will enter. Some provision should be made to keep the groups comparable. Often, this is done by *randomizing,* that is, using an arbitrary method to assign each subject to a treatment.

Because a subject's reactions may be influenced by knowing what treatment he or she is getting, all subjects should be kept in the dark as to which group they are in. This is called *blinding.* As often as possible, the experimenter should also be kept from knowing which subject is receiving which treatment. This is called *double blinding,* and its purpose is to keep the researcher's biases from influencing his or her interpretation of the results. (As a safeguard, someone outside the research group may know which subject is getting which treatment.)

There should be a clear, objective way to measure the results of the treatments. This may require extra tests of some sort, and the tests may add a level of benefit or risk to the experiment. The subject is more closely monitored for complications, but occasionally a test may in itself be somewhat hazardous.

If all these conditions are not met by a trial, it is fair to ask why not. But there are certain circumstances in which it is necessary to give up one or more of them, especially in the earliest phases of testing a new drug, for example, where there usually is no group receiving a placebo. Rather, everyone gets the new treatment but under very close supervision designed to determine the beneficial and harmful effects, if any, of the drug or procedure.

The issue of compensation

Although many people might be more willing to take part in research if they were paid, there are a couple of good reasons for thinking that participation should be voluntary. Results might be distorted if subjects were, in effect, "professional" volunteers. And, when money changes hands, it's hard to say that participation is fully voluntary. Paying someone creates a sense of obligation. However, if a trial creates extra expenses that the participant would not normally incur, it is reasonable for those to be paid.

A related question is whether a subject who is injured should be entitled to collect damages (over and above the medical care required to take care of the injury.) In general, at least when research is federally funded, the answer appears to be no. By giving informed consent, the subject agrees to take the necessary risks. Of course, the experimenters take responsibility for giving proper care; if they are negligent, they are liable for the consequences.

Living Wills

Along with an increased capacity to prolong life, medical technology also has the capacity to prolong the process of dying. The "living will" has been devised as a means by which people can set limits on the effort to keep them alive beyond the point they would themselves choose. But straightforward as the idea seems, the living will has limitations as well as advantages.

The purpose of a living will

Unlike a traditional will, a living will commands an action while a person is still living—but no longer able to manage his or her affairs. It is a concept that was formally proposed in 1968 at a meeting of the Euthanasia Educational Fund. The living will was a response to the perception that control over the dignity of death was coming to be further and further removed from the dying person. The intention of such a will is to assure that the patient's wishes regarding "extraordinary" medical care, or care during a terminal illness, will be followed.

Yet the ability of a written document to cover all possible situations is severely limited. So the living will should be seen as only a part of the effort to communicate one's wishes. Family members and, even more importantly, a sympathetic personal physician must be fully informed if the living will is to be carried out not only in letter but in spirit. It should be recognized that a living will can only guide decision making. If physicians and family members are at odds with each other over the goals of treatment, and the patient cannot communicate his or her own wishes, members of either party may be able to interpret the will as supporting their own point of view.

Living wills have become more common for a number of reasons. Technology is an obvious one. Our ability to delay the inevitable is remarkable—not always good, but always remarkable. Intravenous feedings, dialysis, mechanical respiration, and powerful antibiotics are all commonly used tools of treatment, and they are sometimes used at times when there is no real hope of recovery to a "meaningful existence." Situations are rarely clear-cut, however, and therefore judgments about the outcome of illness usually turn on the question of odds. If there is a 50% chance of recovery, should life-support measures be undertaken? How about a 1% chance—or a tenth of that, or a hundredth? At what point should we decide the chances are so slim that life-support measures are not warranted? What do we decide when we don't know the odds with any accuracy?

And what if recovery can only be partial? Sometimes a patient's life can be saved, but he or she is likely to remain severely impaired. In the past, such sick patients usually couldn't be supported through the acute phase of their illness. The ethical dilemma of saving the life of someone with no further ability to live that life was generally theoretical. Now it is often very real.

As medical technology has changed, so has the social structure of medical care. What is thought of as the traditional doctor–patient relationship has diminished in strength. Physicians and patients can become distanced from one another in large group practices, or when care becomes fragmented by the need for specialization and high technology. No physician may be identified as the primary, personal doctor. The opportunity to discuss and understand issues related to a dignified death may not come up, and no one doctor may feel confident that he or she knows the patient's preferences. In this circumstance, a living will can be helpful. When there is a close, long-standing relationship with a doctor who understands the patient's desires, a living will may still be helpful, but it is certainly not a necessity.

Though requirements vary from state to state, most states require that the person making such a will be at least 18 years of age, be of sound mind at the time of drafting, and have two witnesses to his signature (witnesses cannot be the attending nurse or physician or a potential heir). In general, where it has been addressed by legislation, a living will cannot be acted upon unless the person is terminally ill. The person with a living will can revoke it while still legally competent to act on his own behalf. In some states a parent or guardian is allowed to act for a minor. Only rarely will a state honor a living will if the patient is pregnant.

The pitfalls

Having a living will does not guarantee a passing free of turmoil. It is impossible for any statement of intent (of which a living will is one form) to cover every conceivable combination of events that might occur. There is usually enough ambiguity in any living will to leave any disagreement between physician and family unsettled.

For example, there is always a question of when to activate the living will. Is it when the patient becomes incompetent? If so, who defines incompetence? Is it when the patient goes into a coma, or when he is deemed terminally ill? What if the patient is not terminally ill but is severely brain-damaged, without hope for neurological recovery? If the circumstances under which a will is activated are not defined very clearly, the document may be more trouble than help.

Another pitfall is the definition of "heroic" measures. Antibiotics, feeding tubes, oxygen, and intravenous fluids are part of everyday hospital care. If the use of these will prolong life, do they automatically become "heroic"? Again, an explicit statement as to what is meant by treatment and what is to be avoided can help to limit the uncertainties of interpretation.

One argument against living wills is that they may discount the future. Some critics contend that a healthy person cannot predict his frame of mind when illness becomes a reality. The argument has also been made that a patient may, at the last minute, wish to change his instructions but, because of intermittent delusions, be declared incompetent and thus not permitted to do so.

A measure that can help circumvent some of these criticisms is to delegate to a friend or family member *durable power of attorney*. This role differs from normal power of attorney in that it does not lapse after a specified period of time, or when the person granting it becomes incompetent. The person with power of attorney can help interpret the patient's probable wishes when the circumstances are not covered in the will.

A living will is certainly helpful if a person wants to be sure of maintaining some control over the type and intensity of medical care he receives in his final days. But it should not replace personal discussions with family or a trusted physician.

What Do You Do, Doctor?

Patients confronting difficult decisions, such as those involving major surgery or risky procedures, often pose that seemingly ultimate question to their physician: "What would you do if it were you, doctor?" This question, so frequently asked during a crisis, may be even more to the point when directed to daily practices that are known or alleged to prevent disease. How seriously do doctors take the warnings about cigarettes? What about vitamin C to prevent colds? Is bran important?

The idea for the faculty health-practice survey came up a few years ago when we read a letter from a Texas physician who objected to a somewhat equivocal position expressed in the *Harvard Medical School Health Letter* on the daily use of aspirin to prevent vascular disease. "Every doctor down here is doing it," he said. This stimulated the thought of surveying the Harvard Medical School faculty, not only about aspirin use but about many other items as well. The survey was developed and implemented shortly thereafter.

. Who responded? .			
Age of responders		*Sex of responders*	
Under 30	1%	Male	90%
30 – 39	36%	Female	10%
40 – 49	32%		
50 – 59	19%		
Over 60	12%		
Practice specialty			
Anesthesia	4%	Ear, nose, throat	2%
Dermatology	1%	Pathology	4%
Internal medicine	27%	Pediatrics	10%
Neurology	4%	Psychiatry	20%
Obstetrics/		Radiology	6%
gynecology	5%	Surgery	8%
Ophthalmology	2%	Other	1%
Orthopedics	3%		

The response rate was 60%, a highly respectable one—especially for a single mailing (*see box*). Follow-up reminders to nonresponders were not possible because we felt it important to have the responses submitted anonymously.

The percentage of psychiatrists is disproportionately high in comparison with the entire population of doctors, but no important differences emerged when the answers were tallied after removing the psychiatrists' responses.

Surveys such as these are a natural target for any Doubting Thomas, and the skeptic will ask a few questions about this one. Do the 40% who didn't respond lead lives as seemingly "healthy" as those who sent their answers in? Possibly not, but then again there's no real way of knowing. It is as likely that lack of time due to busyness, rather than embarrassment, was the main reason for failure to respond. A second obvious question is: How truthful are the answers, especially when it's known that the results will reach a national audience? While it's hard to give an iron-clad guarantee for the accuracy of the answers, a few observations drawn from our personal experience are worth reporting. At large gatherings of our faculty—be they in the cafeteria, attending academic conferences, or at relaxed social receptions—cigarette smoking is very rare. Joggers are ubiquitous. And seat belts are usually fastened when colleagues are driving. Although we have not had the chance to make such observations on the use of margarine, laxatives, contraceptive pills, and the like, it's hard to imagine why erroneous claims might be made for these items.

There was actually another feature of the questionnaire that could have been used as a "fall back" measure by someone concerned by a particular response. We asked the doctors to circle any answer if the habit in question worried them, or if they would be embarrassed for it to be known to their patients. Relatively few answers were circled when a deviant response was given (eating red meat, not exercising, not undergoing periodic health checkups). For all but one question, fewer than 20% of the doctors admitting a potentially "unhealthy" practice indicated worry or embarrassment. However, this was not true for cigarette smoking. Thirty-five per cent of all smokers worry about their habit, and 70% of those who smoke a pack a day or more are worried.

In summary, our clinical faculty practice a high level of "preventive medicine" on themselves. Cigarette smoking is very low; three quarters of us use seat belts; there is a fair amount of restriction of red meat, eggs, and butter; and periodic check-ups are sought much more frequently than one might have guessed. There also seems to be a reluctance to take medication without substantial reason, as judged by the negative responses to questions about laxatives, vitamin C, multivitamins, and antibiotics for minor colds. And—to get back to where it all started—unlike Texas doctors, we're not taking aspirin on a daily basis to prevent heart attacks and strokes.

The question, please

1. Do you smoke cigarettes?   *Yes* 8%   *No* 92%
   If not, are you a former cigarette
   smoker?   *Yes* 38% *No* 62%

There's no question that doctors have not only read the warnings but have also seen the consequences "close up" among their patients with heart disease, cancer, and emphysema. Eight percent still smoke cigarettes, as compared with 32% of the general population. And only 13 of 49 reported smokers exceeded one pack a day. The number of *former* cigarette smokers—34% of all responders—is also impressive.

2. Do you use tobacco in any other form
   on a daily basis? *Yes* 11%   *No* 89%

Pipes had it over cigars by 3 to 1. No one chewed tobacco and 2 used snuff. So long as inhaling is avoided, the danger of lung damage is considerably reduced.

3. Do you use a sleeping pill more than
   three times a week? *Yes* 2%   *No* 98%

While the low use of sleeping pills might suggest a high level of serenity, we've been at too many faculty meetings to believe that. More likely, it's a healthy desire to avoid drugs that can be habit-forming. The frequent use of some sleeping pills can even interfere with normal sleep patterns.

4. Have you had a routine health examination during the past two years? *Yes* 54%   *No* 46%

We were surprised to find that so many have, given the common notion that doctors are the last ones to seek a routine check-up. As might be guessed, older physicians did so more frequently. Regular health examinations were obtained by 41% of our faculty in their 30s, 54% in their 40s, 65% in their 50s, and 80% of those over age 60.

5. Do you use seat belts routinely? *Yes* 73%   *No* 27%

Hooray! While hardly perfect, the high rate of seat-belt use is testimony that at least some common sense prevails in ivory towers. And our guess is that doctors who work in emergency rooms that receive auto accident victims approach 100% in *their* seat-belt use.

6. Do you take aspirin on a daily basis
   to protect against vascular disease? *Yes* 7%   *No* 93%

It has been proposed that aspirin taken in low dosage will prevent heart disease and strokes by inhibiting blood clotting. However, few of our faculty seem to act on what remains an unproven hypothesis for otherwise healthy people.

7. Do you usually take an antibiotic
   when you develop an upper respiratory infection? *Yes* 3%   *No* 97%

So much for how we treat our own common colds. We hope that our readers will feel secure without antibiotics for theirs. (Chicken soup has a lower incidence of side effects.)

8. Do you jog or do equivalent aerobic exercise for 20 minutes (or more) at least three times a week?   *Yes* 49%   *No* 51%

Vigorous exercise is popular among faculty of all ages and both sexes. While "feeling good" and "looking good" are important reasons for exercise, the kind of exercise we asked about is also believed to promote cardiac fitness.

9. If practicing contraception, do you (or your partner) use contraceptive pills?   *Yes* 5%   *No* 95%

Among the two-thirds of our responders who practice contraception, the use of the pill by the female partner is strikingly low. One reason, given that 99% are beyond age 30, is that they have probably completed their families, making tubal ligations and vasectomies more acceptable. Also, vascular complications from the pill are higher in older women, an additional reason for seeking other measures.

10. If female, do you routinely perform self-examination of your breasts?   *Yes* 36%   *No* 64%
   If male, do you routinely perform self-examination of your testes?   *Yes* 72%   *No* 28%

Early detection of these cancers leads to earlier treatment and a greater number of cures. Self-examination is easy. We'd like to see both men and women achieve 100% on this one.

11. Do you eat breakfast?   *Yes* 78%   *No* 22%

A point of interest for some, perhaps. It may not be crucial to start the day off with a good meal, but it may indicate a greater awareness of the importance of nutrition.

12. Do you weigh more than 10 pounds above what you'd like to weigh?   *Yes* 29%   *No* 71%

While 29% of our faculty are not as trim as they'd like to be, in most cases it's apt to be more a concern for appearance than for health. A few extra pounds are usually not a health hazard.

13. Do you take more than 2 alcoholic
drinks a day? *Yes* 7%   *No* 93%

Not a bad record. We'd be especially concerned about any who may be taking 4 or more drinks a day.

14. Do you restrict your consumption of
red meat to 3 times a week or less? *Yes* 44%   *No* 56%

A large number of faculty restrict red-meat consumption, probably because of evidence linking red-meat consumption to bowel cancer and high cholesterol levels.

15. Do you try to maintain a high bran or
fiber content in your diet? *Yes* 41%   *No* 59%

High-fiber diets clearly help constipation. Such diets may also decrease the risk for bowel cancer by promoting more rapid evacuation of carcinogens from the colon.

16. Do you drink coffee? *Yes* 83%   *No* 17%

Of those who drink coffee, 47% have 2 cups or fewer a day, 45% average 3 to 5 cups, and only 8% exceed 5 cups. Many of the health problems purportedly linked to coffee remain in question on careful study—but all would agree that too much coffee can cause jitteriness, palpitations, and insomnia.

17. Do you restrict your egg intake to 3
per week or fewer? *Yes* 79%   *No* 21%

A surprisingly high degree of egg restriction, we thought, presumably due to concerns about cholesterol.

18. Does your household use margarine
(as opposed to butter)? *Yes* 69%   *No* 31%

Again, it's probably concern for cholesterol levels that prompts the use of margarine. Soft margarine, also known as "tub" margarine, is better than stick margarine because soft margarine has a higher content of unsaturated fat.

19. Do you visit your dentist at regular
        intervals?   *Yes* 84%   *No* 16%

Good sense. Fewer root canal jobs, we hope.

20. Do you floss your teeth daily?   *Yes* 41%   *No* 59%

The greatest cause of tooth loss among adults is periodontal disease,
not caries. And flossing should help remove the plaques that contribute to periodontal disease.

21. Do you take vacations during which
        no work is done?   *Yes* 83%   *No* 17%

Probably a healthy practice, but hardly an essential one. Several
responders described their golf games as more work than play.

22. Do you take a daily multivitamin?   *Yes* 14%   *No* 86%

There's no real need for vitamin supplementation if one's diet is
normal and special circumstances (such as pregnancy or digestive
disorders) are not present.

23. Do you ever make purchases at
        stores devoted exclusively to health
        foods?   *Yes* 25%   *No* 75%

Many "health foods" are overpriced relative to their true nutritional value. At times, they may produce a positive placebo effect of
"feeling good."

24. Do you use vitamin C to protect
        against colds?   *Yes* 14%   *No* 86%

Few seem to believe that vitamin C really works. Or else they find
that daily pill taking is more bothersome than a few days of sneezing and dripping.

25. Do you take a laxative or enema if
        you don't have a bowel movement
        for 2 days?   *Yes* 3%   *No* 97%

There's wide variation in bowel habits among normal people, and
apparently few of our faculty believe the ads promoting medications to achieve "regularity."

Acknowledgments

This book grew out of material prepared originally for the *Harvard Medical School Health Letter,* a publication that is received each month by 300,000 subscribers. For twelve years, the *HMS Health Letter* has enjoyed warm support not only from its readers but also from the faculty of Harvard Medical School.

Our mainstays have been the members of the *HMS Health Letter's* Advisory Board. Representing various fields of medicine and surgery, they review every article in every issue. In addition, they have served as consultants, authors of articles, guides, and friends. We are grateful for their year-round, unflagging efforts on behalf of this publication.

Current members of our Advisory Board are: Ronald Arky, M.D. (internal medicine); Kenneth Arndt, M.D. (dermatology); Peter Braun, M.D. (internal medicine); Thornton Brown, M.D. (orthopedics); Paul Goldhaber, D.D.S. (dental medicine); Lester Grinspoon, M.D. (psychiatry); B. Thomas Hutchinson, M.D. (ophthalmology); David Link, M.D. (pediatrics); Robert J. Mayer (oncology); John Tobias Nagurney, M.D. (emergency medicine); Stephen Schoenbaum, M.D. (internal medicine); Ruth Tuomala, M.D. (obstetrics and gynecology); Andrew Warshaw, M.D. (surgery); and Edward Wolpow, M.D. (neurology).

We are equally thankful to former members of the Advisory Board, who helped nurture the *HMS Health Letter* through its early years and give it its current form: Mary Ellen Avery, M.D. (pediatrics); Leon Eisenberg, M.D. (psychiatry); Reginald Greene, M.D. (radiology); Walter Guralnick, D.M.D. (oral surgery); the late Rita Kelley, M.D. (oncology); Barbara McNeil (radiology); Johanna Perlmutter, M.D. (obstetrics and gynecology); Marshall Strome, M.D. (otorhinolaryngology); David Wegman, M.D. (occupational health); and Judith Wurtman, Ph.D. (nutrition).

Susan Wallace made this book possible. We have relied on her creative insight and organizational skill, her sense of language, and her gentle insistence that we do what we promised to do, more or less when we promised to do it. As manuscript editor of the *HMS Health Letter* and of this book, she has been a valued colleague and delightful friend. Her editorial contribution to this volume has far exceeded any that we might reasonably have asked. Her intelligence and graciousness have illuminated both our writing and our lives.

A colleague who has joined us in the last few years as assistant editor of the *HMS Health Letter,* Britain Nicholson, M.D., has contributed not only his prose to this book but his good sense, good humor, and medical experience to our planning and editorial efforts.

Michele Markatos, as editorial coordinator of the *HMS Health Letter,* not only ties together a sprawling operation but sees to quality control throughout our editorial and production process. Her warmth and commitment are deeply appreciated.

Stephen Hoffmann, M.D., as a contributing editor in the past couple of years, has produced a number of provocative and thoughtful articles. Robert N. Ross played a most useful role in shaping disparate elements from a monthly publication into cohesive sections of a book. Ellen Barlow, who has consulted with us on the design and layout of the *HMS Health Letter,* also has assisted in research on material incorporated into this book.

Andrea Porth Graham, the general manager of the *HMS Health Letter,* has helped us to understand the world of publishing and has contributed her sane counsel at innumerable points along the way.

Harriet Greenfield, a gifted medical artist and our illustrator from the beginning, teaches us and our readers in ways that no amount of words (certainly not a thousand) could ever accomplish. Her instructive drawings are supplemented in this book by Lee Lorenz's wry cartoons.

Many sections of this book are based on expert knowledge contributed by the following thoughtful and generous colleagues. We name the following people in the hope of completeness and the dread of an unintended omission:

James Adelstein, M.D.	Low-level radioactive waste
Kenneth Arndt, M.D.	Skin care, acne, hair care, nail care, safety of cosmetics

Jerry Avorn, M.D.	Drugs and the elderly
James Bakalar, J.D.	Cocaine
Jeffrey Bernhard, M.D.	Psoriasis
Andrew Bodnar, M.D.	Living wills
Mimi Thompson Breed	Vaginitis
Arline Bronzaft, Ph.D.	Noise pollution
Robert Buxbaum, M.D.	Exercise and aging, alternatives to jogging
Paul Casale, M.D.	Aortic stenosis
Gregory Curfman, M.D.	Exercise and the heart
Victor De Gruttola, Ph.D.	AIDS
Leon Dogon, D.M.D.	Dental sealants
Samuel Doppelt, M.D.	Osteoporosis
Carla Evans, D.D.S.	New techniques in orthodonture
Daniel Federman, M.D.	Impotence and erectile dysfunction
George Garcia, M.D.	Contact lenses
Barbara Gastel, M.D.	Urinary tract infections
Paul Goldhaber, D.D.S.	Periodontal disease
Reginald Greene, M.D.	Medical x-rays
Lester Grinspoon, M.D.	Cocaine
Thomas Hackett, M.D.	Sex after a heart attack
Stephen Hoffmann, M.D.	Chlamydia infections, vitamin C, smokeless tobacco, clove cigarettes, coffee, pregnancy and age
B. Thomas Hutchinson, M.D.	Glaucoma and cataracts
J. Philip Kistler	Strokes
Daniel Kopans, M.D.	X-ray mammography
Alexander Leaf, M.D.	Fish oil and the heart
Susan Love, M.D.	Lumpy breasts
Andrew Marks, M.D.	Drugs for angina pectoris
Robert Mayer, M.D.	Cancer treatments
Kenneth McKusick, M.D.	Low-level radioactive waste
Martin C. Moore-Ede, Ph.D.	Time-shifts and health
Britain Nicholson, M.D.	Choosing a health plan, hiccups, treadmill testing, infertility, nicotine chewing gum, night sweats, radon in houses, hemorrhoids
Patrick O'Connor, M.D.	Arrhythmias

Wayne Peters, M.D.	Cholesterol
Julie Fitzpatrick Rafferty	Microwaves
Peter Reich, M.D.	Heart-felt emotions
Julie Schecter, Ph.D.	Premenstrual syndrome
Isaac Schiff, M.D.	Estrogen and menopause
Paul Schnitman, D.D.S.	Dental implants
Stephen Schoenbaum, M.D.	Human experimentation in medicine
David V. Sheehan	Panic attacks
Harvey Simon, M.D.	Exercise
John Spengler, M.D.	Indoor air pollution
John Stakes, M.D.	Sleep apnea
William Stason, M.D.	Communicating with your doctor
George Vaillant, M.D.	Alcoholism
David Wegman, M.D.	Hazards of the workplace
Edward Wolpow, M.D.	Headaches
Randall Zusman, M.D.	Hypertension

To the people we have named and to many others whose personal support and intellectual guidance have made the *HMS Health Letter* and this book possible, we are grateful.

William I. Bennett, M.D.
Stephen E. Goldfinger, M.D.
G. Timothy Johnson, M.D.

Index

AA (Alcoholics Anonymous), 121, 140
Absorptiometry, 296–297
Accidents, 115–116, 169, 440–441
Accutane, 198–199
ACE (angiotensin converting enzyme) inhibitors, 407
Acetaminophen, 114
Acetazolamide (Diamox), 240
Acne, 196–199, 205, 254
Acquired immune deficiency syndrome (AIDS), 138, 264–266
Acyclovir (Zovirax), 195, 262–263
Addiction: to alcohol, 109–116, 118–121; to cigarettes, 96–98; to cocaine, 136–141; to marijuana, 130
Aerobic exercise, 13–17
Aerophagia, 361
Age: and breast cancer, 286; and cancer, 365; and cholesterol, 63–64; and heart disease, 365, 368; and hypertension, 403; and impotence, 307–308; and pregnancy outcome, 276–280; and stroke, 365; and weight, 36
Agoraphobia, 323
AIDS (acquired immune deficiency syndrome), 138, 264–266
Air-conditioning, 151, 154
Air pollution, indoor, 150–162; from asbestos, 158–162; from carbon monoxide, 152–153; from nitrogen oxides, 153; from radon, 155–158; in sick-building syndrome, 154–155; sources of, 151–154; from tobacco smoke, 151–152
Air swallowing, 361
Al-Anon, 120
Albumin, 474
Alcohol, 108–121; accidents from, 115–116; and arrhythmias, 391; blood levels of, 110; calories in, 111; and cocaine, 137; damage from, 111–114; with other drugs, 114; effects of, 110–111; his-

torical use of, 108–109; impotence from, 308; incidence of drinking, 109; metabolism of, 110–111; and migraines, 347; mortality from, 116–118; physician abuse of, 452, 454, 489; protective effect of, 116–118; and sleep disturbances, 334, 337–338; and toxic chemicals, 164; treatment of problem drinkers, 118–121; types of drinkers, 109–110, 116–117, 119–120; and weight control, 47
Alcoholics, 109–110; controlled social drinking for, 118–121; denial in, 120; drug for, 110–111; treatment for, 121
Alcoholics Anonymous (AA), 121, 140
Aldomet, 407
Alkaline phosphatase, 474–475
Alprazolam, 323
Aluminum chloride, 193
Amenorrhea, 31–32
Ames test, 412–414
Amniocentesis, 277–278
Amphetamines, 48–49
Ampicillin, 299
Amylase, 475
Anemia, 31, 112
Angina, 136, 366, 370
Angiography, 372, 397
Angioplasty, balloon, 378–380, 385
Angiotensin converting enzyme (ACE) inhibitors, 407
Animal testing, 411–412
Antabuse (disulfiram), 110–111, 454
Anthralin, 201
Anti-anxiety medications, 321–322
Antibiotics, 198, 203, 255–256, 487–488
Anti-cholinergic drugs, 362
Antidepressants, 323, 325–326, 341, 347
Antihistamines, 114, 337
Antioxidant nutrients, 81–82
Antiperspirants, 192–194
Anti-platelet drugs, 371, 399–400

Anti-prostaglandin drugs, 283
Anxiety, 12, 136, 320–323
Aortic stenosis, 383–385
Apnea, sleep, 341–343
Appetite-suppressing drugs, 48–49
Arrhythmias, 387–394; from cocaine, 136; from coffee, 125–126; diagnosis of, 388–389; emotions and, 391–394; and stroke, 401; treatment of, 390–391; types of, 389–390
Arthritis, 13, 69–70, 256
Artificial insemination, 271–272
Artificial sweeteners, 90–92
Art materials, 165–167
Asbestos, 151, 158–162
Asbestosis, 160
Ascorbic acid. *See* Vitamin C
Aspartame, 91
Aspirin, 114, 371, 399–400, 487
Asthma, 13, 131
Astigmatism, 232–233
Atherosclerosis, 10, 257, 290; and coronary artery disease, 366–369; and fish oil, 67–73; and stroke, 394
Athlete's foot, 195
Athletic amenorrhea, 31–32
Atrial fibrillation (AF), 390
Attention deficit disorder, 138, 141
Aversion therapy, 105, 139

Bacitracin, 194
Background radiation, 182–183
Back pain, 348–354; from video display terminals, 174–175
Bacteriuria, 304
Baldness, 208–212
Balloon angioplasty, 378–380, 385
Barbiturates (Seconal, Nembutal), 321, 336–337
Barium enema, 424–425
Basal body temperature (BBT), 248, 270
Basal cell cancers, 417
Bath oils, 191
Behavior modification, 42–45, 105, 121, 338–339, 406
Belching, 360–362
Benzodiazepines (Valium, Librium), 321–322, 336, 340
Benzoyl peroxide, 198
Beta-blockers, 239, 322, 347, 373–374, 407
Beta-carotene, 59, 80–81
Betadine (povidone-iodine), 194

Betagen, 239
Betoptic, 239
Bilirubin, 474, 475
Biofeedback, 406
Biological clocks, 169–170
Biopsy, 476–477; breast, 286–287, 426; endometrial, 272
Bipolar disease, 326
Birth control, 247–258; condoms, 249; contraceptive sponge, 250–251; diaphragm, 250; IUD, 251–253; pill, 253–257; reliability of methods of, 250; rhythm method, 248–249; spermicidal agents, 249–250; sterilization procedures, 257–258
Birth control pills, 253–257; and acne, 197, 199; benefits of, 255–256; and migraine headaches, 347, 401; mini-pill, 256; missed-period pill, 256–257; morning-after pill, 256; side effects of, 254–255, 401
Birth defects, 277–278. *See also* Fetal development
Bladder cancer, 85, 123, 124, 167
Bleeding, abnormal: birth control pill and, 256; in colon cancer, 420, 421–425, 429; in endometrial cancer, 434; from IUD, 252; from running, 31; as warning sign of cancer, 415
Blindness: from cataracts, 240–244; from glaucoma, 236–240; from macular degeneration, 244–245; as warning sign of stroke, 395
Bloating, 360–362
Blood: predonated, 477–478. *See also* Bleeding, abnormal
Blood pressure: diastolic vs. systolic, 402, 403; measurement of, 404, 468–469. *See also* Hypertension
Blood sugar, 291, 473–474
Blood tests, 470, 471–476
Blood urea nitrogen (BUN), 473
Blue Cross/Blue Shield, 442
Body building, 26–29
Body fat. *See* Overweight; Weight control
Borg scale, 15–16
Bowel cancer, 73–78, 84–85, 420–425
Braces, orthodontic, 221–222
Bradycardia, 390
Breast: biopsy of, 286–287, 426; lumpy, 123, 284–288; self-examination of, 426, 427, 488. *See also* Breast cancer
Breast cancer, 425–432; and age of first

pregnancy, 279; alcohol and, 112; biopsy in, 286–287, 426; birth control pills and, 254; coffee and, 123; dietary fat and, 73–74; early detection of, 426–429, 469; estrogen and, 290; incidence of, 425–426; lumpy breasts and, 123, 284–288; treatment of, 429–432; from x-rays, 182

Breast milk, 110, 123, 132

Bronchitis, 95, 131

Bruxism, 340

Bubble, for weight reduction, 51–52

BUN (blood urea nitrogen), 473

Buspirone, 321

Bypass surgery: coronary, 375–378; intestinal, 51

CAD. See Coronary artery disease (CAD)

Cafergot (ergot alkaloids), 347

Caffeine. See Coffee

Calcium: in athletic amenorrhea, 32; and cancer, 78, 81; in coronary artery spasm, 371; and dieting, 32–33; in food, 294; and hypertension, 405; for osteoporosis, 292, 294; serum, 473

Calcium-channel blockers, 347, 371, 374–375, 407

Cancer, 408–434; age and, 365; alcohol and, 111–112; antioxidant nutrients and, 81–82; from asbestos, 160–161; birth control pill and, 254, 255; calcium and, 78, 81; coffee and, 123–124; early detection of, 414–415; environmental factors in, 409–411; epidemiologic studies on, 410–411; estrogen and, 290–291; fat and, 73–74; fiber and, 75–80; fish oil and, 69–70; food and, 73–82; genetic factors in, 408–409; obesity and, 38; stress and, 319; sunscreens and, 192; testing for causes of, 411–414; treatment of, 415–417; vitamin A and, 59; vitamin C and, 84–85; vitamins and, 80–81; warning signs of, 414–415; from x-rays, 182. See also specific types of cancer

Cancer "hotline," 416

Candida, 300

Carbamazepine, 358

Carbohydrates, 46–48, 49, 89

Carbonic anhydrase inhibitors, 240

Carbon monoxide pollution, 152–153

Carcinogens, 409–411; coffee and, 124; in cosmetics, 206; fiber and, 75–78; testing for, 411–414; vitamin C and, 85

Cardiac arrest. See Heart attack

Cardiac catheterization, 384–385

Cardiomyopathy, alcoholic, 113

Cardioversion, 391

Carotenoids, 59, 80–81

Carpal tunnel syndrome, 174

Cataplexy, 341

Cataracts, 172, 177, 240–244; contact lenses for, 235, 243

Cavities, 219–221

CBC (complete blood count), 472

Cerebral embolism, 395

Cerebral thrombosis, 394

Cerebral vascular accidents (CVAs), 394

Cervical cancer, 263, 433–434

Cervical mucus: monitoring of, 248–249; post-coital testing of, 273–274

Cervicitis, 260, 298, 301–302

Check-ups, physical, 467–477, 487; biopsies during, 476–477; lab tests during, 471–476; screening tests during, 468–471

Chelation therapy, 375

Chest x-rays, 471

Chewing tobacco, 102

Chlamydia infections, 259–262

Chlorpromazine, 358

Cholesterol: age and, 63–64; alcohol effect on, 116–119; blood, 469; cigarette smoking and, 103, 106; coffee effect on, 125; diet and, 64–67; drug treatment of elevated, 64; exercise effect on, 10–11, 14, 19; fish oil and, 68–69, 70; in food, 72; HDL, 10, 19, 61–66, 116–119; and heart disease, 60–67, 368, 369; LDL, 61–66; levels of, 62–64; noise pollution and, 147; serum, 473; in stroke, 401; types of, 61–62

Chorionic villus sampling, 278

Chymopapain injection, 353–354

Cigarettes, 94–108; addiction to, 96–98; advertising of, 108; air pollution from, 95–96, 151–152; and arrhythmias, 391; and asbestos, 160, 164; availability of, 98, 107–108; cholesterol and, 64; clove, 102–103; and coronary artery disease, 369; and coronary artery spasm, 370; deaths from, 94–95; effect on children, 151; fires from, 96; inhaling, 100–101; low-tar, 98–101; and lung cancer, 410, 419–420; and migraines, 347; programs against, 107–108; quitting, 103–107; saccharin and, 91; second-hand smoke from, 95–96, 151–152; and stroke, 401; and toxic chemicals, 164

Metabolic rate: effect of diets on, 41–42; effect of exercise on, 45; resting, 41, 45
Metastases, 408
Methotrexate, 201
Methylphenidate (Ritalin), 141, 341
Methylxanthines, 287
Metronidazole (Flagyl), 110, 299, 300–301
Metropolitan Life tables, 33–36, 34
Miconazole (Micatin), 195, 300
Microwaves, 176–179
Migraine headaches, 283, 345–347, 401
Migral (ergot alkaloids), 347
Miltown (meprobamate), 321
Minerals, 57, 78
Mini-pill, 256
Minipress, 407
Minoxidil, 211–212
Miotics, 239
Missed-period pill, 256–257
Mitral valve prolapse (MVP), 385–387
MMR (measles-mumps-rubella) vaccine, 463–464
Modified radical mastectomy, 430, 431–432
Moles, 418–419
Mongolism. See Down's syndrome
Monilia, 300
Monounsaturated fats, 66
Monovision, 236
Morning-after pill, 256
Motrin, 226, 283
MRFIT (Multiple Risk Factor Intervention Trial), 60
MRI (magnetic resonance imaging), 352
Mucopurulent cervicitis, 260
Multiple Risk Factor Intervention Trial (MRFIT), 60
Mumps vaccine, 463
MVP (mitral valve prolapse), 385–387
Mycostatin (nystatin), 300

Nails: brittleness of, 217–218; fungus infections of, 218; funny-looking, 217; normal growth of, 214–217
Narcolepsy, 340–341
Narcotics Anonymous, 140
Nautilus machines, 26, 27
Nembutal, 321, 336–337
Neomycin, 194
Neosporin, 194
Nephritis, 69
NGU (nongonococcal urethritis), 259–262

Nicorette (nicotine chewing gum), 105–107
Nicotine. See Cigarettes
Nicotine chewing gum, 105–107
Nifedipine, 375
Night shift, 168–171
Night sweats, 362–364
Nitrates, 373
Nitrogen oxide pollution, 153
Nitrosamines, 85, 206
Nocturia, 313
Noise, 144–150; reduction of, 149–150; sleep disturbances from, 333; sound vs., 144–147; stress response to, 147–149
Nongonococcal urethritis (NGU), 259–262
Non-REM sleep, 329–330
n-3 fatty acids, 69, 71
Nutra-Sweet (aspartame), 91
Nutrition, 56–92; and behavior, 59; and cancer, 73–82; deficiencies in, 57–58; drug-like effects in, 59–60; essential needs for, 56–57; fat and the heart, 60–67; fish oil, 67–73; and longevity, 58; and mood, 59; sweets, 87–92; vitamin C, 82–87. See also Diet
Nystatin (Mycostatin), 300

Obesity. See Overweight; Weight control
Oils, unsaturated, 66
Olive oil, 66
Omega-3 fatty acids, 69, 71
Oncogenes, 409
Orthodontics, 221–222
Osteomalacia, 293
Osteoporosis, 292–297; back pain from, 350; development of, 292–293; dieting and, 39; estrogen for, 289, 291; exercise and, 32; fractures from, 292; prevention and screening of, 296–297; treatment of, 293–296
Ovarian cancer, 255, 279
Ovarian cysts, 275
Overweight: age and, 36; attitudes about, 38–39; definition of, 33–35; dieting for, 40–52; distribution of body fat in, 36; drastic measures for, 49–52; environmental factors in, 54–55; exercise for, 32, 44, 45–46; fiber and, 79–80; genetic factors in, 36, 53–55; hazards of, 36–38; and heart disease, 369; height and weight tables, 34; and hypertension, 405; incidence of, 33–35; and infertility, 273; safe zone and, 39–40. See also Weight control

Tobacco, smokeless, 102. *See also* Cigarettes
Toenails, 214–219
Tolnaftate (Tinactin), 195
Tonometry, 237–238, 469–470
Tooth care, 219–230; and dental implants, 226–230; and dental sealing, 219–221; and orthodontics, 221–222; and periodontal disease, 223–226; and sugar, 89
Tooth grinding, 340
TOPV (trivalent oral polio vaccine), 462–463
Toric soft lenses, 233
TPA (tissue plasminogen activator), 381–382
Tracheostomy, 343
Tranquilizers: alcohol in combination with, 114; for elderly, 459; for generalized anxiety, 321–322; for panic disorder, 323; for sleep disturbances, 336
Transaminases, 475
Transfusions, 477–478
Transient hemispheric attacks, 395–397
Transient ischemic attacks (TIAs), 345, 395–398
Transient monocular blindness, 395
Transurethral resection (TUR), 313
Trials, clinical, 478–481
Trichomonas vaginitis, 300–301
Tricyclic antidepressants, 325–326
Triglyceride, 62, 69, 113, 473
Trinitroglycerol (TNG), 373
Trivalent oral polio vaccine (TOPV), 462–463
L-Tryptophan, 337
Tubal lavage, 275
Tubal ligation, 257
Tuberculosis test, 470
Tumors, 254, 408. *See also* Cancer
"Type A" personality, 318, 369

U-lactin, 191
Ulcers: corneal, 232; peptic, 112, 127, 168; vaginal, 302
Ultrasound: in breast-cancer screening, 429; in infertility work-up, 272; in prostate cancer screening, 433; in stroke, 398
Ultraviolet light (UVL), 192, 201–202
Undecylenic acid, 195
Universal machines, 26
Unsaturated fats, 65–67. *See also* Fats, dietary.
Urea, 191

Urethritis, nongonococcal, 259–260
Uric acid, 474
Urinalysis, 475
Urinary pH, 475
Urinary tract infections (UTIs), 302–306; development of, 303–304; diagnosis of, 304; recurrent, 305–306; treatment of, 304–305
Urination, 259, 260, 289, 303, 311, 313
Urine, 31, 475
Uterine cancer. *See* Cervical cancer; Endometrial cancer
UTIs. *See* Urinary tract infections
UVA, 192, 202
UVB, 192, 202
UVL (ultraviolet light), 192, 201–202

Vaccinations. *See* Immunizations
Vaginal atrophy, 289, 291
Vaginal ulcers, 302
Vaginitis, 297–302; atrophic, 302; bacterial, 299; candida, 300; causes of, 298–299; diagnosis of, 298; douching and, 298; gardnerella, 299; hemophilus, 299; nonspecific, 299; prevention of, 301; trichomonas, 300–301
Valium, 321–322, 336, 340
Valproic acid, 358
Variable-resistance exercise, 27, 28
Varicocele, 271
Vasectomy, 257–258
Vaseline (petrolatum), 191, 201, 266
Vasodilators, 407
VDRL test, 472
VDTs. *See* Video display terminals
Vegetable oils, 66–67
Venereal disease. *See* Sexually transmitted diseases (STDs)
Ventricular contractions, premature, 389
Ventricular fibrillation (VF), 382–383, 390
Ventricular tachycardia (VT), 389–390
Verapamil, 375
Very-low-density lipoprotein (VLDL), 62
VF (ventricular fibrillation), 382–383, 390
Video display terminals (VDTs), 171–175; job stress from, 175; musculoskeletal difficulties from, 174–175; radiation exposure from, 172; visual difficulties from, 172–174
Vision. *See* Eye care
Vitamin A, 59, 80–81, 199
Vitamin B6, 282

Vitamin C, 82–87; and cancer, 81–82, 84–85; and colds, 83–84, 490; in cosmetics, 203; dosage of, 82, 85–87; and longevity, 85
Vitamin D, 296
Vitamin E, 81–82, 203
Vitamins, 57, 58, 490
VLDL (very-low-density lipoprotein), 62
VT (ventricular tachycardia), 389–390

Warts, 195
Wasserman test, 472
Weight control, 32–55; through diet, 40–48, 49–50; by dietary supplements, 48; with drugs, 48–49; environmental factors in, 54–55; by exercise, 32, 44, 45–46; fiber and, 79–80; genetic factors in, 36, 53–55; through jaw wiring, 52; nutrition and, 32; through surgery, 50–51. *See also* Overweight

Weight lifting, 26–29
Weight loss, 324, 342. *See also* Weight control
Weight tables, 33–36, 34
Wernicke's disease, 112
White cell count, 472
White cell differential, 472
Whooping cough vaccine, 461–462
Wills, living, 481–484

Xeroradiography, 426–428
X-ray mammography, 426–429
X-rays: chest, 420, 471; mammography, 426–429; radiation exposure from, 179–184

Yeast infection, 300

Zinc pyrithione, 214
Zovirax (acyclovir), 195, 262–263